Neurocognitive Rehabilitation of Down Syndrome

The Early Years

Neurocognitive Rehabilitation of Down Syndrome

The Early Years

Edited by

Jean-Adolphe Rondal
Juan Perera
Donna Spiker

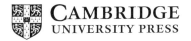

CAMBRIDGE
UNIVERSITY PRESS

CAMBRIDGE UNIVERSITY PRESS
Cambridge, New York, Melbourne, Madrid, Cape Town,
Singapore, São Paulo, Delhi, Tokyo, Mexico City

Cambridge University Press
The Edinburgh Building, Cambridge CB2 8RU, UK

Published in the United States of America by Cambridge University
Press, New York

www.cambridge.org
Information on this title: www.cambridge.org/9781107400436

First published 2011

Printed in the United Kingdom at the University Press, Cambridge

*A catalogue record for this publication is available from the
British Library*

Library of Congress Cataloguing in Publication data
Neurocognitive rehabilitation of Down syndrome : the early years /
edited by Jean-Adolphe Rondal, Juan Perera, Donna Spiker.
    p.   ;   cm.
Includes bibliographical references and index.
ISBN 978-1-107-40043-6 (pbk.)
1. Down syndrome – Patients – Rehabilitation.   2. Preschool
children.   3. Children with disabilities.   4. Learning disabled
children – Identification.   I. Rondal, J. A.   II. Perera, Juan.
III. Spiker, Donna.
[DNLM: 1. Down Syndrome – rehabilitation.   2. Child, Preschool.
3. Disabled Children – rehabilitation.   4. Early Intervention
(Education) – methods.   5. Infant.   WS 107.5.R3]
RJ506.D68N48   2011
618.92′85884203 – dc22   2011005726

ISBN 978-1-107-40043-6 Paperback

To the memory of our friend
Professor Krystina Wisniewski

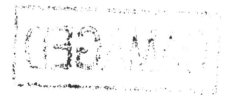

Contents

Contributors

Giorgio Albertini
Child Developmental Department, IRCSS
San Raffaele Pisana, Rome, Italy

Jacob A. Burack
Department of Educational and
Counselling Psychology, McGill University
and Hôpital Rivières-des-Prairies,
Montreal, Quebec, Canada

George Capone
Kennedy Krieger Institute and School of
Medicine, Johns Hopkins University,
Baltimore, Maryland, USA

Katie Cohene
Department of Educational and
Counselling Psychology, McGill University,
Montreal, Quebec, Canada

Jean-Maurice Delabar
Laboratory "Modelling genes
dysregulation: trisomy 21 and
hyperhomocysteinemia," University of
Paris Diderot, Paris, France

Guy Dembour
Department of Paediatric Cardiology,
Cliniques Universitaires Saint-Luc,
Catholic University of Louvain, Brussels,
Belgium

Jamie Edgin
Department of Psychology, University of
Arizona, Tucson, Arizona, USA

Digby Elliott
Department of Psychology, Liverpool John
Moores University, Liverpool, UK

Deborah Fidler
Human Development and Family Studies,
Colorado State University, Fort Collins,
Colorado, USA

Heidi Flores
Department of Educational and
Counselling Psychology, McGill University,
Montreal, Quebec, Canada

Adam Golabek
Pediatric Neuropathology and
Neurogenetic Laboratory, Institute for
Basic Research in Developmental
Disabilities, New York, New York,
USA

Susan L. Hepburn
Department of Psychiatry, University of
Colorado, Denver Health Sciences Center,
Denver, Colorado, USA

Katarzyna Jarząbek
Department of Reproduction and
Gynecological Endocrinology, Medical
University of Bialystok, Bialystok,
Poland

Anne Jobling
School of Education, University of
Queensland, Brisbane, Australia

Elizabeth Kida
Pediatric Neuropathology and
Neurogenetic Laboratory, Institute for
Basic Research in Developmental
Disabilities, New York, New York,
USA

Gerald Mahoney
Mandel School of Applied Social Sciences,
Case Western Reserve University,
Cleveland, Ohio, USA

Deny Menghini
Department of Research and Clinical Care,
Bambino Gesù Children's Hospital, Rome,
Italy

Stephane Moniotte
Department of Paediatric Cardiology,
Cliniques Universitaires Saint-Luc,
Catholic University of Louvain, Brussels,
Belgium

Lynn Nadel
Department of Psychology, University of
Arizona, Tucson, Arizona, USA

Diane Osaki
Osaki Consulting, Denver, Colorado,
USA

Sonia Palminiello
Child Development Department, IRCSS
San Raffaele Pisana, Rome, Italy

David Patterson
Eleanor Roosevelt Institute, Department of
Biological Sciences, University of Denver,
Denver, Colorado, USA

Frida Perales
Mandel School of Applied Social Sciences,
Case Western Reserve University,
Cleveland, Ohio, USA

Juan Perera
Center Príncipe de Asturias, University of
the Balearic Islands, Mallorca, Spain

Michèle Pettinato
Department of Language and
Communication Science, City University,
London, UK

Ausma Rabe
Pediatric Neuropathology and
Neurogenetic Laboratory, Institute for
Basic Research in Developmental

Disabilities, New York, New York,
USA

Alberto Rasore Quartino
Pediatric Department, Ospedali Galliera,
Genoa, Italy

Jean-Adolphe Rondal
Department of Psycholinguistics,
University of Liège and School of
Psychology, Pontifical Salesian University,
Venice, Italy

Goffredina Spanō
Department of Psychology, University of
Arizona, Tucson, Arizona, USA

Donna Spiker
Early Childhood Program, Center for
Education and Human Services, SRI
International, Menlo Park, California,
USA

Stefano Vicari
Department of Research and Clinical Care,
Bambino Gesù Children's Hospital, Rome,
Italy

Naznin Virji-Babul
Down Syndrome Research Foundation,
Burnaby, British Columbia, Canada

Marius Walus
Pediatric Neuropathology and
Neurogenetic Laboratory, Institute for
Basic Research in Developmental
Disabilities, New York, New York, USA

Daniel Weeks
Research Services, University of
Letherbridge, Alberta, Canada

Preface

The study of Down syndrome, the most frequent genetic disorder affecting development, has led to a rich body of interdisciplinary research in genetics, neuroscience, psychology, and education. These collaborations have not only promoted a better understanding of the condition itself, but also favored an increasing recognition that many neurodevelopmental disorders have strong genetic components even though their genetic underpinnings still need to be better understood and the characteristics of their neurocognitive developments better specified. Fifty years of intensive research on Down syndrome following the discovery of the genetic basis of the syndrome have lead to a reasonable understanding of many of its major developmental aspects. On this basis, it has become possible to define an interdisciplinary framework for locating, justifying, and assessing early rehabilitative intervention.

The purpose of this book is to represent some of the major ways in which a comprehensive neurocognitive rehabilitation program may be conceptualized and carried out, taking into account the spectrum of specific knowledge available from the genotype, brain development, and the behavioral phenotype. By comprehensive, we mean a neurocognitive approach connected transactionally with the major therapeutic endeavors in neighboring fields such as neurogenetics, experimental environmental enrichment in animal models, molecular and genic therapies (viewed as synergistic with neurocognitive rehabilitation), pharmacology, pediatrics, and cardiology for infants with Down syndrome.

The book is divided in five sections with the aim of helping to orient the reader and classify the wealth of information provided. Each chapter is followed by a summary and a complete list of references.

Section 1 deals with definition, methodology, and assessment issues. Chapter 1 proposes a definition of early rehabilitative intervention, its age limits, objectives, models of action, and target groups. It also examines the practical challenges that early rehabilitation presents in the short and medium term. Chapter 2, summarizes 50 years of practice of rehabilitative intervention for infants and children with Down syndrome and the changes and progress witnessed in this evolution. Chapter 3 reviews current knowledge of the cognitive profile of Down syndrome, discusses recent advances in our understanding of the pathways that may be potential targets for treatment, and details the ideal properties of assessments for these interventions. It also presents the Arizona Cognitive Test Battery, a set of primarily nonverbal neuropsychological assessments, and details additional assessments that could be included in the context of a clinical trial.

Section 2 deals with genetics, brain, and animal models relating to early neurocognitive rehabilitation. Chapter 4 exposes and discusses new experimental perspectives of molecular and genic therapies in Down syndrome. Chapter 5 analyzes the outcomes of a number of recent works on animal models in Down syndrome. The authors discuss the effect of environmental enrichment for alleviating some of the molecular abnormalities found in Ts65Dn mice, suggesting that it might also have therapeutic potential in children with Down syndrome. Chapter 5 examines the question of adequate nutrition and food supplement in the mother and the fetus during fetal (and before for the mother) and postnatal development, showing that it has profound influences on brain and nervous system development.

Section 3 is devoted to pharmacological and medical management and treatment. Chapter 7 analyzes recent advances in pharmacotherapy for children with Down syndrome, dealing particularly with cognitive enhancement. Pharmacological agents targeting GABA and glutamate receptors and dopamine transporters hold promise for advancing toward clinical testing. Chapter 8 centers on early medical caretaking and following up of children with Down syndrome. Chapter 9 discusses the pros and cons of cardiac surgery in infants with Down syndrome in the light of recent progress in surgical techniques and postoperative intensive care. It appears that congenital heart defects in babies with Down syndrome can be repaired with a very low risk of mortality and morbidity.

Section 4 is concerned with an analysis of key aspects of early neurocognitive rehabilitation. Chapter 10 exposes the basic principles of the developmental theoretical approach, which provides a relevant conceptual instrument for assessing development and interpreting the impact of neurocognitive rehabilitation with children with Down syndrome. Chapter 11 is concerned with motor development and rehabilitation. The difficult problem of hypotonia in children with Down syndrome is addressed together with an analysis of technical ways for reducing its negative incidence on neurocognitive development. Chapter 12 focuses on the characteristics of long- and short-term memories in children with intellectual disability and, particularly, children with Down syndrome. Findings suggest that specific intervention procedures can markedly improve their memory development and functioning. Chapter 13 draws on the research literature on typical development to recommend a number of steps and strategies in the very early training of babies and children with Down syndrome and corresponding congenital genetic conditions leading to intellectual disability and language difficulties. The chapter also deals with conventional aspects of language development in children with Down syndrome, such as prelexical and early lexical development, pragmatics, and grammatical patterning. Chapter 14 explores the work relating to speech perception in Down syndrome and argues that in order to be able to design effective early rehabilitation methods, speech perception in this population needs to be more comprehensively investigated. Chapter 15 stresses temperament and character issues in designing effective early rehabilitation programs for infants and children with Down syndrome. Chapter 16 analyzes the roles of parents in participating actively in the training and education of their Down syndrome children, given that the effectiveness of early rehabilitation is highly associated with the impact it has on parents' level of responsiveness to their children. The ways parents interact with young children with Down syndrome account for a major portion of the variability of the cognitive and communication outcomes these children attain during the first years of their lives.

Lastly, *Section 5* is on therapeutic perspectives. Chapter 17 analyzes the prospects for genetic therapies in Down syndrome and stresses the necessity to keep providing strong neurocognitive rehabilitation in a future interdisciplinary framework labeled "hybrid genetic–neurobehavioral strategies," meant to improve decisively the biological and psychological functioning of the person with Down syndrome.

Acknowledgments

We should like to express our gratitude to the following people and institutions for gener-
ously helping to support financially the preliminary meetings and the editorial work involved
in the realization of a comprehensive and internationally based text of the kind: especially
Gabriel Escarrer, chairman of the Sol Meliá chain; Miguel Fluxá, chairman of Iberostar; Carmen and Luis Riu, chairmen of RIU Hotels & Resorts; the SA NOSTRA savings bank; and
to those who have helped prepare this text for publication: Carmen Crespo, Raquel Marín,
and all the ASNIMO staff in Palma de Mallorca, and Marie-Thérèse Lysens, APEM-T21,
Heusy-Verviers, Belgium. We are also grateful to Richard Marley, Publishing Director, Life
Sciences and Medicine, to Joanna Souter, Assistant Editor, Medicine, Cambridge University
Press, and Lucy Edwards, Production Editor, Science, Technology and Medicine, Cambridge
University Press, for their assistance and support in planning the volume, preparing the final
manuscript, and supervising the production of the book.

Jean-Adolphe Rondal, Juan Perera, Donna Spiker

Early rehabilitative intervention
Definition, objectives, models, and challenges

Juan Perera

Introduction

Realistic estimations indicate that some 780 million children may experience intellectual disabilities between birth and the age of five years (Olness, 2003). This figure represents the growing number of identifiable biological and environmental factors associated with intellectual disability, as well as those conditions that mean children are placed at risk.

Apart from the growing number of genetic and infectious causes of intellectual disabilities that are now recognized, conditions that can also lead to intellectual disability include: malnutrition, fetal alcoholism, cranial trauma, lead poisoning, low birth weight, and cancer, among many others. Environmental causes include the effects of poverty, the abuse of minors, and child neglect (Guralnick, 2000). These environmental causes often work in conjunction with biological conditions (Msall et al., 1998; Fujiura and Yamaki, 2000; Park et al., 2002). Furthermore, when we consider potential causes or risk factors, it is the cumulative effect that represents the greatest threat to the intellectual development of children (Sameroff et al., 1987; Burchinal et al., 2000). The number of children who are likely to experience intellectual disability in the world is overshadowed only by the diversity and complexity of the developmental patterns (Guralnick, 2005a).

However, expectations are relatively optimistic with regard to what can be achieved during the first six years of life if good early intervention (EI) programs are applied; that is, systematic, multidisciplinary programs based on experimentation (Guralnick, 1998).

Why are we focusing on Down syndrome?

Of the 750 to 1000 genetic–chromosomal disorders that cause intellectual disability, Down syndrome (DS) is the only one with a research record that dates back to the early nineteenth century (Seguin, 1846). As the most frequent genetic cause of intellectual disability, DS has served in numerous studies as the control or contrast group for those analyzing other forms of disability (Hodapp, 2008). DS is also the only genetic disorder for which life expectancy has doubled in the last 30 years (Bittles & Glasson, 2004) and which has been etiologically linked to the neurological modifications of Alzheimer's disease (Zigman & Lott, 2007). Moreover, it is detected at birth and children with DS represent an etiologically homogeneous group, although one of its most notable characteristics is precisely its diversity as regards developmental progress (Perera, 1999).

Neurocognitive Rehabilitation of Down Syndrome, eds. Jean-Adolphe Rondal, Juan Perera, and Donna Spiker. Published by Cambridge University Press. © Cambridge University Press 2011.

This is why we are regarding it here as the paradigm of intellectual disability, because we believe that in general, and without underestimating syndrome specificity (discussed below), the principles and practices of EI are useful for other disorders of genetic origin (fragile-X, Williams, Turner, Cri du Chat, Angelman, Prader-Willi, Asperger syndromes, etc.) that have not been as widely studied as DS.

Definition of early rehabilitative intervention

Since the 1970s in the United States and Europe, especially Spain, numerous definitions of EI have been put forward (Bricker & Bricker, 1971; Hayden & Dmitriev, 1975; Shearer & Shearer, 1976; Villa Elízaga, 1976; Coriat, 1977; Hanson, 1977; Gútiez et al., 1993; Candel, 1998; Dunst, 1998; Guralnick, 1998). From the 1990s onwards, a great deal of research has also been undertaken on how children with DS and other developmental disorders function at various stages of their development, in order to design intervention strategies that are more closely adjusted to their specific needs (Dunst, 1990, 1998; Candel & Carranza, 1993; Spiker & Hopman, 1997; Wishart, 1997; Beeghly, 2000).

In parallel to this, a greater implication of the family has made it possible to design and execute numerous studies that have attempted to investigate the family characteristics of children with DS, their reactions and their ability to adapt to the new situation of having a child with DS, and the relation of a series of family variables with the child's development (Crnic et al., 1983; Erickson & Upshur, 1989; Harris & McHale, 1989; Sloper et al., 1991; Candel et al., 1993; Minnes, 1998; Stoneman, 1998).

Furthermore, on reviewing the research carried out on the plasticity of the central nervous system, two intriguing issues arise: (1) It is clear that neurophysiological events are revealed in response to experience, allowing the brain to organize itself. This is a strong argument in favor of intervention, given that experiences are translated into specific changes at the level of the nervous system and behavior. (2) There is also evidence that modifications of the nervous system are not limited to the first months of life, which raises the question as to whether intervention could be effective at other periods of life (Nelson, 2000). Indeed, there are those who claim that intervention should not only be early (i.e. during the first years of childhood) but rather should continue throughout a person's lifetime (Flórez, 2005).

From this, two principal assumptions also arise that provide the basis or reason for EI: on the one hand, the fact that genetic and biological problems can be overcome or minimized; on the other hand, the supposition that early experience is important for the development of children. As a result, there are three theoretical arguments that form the basis of the development of EI programs:

1 Children with developmental problems need more and/or different early experiences compared to children without problems.
2 Programs with specialized personnel are necessary to help provide the early experiences that are required to compensate for developmental difficulties.
3 Developmental progress improves in children with problems who participate in EI programs (Candel, 2003a).

These days, all over the world EI is envisaged as comprehensive care provided to children and their families during the first months and years of life, as a result of disorders in development or because of high-risk situations. Intervention consists of medical, educational, and social treatment that directly or individually influences the functioning of the parents, the family, and the child.

Along this line the Spanish White Paper on Early Intervention (*Libro Blanco de la Atención Temprana*) defines it in Spain as "the set of interventions directed at infants between birth and six years of age, the family and the environment, with the aim of providing as rapid a response as possible to the transitory or permanent needs that the children present, or have the risk of presenting, in their development. These interventions, which have to take the child as a whole into account, must be planned by a team of professionals with interdisciplinary or transdisciplinary training" (GAT, 2000).

Objectives

The following objectives result from the definitions above:

- Reduce the effects of a deficiency or deficit against the child's overall development.
- Optimize, as far as possible, the course of the child's development.
- Introduce the necessary mechanisms of compensation, elimination of barriers, and adaptation to specific needs.
- Avoid or reduce the appearance of secondary or associated effects or deficits produced by a disorder or high-risk situation.
- Attend to and cover the needs and requirements of the family and the environment in which the child lives.
- Consider the child as an active subject in the intervention.
- Consider the family as the main agent of the intervention.

As a result, EI programs aim to:

1 Provide parents and the entire family with the necessary information, support, and advice, so that they can adapt to the new situation and maintain adequate affective relations with the child.
2 Enrich the environment in which the child is going to develop, providing adequate stimuli in all aspects to favor development.
3 Encourage the parent–child relationship, preventing the appearance of inadequate interactive styles.
4 Increase the child's progress as far as possible to achieve independence in the different areas of development.
5 Employ intervention strategies in a natural context and through the child's routine situations, avoiding excessively artificial formulae.
6 Take preventive action as EI programs make it possible to slow down the progressive deterioration of development levels to some extent, thereby preventing the child from presenting more serious disorders in different developmental aspects. This preventive facet also extends to the rest of the family environment, with adequate behavior that is better adapted to the reality of the situation being established from the start.

Early intervention models

Traditional models based on behavioral criteria that inspired EI programs up until the 1980s are now obsolete, and today models are employed that have at least two points in common:

they envisage human development as a transactional process, and they have been widely applied to deficient or high-risk children.

Over the last decade three theories have been proposed that have had a decisive influence on the incorporation of new approaches: the Ecological Systems Theory developed by Bronfenbrenner (1979), the Transactional Model by Sameroff and Chandler (1975), and Feuerstein's theory of Structural Cognitive Modifiability (Feuerstein, 1980).

The ecological model underlines the complexity of development and the large number of environmental influences on children (Sameroff & Fiese, 2000). Ecological theories posit that ecological frameworks and social units, as well as people and what happens to them, do not operate in isolation, but that each influences the other, both directly and indirectly, so that changes in a unit or subunit have an impact on and influence members of other units (Dunst & Trivette, 1988). The theory of social support attempts to describe the properties of social units, the relations between these and how social support improves the well-being of the individual, family, and community (Cohen & Syme, 1985).

Human ecology places emphasis on the interactions and adjustments between children undergoing development and their animate and inanimate environments, and on how events in different ecological frameworks directly and indirectly affect a person's behavior (Bronfenbrenner, 1979; Cochran & Brassard, 1979). Adaptive theory attempts to explain how ecological influences affect reactions to the birth and upbringing of a child with problems, and how diverse ecological forces have positive and negative influences on the ability of the family to deal with and adapt to the birth and education of a child with developmental difficulties (Crnic et al., 1983).

The Transactional Model is based on the capacity of social response of the environment and on the interactive nature of the child–environment exchange. From this perspective the child's development is the product of constant dynamic interactions between the child and the experiences provided by the family and social context. The innovative aspect of this model, according to Sameroff and Fiese (2000), is that it places equal emphasis on the effects of the child and the environment, so that the experiences provided by the environment are not envisaged as independent from the child. The child may have been a determining factor in current experiences, but developmental performance cannot be described systematically without an analysis of the effects of the environment on the child.

The main consequences of applying this model to the field of EI are as follows: (1) the parent–child dyad must be the objective of home-based intervention; (2) children learn and develop by means of positive, reciprocal exchanges with the environment, especially with their parents; (3) the parents or carers, where appropriate, are the most important figures in the child's environment; (4) childhood is the best time to initiate intervention for children with developmental problems, children with a biological or environmental risk, and their parents, within the context of the family.

The theory of Cognitive Structural Modifiability maintains that by means of systematic, consistent intervention, it is possible to bring about changes of a structural nature that can alter the course and direction of cognitive development. In this context, cognitive development is the result of the combination of the direct exposure of the organism to environmental stimuli, related to maturing processes, and of mediated learning experiences, with all cultural transmission processes being implicated.

With good mediation there are no limits to cognitive development, irrespective of individual deficiencies. What is important is good interaction between the organism and its surrounding environment (Feuerstein et al., 1991).

This theory states that two types of factor have an influence in cognitive development: (1) distal factors, linked fundamentally to genetic, organic, environmental, and maturation factors, which do not cause irreversible damage to people; (2) proximal factors, related to the conditions and contexts of learning. Feuerstein and colleagues claim that it is possible to offer mediated learning experiences successfully to all individuals, whatever their condition or age, as the relevant factor consists only of the use of an appropriate type of mediated learning.

The active modifying environment must have the following characteristics: (1) organize the child's life in such a way that it provokes structural cognitive modification; (2) create positive reinforcements – trigger an imbalance in order to create changes; (3) promote challenges; in other words, planned, controlled confrontations with the new and the unexpected; (4) the heterogeneity of the environment is an important element for the development of higher cognitive processes; (5) individualized mediation.

As well as the three models outlined above, it is also worth making reference to the activity-based approach (Bricker & Cripe, 1992), which is founded on the theory of learning and on the work of various authors, such as Vygotsky, Piaget, and Dewey. It is based on three elements: (1) the influence and interaction of the immediate socio-cultural and larger environments; (2) the need for the active involvement of the child; (3) improvement in learning, occupying children with functional, meaningful activities.

According to this approach, the acquisition of knowledge and learning skills must take place within authentic conditions. These must include activities that reflect the reality and demands of everyday life. Children thus learn and practice skills that will improve their capacity to adapt to the numerous demands of their physical and social environments.

Finally, one of the models that is most widely used today as a result of the solid basis that it offers for intervention is that of early development and risk factors, contributed recently by Guralnick (1998). This model has three main components: family patterns, family characteristics, and potential stress factors. Both the family characteristics and stress factors tend to be distal to the child, while the family patterns are proximal and directly influence the child's development.

The family patterns component consists of three elements: the quality of parent–child transactions, family-orchestrated child experiences, and the environmental measures that improve the child's health and security. These factors are influenced, in turn, by the model's two other components. One of these, family characteristics, includes two wide contextual factors: the personal characteristics of the parents and the characteristics of the child, which are not related to his or her disability. The third component, potential stress factors due to the child's disability, can also distort the family dynamic. Guralnick classifies these factors into four categories: information requirements that arise as a result of the child's disability; interpersonal and family anxiety (reactions that arise as a result of the child's disability, relationship problems between the parents, negative reactions from people who are close to the family); resource requirements; loss of confidence in the ability to bring up a child with problems.

Guralnick (1998) proposes, moreover, that the intervention program should include the following components: resource supports (coordination and access to services); subsidiary supports (financial help, family relief programs); social support (parent groups, family guidance, friends, community networks); and information and services (formal intervention programs, communication between parents and professionals).

All these intervention models have common elements and coincide as regards principles that constitute the basis of the majority of current EI programs: (1) the importance of socio-communicative exchanges between children and their environment is highlighted; (2) children are active learners; (3) emphasis is placed on learning in a natural context; (4) in order to achieve objectives, functional activities are employed that have meaning for children and which are inserted into their daily routine; (5) natural reinforcements are used; (6) the parents are the principal agents of the intervention and not mere recipients.

"Whatever the case, every professional has their own preferences and will have recourse to those premises that best adapt to their personal and professional circumstances. Experience tells us that, with the passing of time, we become eclectic and begin to take the best of the different options available until we create a tailor-made suit. Perhaps the models outlined above may be useful in making this selection" (Candel, 2003b).

The short- and medium-term challenges of early intervention

Challenge 1

Advances in genetic research in animal models and possible application to human beings
Laboratory experiments with trisomic, transgenic, and transchromosomic mice models are attempting to achieve results from three angles: (1) relating the phenotypic characteristics of DS precisely with the genes whose overexpression is responsible for these appearing. Which gene(s) are involved in the appearance, for example, of intellectual disability, cardiopathy, etc.?;(2) discovering the mechanisms as to why this happens: what does the overexpression of a gene do, so that a pathological modification of a specific organ appears at a specific age, in a specific person with DS?; (3) testing therapeutic measures that could be useful in the short and medium term: some gene related (gene therapy), others of a chemical nature (drugs that inhibit the excessive presence of a product caused by the overexpression of a gene), others of an immunological nature (vaccinations that neutralize the negative action of those same products, and others of a general nature (interventions directed at improving the mechanisms of learning or behavior) (Flórez, 2001).

In Chapters 3–6, and the final chapter of this book, extensive information is given about the advances made in genetic research in animal models and its possible application to human beings.

Challenge 2

Early intervention research and praxis have to be established from a multidisciplinary and interdisciplinary perspective Environmental enrichment (the environment is capable of modifying cerebral function and structure), gene therapy (the possible substitution of a damaged gene for a normal one), and health and education programs have to converge necessarily with the objective of understanding the genotype and its specific causes. For many years, in developed countries, EI has been very fragmented and compartmentalized. In many nations controversy still exists regarding powers and jurisdiction (Social Services, Health, Education), which needs to be overcome. It is necessary to join forces. We must try to integrate the knowledge from molecular genetics, animal models and their experimental manipulation, new science, medicine, developmental psychology, cognitive science, family therapy and systemic practice, educational technology and school integration – and this can only be achieved by well-trained multidisciplinary teams with an open outlook, which are capable of synthesizing current knowledge and establishing new joint objectives for research and intervention.

Challenge 3

The urgent translation of growing scientific findings into specific intervention programs We need good intervention programs that are backed up by serious, verified scientific research and which, therefore, serve to alleviate or cure what they say they do.

In EI, the strategy consists of taking advantage of early childhood to activate, boost, and optimize neurobehavioral structures and processes that would remain undeveloped owing to adverse genetic effects in neurobehavioral genesis (Rondal & Perera, 2006).

There are various reasons for carrying out this systematic strategy. In the case of a congenital intellectual disability (DS), assuming early diagnosis, it is advisable to begin intervention during the weeks following birth in order to reduce, as far as possible, retardation in the socio-personal, physical, and cognitive aspects of development. Ontogenesis is highly accumulative. This means that the earliest acquisitions serve as the basis for later development. The sooner the basic structures are established, the better the prognosis for subsequent progress and, assuming continuous training, the greater the probability that the highest levels of development permitted by the condition can be reached.

A second reason is that neuroplasticity, as we know, is greater during the first years of life, and this also applies to children with intellectual disability; in this way a more fertile terrain is provided, as it were, for the undertaking of well-designed interventions.

The two reasons mentioned above suggest that the application of EI is probably more beneficial than any other intervention carried out at a later stage in life. However, this does not mean that the latter is not important or that intervention in children with DS should stop after the age of six (Perera, 1995).

Guralnick (1997, 2005b) has evaluated underlying current knowledge in a series of dimensions that improve development, and concludes that decades of study on a large and small scale indicate that we are capable of modifying individual development as a result of good EI programs, and that comprehensive EI programs have demonstrated that we are capable of preventing, to a large extent, the decline in cognitive development in children with DS that typically appears during their early years.

Although demonstration of the long-term effects still represents a methodological challenge, long-term results have also been documented for various developmental conditions, including DS.

Finally, the challenge lies in the need to translate scientific findings into specific intervention programs, strategies, and therapeutic methods that can be used in EI services and in educational classrooms to improve maturity, health, and cognitive, memory, linguistic, and behavioral aptitudes of children with developmental problems of a genetic origin (Perera, 2007).

Challenge 4

The need to gain further insight into the "specificity" of each syndrome The scientific approach to intellectual disability needs to take into account the etiological dimension (Rondal & Perera, 2006). For theoretical and clinical reasons it is necessary to gain further insight into knowledge of various types of intellectual disability, beginning with those of genetic origin, and to determine, with a firmer empirical base, which traits are different in one entity and another and to what extent, and which symptoms are found in various or all syndromes (Rondal et al., 2004).

The perspective of specificity seems to be clearer at the systemic level. Recent research has revealed a high number of symptomatic characteristics in DS which, together, show a specific picture of the syndrome that some have called partial specificity (Dykens et al., 2000), and others syndromic specificity (Perera, 2006).

The key methodological dimension for the study of specificity must focus on inter-syndromic comparison, as it is not possible to discuss specificity in any syndrome without carrying out systematic comparisons with other syndromes.

The theoretical and practical implications of the existence of behavioral phenotypes and their possible specificity are of the highest importance. On the theoretical side, the evidence of partial specificity between genetic syndromes, or those associated with intellectual disability, seems to indicate that there are certain shared relations between particular genes and some behavioral development patterns with important variations. On the practical side, the verification of specific development and functioning patterns leads to the strategic question of whether single or different intervention methods should be used.

The consequence of this is that if at least partial specific patterns can be demonstrated in individuals with different genetic syndromes, then intervention strategies would have to be designed precisely around the particular needs of the genetic group, leaving only functional characteristics shared with other groups to common rehabilitative strategies (Hodapp, 2008). In addition, the most reasonable criterion is that "Specific aspects require particular intervention methods, non-specific aspects require more general methods that can be extended to various entities" (Rondal & Perera, 2006).

It therefore seems evident that good intervention has to follow this criterion, because if programs, strategies, therapeutic methods, and didactic instruments used in EI or educational classrooms are designed by taking into account these specific aspects that pertain to certain syndromes and which refer to specific forms of capturing, processing, and assimilating information (in their cognitive, linguistic, perceptive, memory, sensory aspects, etc.), they would be more direct and effective at teaching children to think, speak, read, write, etc.

Challenge 5

Promote the role of parents (especially the mother) as principal agents of EI This is because it has been demonstrated that the effectiveness of EI is closely linked to the level of responsiveness to and good intervention of the parents with their children.

Mahoney, in Chapter 16 of this book, presents the results of his longitudinal studies and research on the role that parents play in EI in children with DS and other developmental conditions. His findings were, among others, as follows:

1 That the way in which parents interact with their young children with DS has an effect on much of the variability in cognitive and communicative outcomes that these children achieve during their first three years of life.
2 That this is also linked to academic and developmental achievements in the years following infancy.
3 That the outcomes in development that children reach in EI programs that do not work with their parents are related with the parents' style of interacting with their children, but not with the type of intervention the children receive.
4 That the effectiveness of EI is very closely linked to the impact it has on the degree of acceptance and responsiveness of the parents toward their children.

5   That the only way of involving parents in EI that systematically improves the development of their children and their emotional and social functioning is that which encourages parents, through their coaching, to learn and use responsive interactions with their children. The term responsive interactions means following the children's interests, responding to their needs, adapting to their rhythms, and gently correcting their errors. This focus has served to improve children's cognitive, communicative, social, and emotional functioning (Mahoney et al., 1998).

All this should probably lead us to insist less on standardized programs and focus much more in the future on the interaction between parents and children.

Challenge 6

Encourage governments and political representatives to trust and invest in EI services I am not going to linger over this point, but convincing politicians wherever we live is a responsibility that involves us all. The effectiveness of programs during the early years of life has been scientifically proven, even though there are still methodological challenges to demonstrate their long-term effectiveness, as has been stated previously.

We can probably do more for people with DS during the first six years than during the rest of their lives. If good EI is provided, we will be able to compensate for their limitations and strengthen their skills, which will mean that children will come to be active, independent, autonomous individuals, rather than passive, dependent people. It is therefore necessary to convince governments to prioritize EI in their medical, educational, and social programs.

Challenge 7

Professional qualification and teamwork The concept of interdisciplinarity goes beyond a simple parallel sum of different disciplines. The preparation of professionals who are involved in EI implies both training in a specific discipline and in a conceptual framework common to all these disciplines that should have its own space for development through reflection and teamwork. The drawing up of regular training plans and the need for continued supervised professional experience is an essential condition for the organization of qualified EI services, at a level in accordance with their responsibility (GAT, 2000).

Quality It is not enough to say that we are good. It is necessary to prove it. In the business world, this is demonstrated by means of external certificates that make it possible to use rigorous controls to analyze the compliance of internationally approved regulations with criteria of continuing improvement, client satisfaction, efficacy, and efficiency.

Quality in EI services is a right and guarantee for the user and an obligation for the professional team. Furthermore, it has special significance and importance in situations with children who have developmental disorders where the application of good or bad practices can seriously affect their biological, psychological, or social progress.

In the concept of intellectual disability (AAMR, 2002), developmental disorders go from being considered an absolute trait of an individual to being the result of interaction between a person with specific limitations and his/her surroundings. This concept, moreover, is not limited to studying children and intervening in their environment, but rather raises the need to evaluate and intervene where children develop. This is why the so-called supports acquire such special significance.

Early intervention is not a refuge for beginners. It requires solid multidisciplinary training, demonstrated experience, systematic continuity, rigor in procedures, and continuing evaluation of results (Grupo PADI, 1996; GAT, 2000; ICASS, 2001; European Organization for Quality, 2002; Millá, 2003; Ponte et al., 2004).

A key challenge therefore is to demand an international quality standard for EI.

Conclusion

To conclude, I would like to sum up and present three future perspectives which, in the short and medium term, could introduce important improvements in the results of EI.

The first is current and future research in genetic intellectual disability using animal models, which is extremely important, as has been explained previously. In addition, very important is the difficult matter of extrapolating the relevant data and findings from lower order mammals (mice, etc.) to human beings. This research will promote better understanding of some of the organic difficulties and limitations that are important in DS and, furthermore, will make it possible to define the drugs and early environmental enrichment that can best help to improve developmental results and compensate for deficits.

The second is the stimulation that may soon be possible to carry out in the uterus – especially auditory stimulation if the fetus is detected to be at a disadvantage as regards commencement of early language acquisition compared to babies that develop normally.

Advances that have been made over the last few decades have transformed neonatology. Changes in therapy and in the development of newborn babies, and other groups, with a very low weight have been very important.

Treatments carried out on the fetus before birth represent one of these advances. The induction of the maturation of fetal tissues by means of the use of corticoids has been shown to be effective at preventing not only hyaline membrane disease, but also cerebral hemorrhage and necrotizing enterocolitis which, when they occur, represent a risk to survival and later development of the newborn.

Postnatal handling of these patients has also changed. Better knowledge of the pathophysiology of diseases typical of prematurity has made it possible to introduce new treatments.

In the 1980s, it would have been difficult for a newborn with a weight below 800 grams to have been viable. These days the viability thresholds that are established are a gestational age of 24 weeks and 400 grams in weight. However, these limits become blurred in the face of the need to individualize each situation.

In this context, as well as in specific therapeutic guidelines, there has been an increase in the measures aimed at improving the development of the newborn through interventions that favor the infant and the family, with the understanding that, in actual fact, both constitute a whole. Such measures are known as "care focused on development and the family." This represents a radical change, not so much of a technological nature, but in the involvement of health personnel and the family of each infant in such care. It is a question of trying to create as favorable an environment as possible by reducing macroenvironmental noxae (noise, light) and microenvironmental noxae (posture, handling, pain), and attempting to involve the family in the infant's care, promoting breast feeding and skin-to-skin contact between the infant and parents, and allowing families entry into care areas as far as possible. This philosophy should be understood as a form of EI which, through improvement to the relationship between the infant and its carers and to the environment, attempts to prevent the appearance of less serious morbidities but which can determine limitations in the long term.

This way of acting is going to be introduced slowly in developed countries and represents a considerable cultural change for neonatal units that are, at times, restricted by structural limits.

The third is that I would like to emphasize the future possibility, which is no longer science fiction, of anticipating within our lifetimes the arrival of a strong convergence between gene therapies and neurobehavioral intervention; that is, what Rondal and I call hybrid therapeutic strategies in this book. There may still be a long way to go before we see gene therapy for intellectual disabilities materialize, although it will probably be shorter for monogenic syndromes such as fragile-X syndrome and others, and longer for multigene disorders such as DS or Williams syndrome. However, a gradual gene-by-gene strategy that is effective with regard to organic disorders may be appropriate. When this moment arrives, far from eliminating the need for neurobehavioral rehabilitation measures, these will be more necessary in order to combine the two strategies (gene therapy and behavioral intervention) and achieve maximum efficacy. Moreover, early diagnosis (once this has become completely safe, noninvasive, and error free) will have all the positive connotations – it will allow the initiation of a genuine cure for the real benefit of the child instead of being, as unfortunately happens today in too many cases, the prelude to an abortion.

Summary

This chapter proposes a definition of early intervention (EI) and its limitations, objectives, and target groups. It reviews the main intervention models: Brofenbrenner's Ecological Systems Theory (1979), Sameroff and Chandler's Transactional Model (1975), Feuerstein's theory of Cognitive Structural Modifiability (1980), and Guralnick's Model of Early Development and Risk Factors (1998). All these models have common elements and coincide with regard to the principles that represent the basis for the majority of current EI programs: (1) intercommunication between the child and the environment; (2) the child as an active learner; (3) learning in a natural context; (4) the use of functional activities that have meaning for the child and which are inserted into the daily routine; (5) the use of natural reinforcements; (6) the parents as the principal agents and not mere recipients of the intervention. Finally, the short- and medium-term challenges that EI presents are analyzed and conclusions are reached.

References

American Association on Mental Retardation (AAMR). (2002). *Mental Retardation: Definition, Classification and Systems of Supports*. (10th edn.). Washington DC: AAMR.

Beeghly, M. (2000). El temperamento en los niños con síndrome de Down. In J. A. Rondal, J. Perera, L. Nadel (eds.), *Síndrome de Down. Revisión de los últimos conocimientos*, pp. 167–183. Madrid: Espasa Calpe.

Bittles, H. A. & Glasson, E. J. (2004). Clinical, social and ethical implications of changing life expectancy in Down syndrome. *Developmental Medicine and Child Neurology*, 46, 282–286.

Bricker, D. D. & Bricker, W. A. (1971). *Toddler, Research and Intervention Project Report, Year I*. IRMID, Behavioral Science Monograph, 20. Nashville, TN: Institute on Mental Retardation and Intellectual Development.

Bricker, D. D. & Cripe, J. (1992). *An Activity-based Approach to Early Intervention*. Baltimore: Brookes.

Bronfenbrenner, U. (1979). *The Ecology of Human Development*. Cambridge: Harvard University Press.

Burchinal, M. R., Roberts, J., Hooper, S., Ziesel, S. A. (2000). Cumulative risk and early cognitive development: a comparison of statistical risk models. *Developmental Psychology*, **36**, 793–807.

Candel, I. (1998). Atención temprana. Aspectos teóricos y delimitaciones conceptuales. *Revista de Atención Temprana, 1, abril,* 5–9.

Candel, I. (2003a). Aspectos generales de la atención temprana. In I. Candel (ed.), *Atención Temprana. Niños con Síndrome de Down y otros Problemas del Desarrollo,* pp. 7–17. Madrid: FEISD.

Candel, I. (2003b). Propuestas de organización del servicio de atención temprana. In: I. Candel (ed.), *Atención Temprana. Niños con Síndrome de Down y otros Problemas del Desarrollo,* pp. 19–27. Madrid: FEISD.

Candel, I. & Carranza, J. A. (1993). Características evolutivas de los niños con síndrome de Down en la infancia. In I. Candel (ed.), *Programa de Atención Temprana. Intervención en niños con Síndrome de Down y otros Problemas del Desarrollo,* pp. 55–87. Madrid: CEPE.

Candel, I., Carranza, J. A., Galiana, R., et al. (1993). Interacción Padres – Hijos. In I. Candel (ed.), *Programa de Atención Temprana. Intervención en niños con Síndrome de Down y otros Problemas del Desarrollo,* pp. 30–31. Madrid: CEPE.

Cochran, M. & Brassard, J. (1979). Child development and personal social networks. *Child Development*, **50**, 601–616.

Cohen, S. & Syme, S. L. (eds.) (1985). *Social Support and Health,* pp. 132–143. New York: Academic Press.

Coriat, L. (1977). Estimulación temprana: la construcción de una disciplina en el campo de los problemas de desarrollo infantil. *Escritos de la Infancia, 8,* 29, Buenos Aires: Fundación para el Estudio de Problemas de la Infancia.

Crnic, K. A., Friedrich, W. N., Greenberg, M. T. (1983). Adaptation of families with mentally retarded children: a model of stress, coping and family ecology. *American Journal of Mental Deficiency,* **88**(2), 125–138.

Dunst, C. J. (1990). Sensorimotor development of infants with Down syndrome. In D. Cichetti & M. Beeghly (eds.), *Children with Down Syndrome. The Developmental*

Perspective, pp. 180–230. New York: Cambridge University Press.

Dunst, C. J. (1998). Sensorimotor development and developmental disabilities. In J. A. Burack, R. M. Hodapp, E. Zigler (eds.), *Handbook of Mental Retardation and Development,* pp. 135–182. New York: Cambridge University Press.

Dunst, C. J. & Trivette, C. M. (1988). A family system model of early intervention with handicapped and developmentally at risk children. In D. R. Powell (ed.), *Parent Education as Early Childhood Intervention: Emerging Directions Theory, Research and Practice,* pp. 131–179. Norwood: Ablex Publishing Corporation.

Dykens, E. M., Hodapp, R., Finucane, B. (2000). *Genetics and Mental Retardation Syndromes,* pp. 125–135. Baltimore: Brookes.

Erickson, M. & Upshur, C. C. (1989). Caretaking burden and social support: comparison of mothers of infants with and without disabilities. *American Journal on Mental Retardation,* **94** (3), 250–258.

European Organization for Quality (2002). *Modelo Europeo de Excelencia EFQM.* Bruselas: Unión Europea.

Feuerstein, R. (1980). *Instrumental Enrichment: an Intervention Program for Cognitive Modificability.* Baltimore: University Park Press.

Feuerstein, R., Klein, P., Tannebaum, A. (1991). *Mediated Learning Experience. Theoretical Psychosocial and Learning Implications.* Tel Aviv: Freund.

Flórez, J. (2001). Los modelos animales en el síndrome de Down. In *Canal Down 21.* Available from: http://www.down.21.org/salud/genetica/modelos_animales.htm

Flórez, J. (2005). La Atención Temprana en el síndrome de Down: bases neurológicas. *Revista Síndrome de Down de Cantabria.* 22(4), 132–142.

Fujiura, G. T. & Yamaki, K. (2000). Trends in demography of childhood poverty and disability. *Exceptional Children,* **66**, 187–199.

Grupo de Atención Temprana – GAT. (2000). *Libro Blanco de la Atención Temprana.* Real

Patronato de la Discapacidad. Serie Documentos n 55. Madrid: Genysi.

Grupo PADI. (1996). *Criterios de Calidad en Centros de Atención Temprana*. Madrid: Genysi.

Guralnick, M. J. (1997). *The Effectiveness of Early Intervention*. Baltimore: Brookes.

Guralnick, M. J. (1998). The effectiveness of early intervention for vulnerable children: a developmental perspective. *American Journal on Mental Retardation*, **102**, 319–345.

Guralnick, M. J. (2000). The early intervention system and out-of-home childcare. In D. Cryer & T. Harms (eds.), *Infants and Toddlers in Out-of-home Care*. Baltimore: Brookes.

Guralnick, M. J. (2005a). An overview of the developmental systems approach to early intervention. In M. J. Guralnick (ed.), *The Developmental Systems Approach to Early Intervention*, pp. 3–28. Baltimore: Brookes.

Guralnick, M. J. (2005b). Early intervention for children with intellectual disabilities: current knowledge and future prospects. *Journal of Applied Research in Intellectual Disabilities*, **18**, 313–324.

Gútiez, P., Saez-Rico, S., Valle, M. (1993). Proyecto de atención temprana para niños de alto riesgo biológico-ambiental con alteraciones o minusvalías documentales. *Revista Complutense de Educación*, **4**(2), 113–129.

Hanson, M. J. (1977). *Teaching your Down's Syndrome Infant. A Guide for Parents*. Baltimore: University Park Press.

Harris, V. S. & McHale, S. M. (1989). Family life problems, daily caregiving activities and the psychological well-being of mothers of mentally retarded children. *American Journal on Mental Retardation*, **94**(3), 231–239.

Hayden, A. H. & Dmitriev, V. (1975). The multidisciplinary preschool program for Down's syndrome children at the University of Washington Model Preschool Center. In B. Z. Frienlander, G. M. Sterriff, G. E. Kirk (eds.), *Exceptional Infant: Assessment and Intervention*, **3**. New York: Brunner/Mazel.

Hodapp, R. M. (2008). Familias de personas con síndrome de Down: perspectivas, hallazgos,

investigación y necesidades. *Revista Síndrome de Down de Cantabria*, **25**(96), 17–30.

Institut Català d'Assistençia i Serveis Socials. (2001). *Indicadors d'Evaluació de la Qualitat. Centres de Desenvolupament Infantil i Atenció Precoç*. Barcelona: ICASS.

Mahoney, G., Boyce, G., Fewell, R., Spiker, D., Wheeden, C. A. (1998). Early intervention effectiveness depends upon parental involvement/responsives. *Topics in Early Childhood Special Education*, **18**(1), 5–17.

Millá, M. G. (2003). La calidad en Atención Temprana. *Revista Minusval*, **3**, 71–74. Madrid: IMSERSO.

Minnes, P. (1998). Mental retardation: the impact upon the family. In J. A. Burack, R. M. Hodapp, E. Zigler (eds.), *Handbook of Mental Retardation and Development*, pp. 693–712. New York: Cambridge University Press.

Msall, M. E., Bier, J., Lagasse, L., Tremont, M., Lester, B. (1998). The vulnerable preschool child: the impact of biomedical and social risks on neurodevelopmental function. *Seminars in Pediatric Neurology*, **5**, 52–61.

Nelson, C. A. (2000). The neurological bases of early intervention. In J. P. Shonkoff & S. J. Meisels (eds.), *Handbook of Early Childhood Intervention*, pp. 204–227. New York: Cambridge University Press.

Olness, K. (2003). Effects on brain development leading to cognitive impairment: a worldwide epidemic. *Journal of Developmental & Behavioral Pediatrics*, **24**, 120–130.

Park, J., Turnbull, A. P., Turnbull, H. R. (2002). Impacts of poverty on quality of life in families of children with disabilities. *Exceptional Children*, **68**, 151–170.

Perera, J. (1995). Intervención temprana en el síndrome de Down: estado de la cuestión y aspectos específicos. In J. Perera (ed.), *Síndrome de Down. Aspectos específicos*, pp. 75–85. Barcelona: Masson.

Perera, J. (1999). People with Down syndrome: Quality of life and future. In J. A. Rondal, J. Perera, L. Nadel (eds.), *Down Syndrome. A Review of Current Knowledge*, pp. 9–26. London: Whurr.

Perera, J. (2006). Specificity in Down syndrome: a new therapeutic criterion. In J. A. Rondal &

J. Perera (eds.), *Down Syndrome Neurobehavioral Specificity*, pp. 1–16. Chichester: Wiley.

Perera, J. (2007). Professional inclusion as global therapy for the individual with Down syndrome. In J. A. Rondal & A. Rassore Quantino (eds.), *Therapies and Rehabilitation in Down Syndrome*, pp. 181–194. Chichester: Wiley.

Ponte, J., Cardama, J., Arcanzon, J. L. et al. (2004). *Guía de Estándares de Calidad en Atención Temprana*. Ministerio de Trabajo y Asuntos Sociales. Madrid: IMSERSO.

Rondal, J. A., Hodapp, R., Soresi, S., Dykens, E., Nota, L. (2004). *Intellectual Disabilities, Genetics, Behavior and Inclusion*. X Preface. London and Philadelphia: Whurr.

Rondal, J. A. & Perera, J. (2006). Specific language profiles. In J. A. Rondal & J. Perera (eds.), *Down Syndrome Neurobehavioral Specificity*, pp. 101–103. Chichester: Wiley.

Sameroff, A. J. & Chandler, M. J. (1975). Reproductive risk and the continuum of caretaking casuality. In F. D. Horowitz, E. M. Hetherington, S. Scarr-Salapatek, G. Siegel (eds.), *Review of Child Development Research*, **4**, 187–244. Chicago: University of Chicago Press.

Sameroff, A. J. & Fiese, B. H. (2000). Transactional regulation: the developmental ecology of early intervention. In J. P. Shonkoff & S. J. Meisels (eds.), *Handbook of Early Childhood Intervention*, pp. 135–159. New York: Cambridge University Press.

Sameroff, A. J., Siefer, R., Barocas, R., Zax, M., Greenspan, S. (1987). Intelligence quotient scores of 4-year-old children: social-enviromental risk factors. *Pediatrics*, **79**, 343–350.

Seguin, E. (1846). *Idiocy: It's Treatment by Physiological Method*. New York: Wood.

Shearer, D. E. & Shearer, M. S. (1976). The portage project: a model for early childhood intervention. In T. D. Tjossen (ed.), *Intervention Strategies for High Risk Infants and Young Children*. Baltimore: University Park Press.

Sloper, P., Knussen, L., Turner, S., Cunningham, C. (1991). Factors related to stress and satisfaction with life in families of children with Down syndrome. *Journal of Child Psychology and Psychiatry*, **32**(4), 655–676.

Spiker, D. & Hopman. (1997). The effectiveness of early intervention for children with Down syndrome. In M. J. Guralnick (ed.), *The Effectiveness of Early Intervention*, pp. 271–305. Baltimore: Brookes.

Stoneman, Z. (1998). Research on siblings of children with mental retardation: contributions on developmental theory and etiology. In J. A. Burack, R. M. Hodapp, E. Zigler (eds.), *Handbook of Mental Retardation and Development*, pp. 669–692. New York: Cambridge University Press.

Villa Elízaga, I. (1976). *Desarrollo y Estimulación del Niño Durante sus Tres Primeros Años de Vida*, pp. 289–291. Pamplona: Eunsa.

Wishart, J. (1997). Learning in young children with Down's syndrome: developmental trends. In J. A. Rondal, J. Perera, L. Nadel, A. Comblain (eds.) *Down's Syndrome Psychological, Psychobiological and Socioeducational Perspectives*, pp. 81–96. London: Whurr.

Zigman, V. B. & Lott, I. T. (2007). Alzheimer's disease in Down syndrome: neurobiology and risk. *Mental Retardation and Developmental Disabilities Research Reviews*, **13**, 237–246.

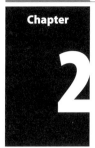

2

The history of early intervention for infants and young children with Down syndrome and their families

Where have we been and where are we going?

Donna Spiker

Fifty years ago, early intervention (EI) for infants and young children with Down syndrome (DS) did not exist in any formalized or universal way. Beginning with a few experimental programs instigated by the advocacy of parents and the forward thinking of researchers, the field of EI for infants and young children with disabilities was born. Since then, steady progress and significant changes have occurred in the practice of EI. Many factors are influencing what we know and how we think about EI – changes in our understanding of and research about the development of infants and young children with DS, research on early development and learning more generally, and significant policy developments and changes in expectations about participation of persons with disabilities, including those with DS, in education and the community.

This chapter presents an overview of the history of EI, with a particular emphasis on EI for infants and young children with DS. The history includes summaries of: (1) the goals of EI for both the children and their families and how they have changed over the past 50 years; (2) research on the efficacy of EI as well as its actual implementation in practice; (3) how research in early childhood and early learning has in the past and will in the future affect the practice of EI; and (4) how research and policy developments concerning older children and adults with disabilities, including those with DS, are influencing the practice of EI. Conclusions about where we have been with research and policy developments are used to discuss implications for the future directions of the EI field.[1]

---

[1] Throughout the chapter, early intervention (EI) is mainly used to refer to programs and services for infants, toddlers, and preschoolers (birth to age 5 years) and their families, although in the United States EI refers to programs for infants and toddlers (birth to age 3 years) and preschool special education for children ages 3–5 years.

Neurocognitive Rehabilitation of Down Syndrome, eds. Jean-Adolphe Rondal, Juan Perera, and Donna Spiker. Published by Cambridge University Press. © Cambridge University Press 2011.

Goals of early intervention

For the past 50 years, the overarching goals of EI have stayed the same: (1) to promote and advance the development and skills of infants, toddlers, and preschoolers; and (2) to support and assist families in promoting the development and skills of infants, toddlers, and preschoolers. However, the goals have become broader and more differentiated. It is now common to think of EI as serving to lay a foundation for the child's life-long learning. This foundation is expected to help the child achieve high levels of functioning; participate fully in family, school, and community life; and have a good quality of life. Similarly, EI lays a foundation for the family to be able to help the child learn and grow; participate fully in family, school, and community activities; and have a good quality of life as a family.

Thus, while the overall goals of EI have stayed the same, what has changed? This chapter discusses changes in: (1) research demonstrating effects of EI on children and families; (2) research on early development of all children and those with DS in particular; (3) views and expectations about how the two goals are defined and about EI practices to achieve those goals; (4) changes in policy regarding expectations about disabilities, particularly relative to services and supports; and (5) changes in policy about early childhood, accountability, and school readiness that are beginning to have significant impacts on EI for children with disabilities, including those with DS.

Changing expectations for children with Down syndrome

Progress in EI for infants and young children with DS and their families has been sustained by an accumulation of research studies, by the active and persistent advocacy efforts of parents and professionals, and by major policy developments concerning the treatment of individuals with disabilities. All three of these activities have steadily and dramatically changed expectations about how children with DS are raised, educated, and participate in family life, schools, and the community.

A major textbook about DS published in 1976 (Smith & Berg, 1976) shows that although raising children in the home rather than in large institutions was taking hold at that time and becoming the norm, the practice still needed to be stated:

Considerable emphasis is now being placed on the advantages to the Down's syndrome child of home or home-like environments. (p. 276)

Likewise, the predominant view about education in the 1970s was that children with DS were quite limited in their ability to benefit from academic training. In the terminology of the last half of the twentieth century, children with DS were referred to as trainable (they could learn low-level, rote skills) but not educable (able to learn academic and abstract skills).

Although the Down's syndrome child generally is not well-suited for a type of education involving many abstract concepts, he or she usually can benefit from appropriate teaching of simple reading, writing, and arithmetic and of many useful self-help skills. (Smith & Berg, 1976, p. 275).

These low expectations about the educability of children with DS led our team, working on a study of EI in Minnesota, to present a counter-argument to the following quotation that appeared in a 1975 *Psychology Today* magazine article:

You show me just one mongoloid that has an educable IQ...I've never seen one in my experience with over 800 mongols. (Cited in Rynders et al., 1978)

Such low expectations and negative attitudes were based on a long history of institutionaliza-tion of children and adults with DS. Even into the 1970s, most parents were routinely told not to take their newborn baby with DS home after birth. EI and early education services were not widely available, and expectations for participation in home, school, and community life were low. These low expectations were unfortunate because they served to limit educa-tional policies, available services and programs, and the kind of research that was funded and conducted.

The social and political context has had an enormous impact on both policies and research that were even considered for implementation. For example, the disability rights movement and changing terminology have contributed to changes in expectations about how children with DS should be raised, educated, and treated. As evident in the quotations above, in the past 50 years terminology has changed from mongoloid or mongol, to handicapped or disabled child, to Down's syndrome or Down's child, and currently to child with DS. This demonstrates a change of view from the disability defining the child to the child with DS being a child first. Terminology is not trivial; it impacts i.e. expectations, policies, practices, and research.

Research about early intervention: past, present, and future

Early efficacy studies

Research has demonstrated many benefits of EI for infants and young children with DS: (1) acceleration of skill acquisition; (2) prevention of abnormal patterns or functioning; (3) promotion of optimal parent–child interactions; (4) provision of helpful parent support; and (5) encouragement of the child's participation in inclusive settings (Gibson & Harris, 1988; Crnic & Stormshak, 1997; Guralnick, 1997; Spiker & Hopmann, 1997; Bailey et al., 1998; Spiker et al., 2005; Spiker, 2006).

Some of the earliest EI programs were research demonstration projects in the 1960s and 1970s. These early programs tended to focus on promoting language, communication, and motor skills. Training strategies were used that emphasized stimulus–response learn-ing models and behavior modification, with the parents being trained to stimulate the child. Reviews done in the 1990s (Spiker & Hopmann, 1997) indicated that studies conducted in the 1960s, 1970s, and early 1980s showed benefits of EI programs compared with control groups in the United States, England, Canada, and Australia (Guralnick & Bricker, 1987; Gibson & Harris, 1988). The results showed increased rates of development of skills and milestones and slower declines in the rate of development as measured by global developmental or IQ tests.

For example, two early major experimental studies of EI with infants and preschool-ers with DS, Project EDGE in Minnesota and the Model Preschool Program in Seattle, Washington, had positive outcomes in promoting developmental milestones and building individual skills earlier than without EI participation (Hayden & Dmitriev, 1975; Rynders & Horrobin, 1975). In Project EDGE, begun in 1968, the EI group of 17 children with DS in Minnesota was compared with a control group of 18 in Chicago. This experimental EI program used a curriculum delivered by parents that concentrated on developing language and communication skills. Children in the EI group showed significant developmental gains on IQ and motor tests and naturalistic language samples compared with the control group of children (Rynders & Horrobin, 1975). Follow-up at 14–15 years of age showed second-to fourth-grade reading comprehension (Rynders & Horrobin, 1990). The Model Preschool Program, begun in 1971, was a center-based preschool program that began at 18 months and used a behavior modification approach to teach young children with DS. On a variety of standard developmental tests, children in the experimental group attained milestones earlier and showed less decline in development (on pre- to post-tests) than the control group children (Hayden & Dmitriev, 1975). A follow-up study showed that the children in the experimental group had second- to sixth-grade reading comprehension at 11–13 years of age (Fewell & Oelwin, 1991).

These and other studies from this era relied heavily on behavior modification or stimulus–response approaches, also known as applied behavior analysis (Gardner, 2006). Indeed, many would argue that this was the only approach to teaching and to intervention strategies used with young children with DS (Vincent et al., 1990), partly because it had to be established that the children could learn at all. Beginning in the1970s, a great deal of research was published that showed how applied behavior analysis techniques could help establish as well as consolidate and generalize behaviors, using reinforcement principles and stimulus–response models of learning (Cooper et al., 2007). Many studies focused on discrete behaviors of individuals that often were decontextualized. One major criticism of these kinds of studies and this approach was that skills learned in this way did not generalize and were not easily used in everyday situations.

More recent efficacy studies

Concerns about generalization of learned behaviors and skills have led to new approaches to teaching and intervention that address more functional behaviors and more natural contexts. Thus, some recent approaches involve more contextualized learning and focus on more meaningful behaviors such as errorless learning, chaining, functional analysis, naturalistic teaching, and pivotal response training (Hepburn, 2003; Koegel & Koegel, 2006). For instance, pivotal response training, particularly developed for use with young children with autism but applicable to all young children with disabilities, aims to intentionally teach children key behaviors that help them learn to learn, emphasizing a child's motivation to learn by explicitly teaching behaviors relevant for initiating and maintaining social interactions, using joint attention skills, being responsive to multiple cues, and learning other attention and self-regulation behaviors (Koegel & Koegel, 2006). This and other recent naturalistic learning approaches: (1) emphasize teaching functional behaviors in natural settings rather than using isolated, rote-learning approaches; (2) have a large and growing research base to support their efficacy for promoting children's early academic, language, and social skills; and (3) have an explicit goal of supporting the inclusion of young children with disabilities in settings with typical peers (Wolery, 2000; Koegel & Koegel, 2006).

By the 1980s and 1990s, a growing set of studies about EI showed benefits for both children and families (Spiker & Hopmann, 1997). Service provision in EI had moved toward individual intervention plans that involved a combination of services and supports. In a review about EI for young children with disabilities, Spiker et al. (2005) noted that the constellation of services and supports might include:

- Information about the child's disability
- Ongoing health monitoring to meet both routine and specialized medical needs
- Individualized one-to-one services and therapies targeted to promote specific skill acquisition and improvements in functioning
- Parent education and training that focuses on optimal responsivity to promote the child's learning and participation in daily activities and routines
- Opportunities for interactions with peers in group settings. (pp. 316–317)

Exhibit 2.1 History of US federal legislation

- 1967 – Federal legislation for education of handicapped children includes research
  - First experimental EI programs
- 1975 – PL 94–152 – Education for All Handicapped Act
  - Denied public education before this time
  - Landmark legislation
- 1983 – Amendments to PL 94–152 – state to develop birth to three years system
- 1986 – Mandates for 0–3 years EI system
- 1990 – Legislation retitled Individuals with Disabilities Education Act (IDEA) of 1990
- Included all preschool-age children
- 1997 – Reauthorization of IDEA
- Established a framework for policies and services

Based on Gallagher (2000), Hanson (2003).

Research continued to focus on accelerating skill acquisition and attainment of early developmental milestones, as well as preventing abnormal patterns or functioning (e.g. therapies to normalize the effects of hypotonia on motor and language development) (Spiker et al., 2005). Increasing attention was given to promoting optimal parent–child interactions by providing parents with information about both DS and early development, by modeling of stimulating interactions, and by providing positive emotional support (Dunst et al., 1997; Spiker et al., 2002; Kelly et al., 2005).

With an increased understanding of how young children with DS may show reduced social engagement and arousal, researchers sought to develop more tailored parent–child interaction intervention models to address these learning styles (Warren, 2000; Roper & Dunst, 2003; Yoder & Warren, 2004; Mahoney & Perales, 2005). Basic research about normal social and language development indicated that encouraging young children's active learning and ability, and disposition to actively initiate social interactions is critically important to early language acquisition and cognitive development (Bowman et al., 2001). More recent research about EI from the 1990s to the present has continued to focus on language and communication, building on this early childhood research.

One of the major issues addressed in more recent studies is how to best encourage participation in inclusive settings (Guralnick, 2001, 2005). Such a strategy gives young children with DS access to early childhood curricula, typical peers, and more of the usual activities available to all other children. This issue is addressed more fully in the following sections.

Early education policy and practice for children with disabilities

In the United States, the early research from the 1960s led to federal legislation that advanced educational opportunities for all children with disabilities (Exhibit 2.1). Parents were the driving force behind these educational policy developments, now codified in the Individuals with Disabilities Education Act (IDEA) of 1990. Although education for school-aged children with disabilities was mandated in 1975, legislation to include preschoolers did not go into effect until 1983 and infants and toddlers were not included until 1986.

The framework underlying IDEA comprised six core principles (Exhibit 2.2). This groundbreaking legislation made it possible for children with disabilities to participate in

Exhibit 2.2 The framework underlying the Individuals with Disabilities Education Act (IDEA)

Six core principles:

- Free appropriate public education (FAPE)
- Appropriate evaluation
- Development of an Individualized Education Program (IEP)
- Education in least restrictive environment
- Parent and student participation in decision making
- Procedural safeguards to protect rights

Adapted from Hanson (2003).

public education, and its evolution has been supported and advanced by research about the unique learning needs and unique and special approaches required to support the education of children with disabilities, including children with DS. The legislation strongly articulated principles, seen as rights, that acknowledge a wide range of functioning and needs of children with disabilities requiring individualized education plans as well as parent and student participation in decision making and in assessment activities. Particularly far reaching is the concept of least restrictive environment, which has advanced the agenda of full inclusion of children with disabilities, discussed in the next section.

Promoting inclusive educational programming

The inclusion of children with disabilities in programs that serve typically developing children is perhaps the most remarkable change in education, brought about by parent advocacy and a legislative expectation that children with disabilities have a right to be educated in the least restrictive environment (Fuchs & Fuchs, 1994; DEC/NAEYC, 2009). Inclusion meant moving from segregating and isolating children with disabilities to including and promoting their full participation (Guralnick, 2001, 2005). Beginning in the 1980s, experimental inclusion programs began to demonstrate that it was possible to offer inclusive programs and that children with disabilities could make good progress in them (Bricker, 2000; Guralnick, 2005). More recently, research has been increasing to show how inclusive early childhood programs can be implemented successfully (Wolery & Wilbers, 1994).

Recent developments in mainstream early childhood policy are affecting how we think of and implement preschool special education. In the 1990s in the United States, a significant expansion of community-based preschool and public school prekindergarten programs occurred, driven by concerns about an achievement gap between children from low-income families and their more affluent peers (McLanahan, 2005) and a growing research base showing that young children's school readiness is the outcome of all their experiences over the first five years of life (and prenatally as well) (National Research Council and Institute of Medicine, 2000). With a surge of research and policy attention cast on school readiness, a broad and comprehensive definition of school readiness became accepted, a definition that included five major domains of functioning: health and physical well-being, cognitive and general knowledge, language and communication development, emotional well-being and social competence, and approaches to learning (curiosity, attention, persistence) (National Education Goals Panel, 1997).

Exhibit 2.3 Issues about preschool inclusion and future directions for research

- Teachers and parents who did not support inclusion
- Special education and support staff who saw inclusion as a mechanism that would remove resources and supports
- Programs with inadequate staff or resources to meet individual needs
- Lack of research on use of mainstream curricula and how accountability affects services
- Lack of good studies on how curricula impact on children with Down syndrome
- Need for more studies about how to work in general education classrooms effectively and how to train teachers well

From Bricker (2000).

The new interest in school readiness had important ramifications for young children with disabilities: it led to more mainstream or inclusive program options, more research on the effects of inclusive settings, more access to early childhood curricula, a new focus on school readiness in preschool programs, and an increasing emphasis on accountability. Summarizing progress in providing inclusive educational programs at the turn of last century Bricker (2000) raised a number of critical issues that arose from early efforts, challenges that need to be addressed with additional research and policy attention (Exhibit 2.3).

Currently, infants, toddlers, and preschoolers (birth to age 5 years) participate in a wide range of early care and education programs, some of which are the same as those that serve typically developing children (e.g. center- and family-based child care, Head Start, state-funded preschool programs) and some of which serve children with disabilities exclusively (e.g. school-based preschool special education programs). Bailey et al. (1998) argued that there is a strong empirical basis for including children with disabilities in programs serving typically developing children. They cited a review of 22 studies that found that preschool-age children with disabilities have better outcomes when served in inclusive rather than segregated settings – better outcomes on standard measures of development, social competence, play behavior, and engagement (Buysse & Bailey, 1993); these findings are supported by more recent data as well (Guralnick, 2001). Bailey and colleagues went on to argue that several values that have driven the history of early intervention and special education programming for young children with disabilities need to be considered in defining the quality of inclusive programs. They proposed that inclusive programs for young children with disabilities need to be "of high-quality, consistent with family preferences, and capable of supporting each child's unique learning needs" (p. 28).

The principle of inclusion is to promote children's full participation rather than segregating and isolating them, and it has legal status in legislation mandating educational services for all children with disabilities from birth on. Inclusion involves "efforts to maximize the participation of children and families in typical home and community activities" (Guralnick, 2005, p. 59), including "full involvement of the child in family routines and in social activities with relatives and friends, as well as taking advantage of the entire array of educational and recreational opportunities that communities have to offer" (p. 59).

In 2009, a joint position statement about early childhood inclusion was distributed by the Division for Early Childhood (DEC) and the National Association for the Education of Young Children (NAEYC) (DEC/NAEYC, 2009). It contains a definition of inclusion that emphasizes high-quality features of inclusive programs, namely, (1) access (i.e. a wide range of typical environments and use of universal design to support full access); (2) participation (i.e. suggested approaches to support and promote the child's full participation, such as embedded instructional approaches); and (3) supports (i.e. infrastructure to support staff, such as appropriate professional development opportunities and specialized services in the setting). For these organizations, the goal of having this statement is to define what is meant by high-quality inclusion, which can influence policies and practices that improve services for young children with disabilities. Continuing progress is still needed in making successful inclusion a reality. For example, a recent research study showed that a significant number of children with mild developmental delays who were fully included in preschool and kindergarten were not in an inclusive placement by first and second grade (Guralnick et al., 2008).

With the growing trend to serve young children with disabilities in preschool inclusive environments, future research needs to advance the goal of meaningful and successful inclusion in natural settings. To do this successfully, early care and education programs should use approaches that target functional and developmentally appropriate goals and objectives. Further, they should effectively implement intervention activities within the context of ongoing classroom activities and routines. Finally, teaching approaches should focus on acquiring, generalizing, and maintaining skills. A number of innovative approaches fit these criteria, including response-prompting, naturalistic teaching, and use of embedded instruction, all of which incorporate instruction into classroom routines, not as a single isolated activity (Hemmeter, 2000).

Child characteristics that impact on inclusion

Spiker (2006) summarized how infants and young children with DS may have unique characteristics and needs related to the five domains of school readiness that must be addressed to promote their readiness for and their ability to successfully participate in inclusive programs. Basic research studies of young children with DS have documented learning styles that can interfere with and limit the child's ability to succeed in inclusive settings. These include tendencies to be less persistent and goal directed in problem solving and exploration situations, to use avoidance strategies in learning contexts or be less open to trying new tasks, and to use social ploys to avoid difficult tasks (e.g. frequent off-task behavior combined with social smiling and looking) (Wishart, 1993, 1996, 2001; Linn et al., 2000; Fidler, 2006). This less than optimal learning style or reduced mastery motivation, described as a lower motivation to explore and be goal directed (Niccols, et al., 2003), may be a result of adults' lower expectations for mastery and sustained engagement in problem solving, more failure experiences that contribute to avoidance of challenging tasks, less frequent reinforcement for independent efforts, or all three factors (Glenn et al., 2001). This reduced goal-directedness can also affect how adults interact with the child, making it harder for them to keep the child engaged for sustained periods of time in learning situations (Landry et al., 1998).

Such basic research that explicates unique learning tendencies in young children with DS is providing the crucial data needed for developing specific instructional strategies that are better tailored for these children. For instance, mindful of this basic research data, Hepburn (2003) has suggested a number of specific strategies for interactions and learning situations with young children with DS that can limit this counter-productive learning style and encourage a more active goal-directed learning. These include:

- determining activities that sustain the child's engagement and interest and using them to increase learning

- practicing with well-developed skills the child has already mastered
- using errorless teaching techniques
- reinforcing the child's attention when engaged in tasks that interest the child
- using a visual schedule
- pacing tasks with work and breaks.

Many of these suggestions are congruent with the recommendations that emerge from research about responsive teaching and strategies to promote early language and communication skills, as described below (see also Mahoney and Perales, Chapter 16 of this book).

Strategies for promoting language, communication, and social development

As described earlier, from the very beginning of the history of EI for children with DS, language and communication have been emphasized as key skills to target. This has been the case because children with DS have such significant deficits in this area (Chapman, 1995) and because these skills are essential for school and life success and to promote the full participation goals of inclusion. The earliest studies examining how to promote speech and communication skills tended to focus on interventions to teach children sounds, words, etc., and use operant or stimulus–response training methods. Recent advances in the understanding of prelinguistic and language and communication acquisition have led the field away from using decontextualized, nonfunctional approaches for teaching and supporting young children's communication skills. For instance, until the 1980s and 1990s, we did not have a rich research base for prelinguistic communication with infants and toddlers. This research has demonstrated how the amount and quality of language input are important for children's language development (Hart & Risley, 1995). Some studies suggest that for infants and young children with DS who may have a higher tendency to be passive or unresponsive in social interactions, language input may be reduced and may be qualitatively different from the input received by typical peers (Chapman, 1995).

The movement toward inclusion in settings with typical peers also gives children opportunities in their peer interactions that are beneficial to acquiring and using language. Newer studies have been showing the importance of reciprocal communication in everyday life in a functional way (McCathren et al., 1995; Roper & Dunst, 2003). Highly responsive conversations that will help consolidate and extend communication and general knowledge focus on interventions to help child communicate; use interaction approaches and more evidence-based communication approaches; draw from a rich research base about prelinguistic communication and language development; use more contextualized, functional approaches to teaching; and include use of typical peers as models and communication partners.

Increasingly, research and practice have been addressing the features of communication interventions that encourage the use of speech, language, and nonverbal communication to engage in meaningful conversations and social interactions, both with adults and peers (Chapman, 1995; Ramruttun & Jenkins, 1998; Warren, 2000; Wishart, 2001; Kim & Mahoney, 2004). The research about prelinguistic communication and early language acquisition suggests that adult–child interactions in which the adult follows the child's lead to topic and activity, uses a variety of child-centered activities (e.g. toy play, motor games), and aims to increase the number of communication opportunities, particularly by using natural contexts, facilitate language and communication development (Warren, 2000; Spiker et al.,

Exhibit 2.4 Family-centered practice: current conceptualizations

- Families viewed as competent, not deficit oriented
- Family-centered approaches that take into account families' needs, concerns, resources, priorities, and their goals for the child and their family
- Individualization of service plans to meet family needs
- Coordination of services that accommodate family schedules
- Services delivered in natural environments to maximize meaningful and functional adaptation
- Emphasis on positive interactions with families to support competence
- Family focus that is central to the program's philosophy
- Intervention activities that can be integrated into typical daily routines
- Use of effective help-giving practices (e.g. active listening)
- Parents working with professionals as partners in decision making
- Parents assisted in accessing support systems and typical supports (e.g. child care)
- Emphasis on supports that advance child and family quality of life

2002; Roper & Dunst, 2003; Walker et al., 2008). Other work suggests that the use of signs and gestures early in the acquisition process can promote speech development, not hinder it as formerly believed (Clibbens, 2001). Furthermore, it is now well understood that language development can also be facilitated by focusing on important core skills, such as imitation and joint attention (Kasari et al., 1995; Fidler, 2006). Additionally, recent reviews show that early social interactions that provide the context for language acquisition are predictive of more positive outcomes for children participating in EI (Mahoney et al., 1998).

One particularly promising intervention model to encourage communication development is relationship-focused intervention (Mahoney & Perales, 2003; Kelly et al., 2008; Mahoney and Perales, Chapter 16 of this book). This approach is based on more than two decades of research about parent–child interactions showing that young children with DS have social and emotional difficulties that may make them difficult social partners. Such difficulties are briefer and less intense emotional expressiveness, reduced tendencies to take the initiative in social interactions and to sustain reciprocal interactions, less predictability, and less persistent and goal-directed social interactions (Spiker et al., 2002). Relationship-focused intervention seeks to address these difficulties by explicitly increasing contingency and responsiveness in parent–child interactions; addressing the child's social responsiveness; encouraging active and self-directed learning, exploration, and communication; and managing feelings that can interfere with sustained social interactions.

Changing perspectives about parent participation in early intervention

As described earlier, one of the major goals of EI is to support and assist families so they can support and assist their child. From the beginning, EI professionals have recognized the importance of parent involvement in EI, emphasizing specific training and parent education and needs for emotional support. While the reciprocity in parent–professional relationships has been the subject of much research over the years, increasingly parents are being seen as partners with professionals in assessment, program planning and implementation, and advocacy efforts (Turnbull et al., 2000; Bailey & Powell, 2005). Some of the important changes in family-centered practices that have taken place in the past 50 years are identified in Exhibit 2.4.

Remarkable changes in the availability of support for families of infants and young children with DS have occurred over the past 50 years (Orsmond, 2005). Whereas 50 years ago, after the child's birth, parents were routinely encouraged to place the child in an institution, it is now routine for parents to receive in-hospital support after the birth, and birth announcements specifically for families with an infant with DS are available (an example of resources for new parents can be found at http://www.mhdsa.org/NewParentsRaisingChild.htm). Parent-to-parent support groups and information are available from EI programs, community-based agencies, and online. Not only have children with DS been receiving the same types of routine well-child medical care expected for all children, but medical clinics specifically devoted to DS also exist now (for listings of such clinics, refer to http://www.ndsccenter.org/resources/clinics.php).

US national data on early intervention and preschool special education

Until recently, no national data were available in the United States about the EI and preschool special education service systems. In the 1990s, the Office of Special Education Programs (OSEP) in the US Department of Education funded two studies, the National Early Intervention Longitudinal Study (NEILS) about EI for infants and toddlers ages 0–3 years (Scarborough et al., 2004, 2006; Hebbeler et al., 2007) and the Pre-elementary Education Longitudinal Study (PEELS) (Markowitz et al., 2006). The NEILS data, although not broken down specifically for children with DS, showed that EI consists mainly of home-based services (for 76% of all children), with a core set of six services for most children [service coordination (78%); speech therapy (52%), special instruction (43%); occupational therapy (39%), physical therapy (39%), and developmental screening (37%)] (Hebbeler et al., 2008). Furthermore, the median amount of service received is 1.5 hours per week, with 63% of children receiving 2 or fewer hours per week and 84% receiving less than 4 hours per week. This relatively small amount of service suggests how critical it is for EI to focus on assisting parents and other regular caregivers in learning how to maximize all daily activities as learning opportunities, and to teach parents and other caregivers how to use daily activities and routines as occasions for learning (Bruder & Dunst, 1999; McWilliam, 2005; Dunst et al., 2006).

In the PEELS study of preschool special education (ages 3–5 years) in the United States (Markowitz et al., 2006), data showed that preschool-aged children receive about 15 hours of services per week, with 85%–90% receiving speech therapy. Of the reasons for eligibility, speech delays (49%) and developmental delays (27%) were the most common, with 4% eligible because of mental retardation (a category that includes many of the children with DS). Child outcome data, based on scores on standard tests (Peabody Picture Vocabulary Test, Woodcock-Johnson Test) varied by groups, with the mean for those with developmental delay being about 85 [1 standard deviation (SD) below the mean] and those with mental retardation being about 60–70 (2 SDs below the mean). The latter groups also scored about 1 SD below the mean on behavior assessments and 2 SDs below the mean on motor assessments. Not surprisingly, children with mildest delays made the most progress while in preschool special education programs.

The findings from these two large national studies provide an important snapshot of EI services. The amount of service provided strongly suggests that involving parents and other caregivers in encouraging young children's learning is imperative to achieve the best outcomes for the children. The findings also give a baseline for tracking trends in service delivery and outcomes in future research studies (e.g. the question is: does the more recent focus on school readiness lead to better early literacy outcomes in preschoolers with disabilities?). Finally, they also provide data that can be used to generate hypotheses for future in-depth studies.

Changes in assessment: research and practice and future directions

One of the most significant changes over the past 50 years that is having an impact on services and education for children with DS has been in early childhood assessment. Rather than earlier uses of assessment to exclude, isolate, and separate children with disabilities and to focus on deficits, assessment now has new purposes:

- identify concerns for further intervention
- make sound decisions about teaching and learning
- help programs improve their developmental and educational interventions.

These new uses are exemplified in a new and broad definition of assessment: "Assessment is a generic term that refers to the process of gathering information for decision-making" (McLean et al., 2004). Within the early childhood field more broadly and for young children with disabilities specifically, position statements by major early childhood professional organizations are defining assessment as being used in the service of goals that support young children, such as to:

- promote full participation
- promote school readiness
- link assessment information to curriculum and services
- promote functional child outcomes
- assist in assessing children's learning styles, strengths, challenges [DEC, 2007; NAEYC & National Association of Early Childhood Specialists (NAECS) in State Departments of Education, 2003].

These position statements identify recommended best practices for an assessment process that advocates the use of multiple sources of information and informants, including parents, and multiple methods to gather assessment information (e.g. tests, observations, checklists, portfolios/work samples, interviews). Typical questions that need to be asked about assessment practices are shown in Exhibit 2.5.

One critical feature of the newer views about assessment is how to look at functional outcomes, behaviors, and skills used in a variety of natural settings, situations, and daily routines – with family, with siblings, with peers; at the playground, park, grocery store, home, child care; in therapy, etc. (Exhibit 2.6) (McWilliam, 2005). Instead of assessing skills in an artificial and nonfunctional way, recent assessment approaches seek to understand meaningful use of skills in real-life settings and to achieve everyday goals. The next section about accountability has additional discussion of this issue.

Exhibit 2.5 Critical questions about appropriate early childhood assessment

- When, how, and with whom does assessment occur?
- Is it a central part of our program?
- Is it conducted in a way that is developmentally appropriate?
- Is it culturally and linguistically responsive?
- Is it tied to children's daily activities?
- Does it include families in meaningful and respectful ways?
- Does it show strengths, needs, and progress for the child and/or group of children?
- Does our professional development support assessment?

From DEC, 2007; NAEYC & NAECS in State Departments of Education (2003).

Exhibit 2.6 Considerations in assessment of young children's functional skills

- Does the assessment process tap the child's functioning when doing things that are meaningful to the child?
- Do we assess what a child typically does or assess in unusual situations?
- Do we know about the child's actual performance across settings and situations?
- Do we observe how a child uses his/her skills to accomplish tasks?
- Does the assessment go beyond domains to consider integrated functioning?

Accountability in early childhood

A major policy development in the United States in the past decade that is beginning to have a significant effect on programs serving infants and young children with disabilities is the growing calls for accountability. As part of a growing trend in government, all types of agencies and programs are being asked to provide data that demonstrate that the services they provide are having the intended effects. As a result of government reviews beginning in 2002, OSEP now requires all states to submit data about child and family outcomes for programs serving children with disabilities from birth to age 5 years (Hebbeler & Barton, 2007; Hebbeler et al., 2008). OSEP has been funding a national Early Childhood Outcomes (ECO) Center since 2003, to make recommendations about relevant outcomes and to help states develop systems for collecting outcomes data, to report to OSEP annually, and to use in state and local accountability and program improvement efforts (see www.the-eco-center. org for more information and specific papers at http://www.fpg.unc.edu/~eco/papers.cfm).

Stakeholder involvement is central to the mission of OSEP. This stakeholder input has led to agreement that an accountability system should be true to the overarching goal of EI and early childhood special education, which is:

To enable young children to be active and successful participants during the early childhood years and in the future in a variety of settings – in their homes with their families, in child care, in preschool programs, and in the community. (See www.the-eco-center.org.)

Furthermore, stakeholders had a number of key suggestions for OSEP and the ECO Center about how to develop an appropriate accountability system. Stakeholders worried about how an outcome system could do justice to the wide range of types and severities of disabilities and strongly recommended that the system not harm children or their families. They also wanted the child outcomes to be defined functionally and not be domains based, in accordance with

---

Exhibit 2.7   US child outcome and accountability system

Percentage of infants and toddlers with Individualized Family Service Plans (or preschool children with IEPs) who demonstrate improved:

- Positive social–emotional skills (including social relationships)
- Acquisition and use of knowledge and skills (including early language/communication, (Part C); including early language/communication and early literacy (Part B, Preschool)
- Use of appropriate behaviors to meet their needs

See www.the-eco-center.org and http://www.fpg.unc.edu/~eco/index.cfm.
Note: From Part C and Part B State Performance Plan and Annual Performance Report Indicator Measurement Tables (http://www.fpg.unc.edu/~ECO/pdfs/Part_C3_measurement_table. pdf and http://www.fpg.unc.edu/~ECO/pdfs/Part_B_measurement_table.pdf).

---

best practices in early childhood assessment. In addition, they argued that outcomes should be defined in such a way as to reflect best practices toward a more integrated, functional, and inclusive view of young children's development.

Stakeholders urged OSEP to identify outcomes that parents and the general public could easily understand, that reflect the purposes of these programs, and that would not be overly burdensome to services' providers who should be concentrating on serving children and families. Stakeholders also reminded OSEP that young children with disabilities could possibly be participating in several accountability efforts (e.g. assessments done as part of participation in other early childhood programs, such as Head Start or state prekindergarten programs).

After broad input and review by a variety of stakeholder groups, three child outcomes were identified (Exhibit 2.7).

Functional child outcomes in an accountability system

One important feature of the outcomes being used in the US accountability system is the focus on functional child outcomes. Rather than thinking of children's development and learning in terms of domains, milestones, or isolated skills, thinking functionally requires describing development in context and assessing skills that are meaningful to the child in the context of everyday living. Thus, the three child outcomes concern the integration of skills and behaviors in order for the child to participate meaningfully in family, school, and community activities; to use skills to meet needs and accomplish goals; and to generalize across settings and people, adults, and peers. For instance, using a finger in a pointing motion and using two-word utterances are examples of isolated skills, but pointing to indicate needs or wants and engaging in back-and-forth verbal exchanges with caregivers using two-word utterances are examples of functional skills. Functional outcomes emphasize the integration of skills to accomplish a task, not the individual skills themselves.

Family outcomes in an accountability system

The US federal legislation mandating EI and preschool special education is also predicated on the assumption of benefits of EI to families. Much research over the past 50 years has documented the critical role of families in child development, for both typically developing children and those with disabilities such as DS. Earlier research about families tended to focus on outcomes, such as the receipt of services or satisfaction with services rather than

Exhibit 2.8 Family outcomes in an accountability system

- Families understand their child's strengths, abilities, and special needs
- Families know their rights and advocate effectively for their children
- Families help their children develop and learn
- Families have support systems
- Families are able to access desired services, programs, activities in their community

Based on Bailey et al. (1998, 2006); see also Hebbeler & Barton (2007).

Exhibit 2.9 Selected websites about Down syndrome

- National Association for Down Syndrome – www.nads.org
- National Down Syndrome Society – www.ndss.org
- World Down Syndrome Day – www.worlddownsyndromeday.org
- Down Syndrome Research and Treatment Foundation – www.dsrtf.org
- Down Syndrome Association – www.downs-syndrome.org.uk
- Down Syndrome Education International – www.downsed.org
- European Down Syndrome Association – www.edsa.info
- Asociacion Sindrome de Down de Baleares– www.asnimo.com

the benefits families experienced as a result of services and supports received. These newer conceptualizations of family outcomes recognize that helping families attain their goals has a direct bearing on child outcomes (Bailey et al., 1998, 2006). Thus, because parents can be affected by having a child with a disability, EI should promote positive adaptation and reduce potential negative impacts (Exhibit 2.8).

Expectations and information about Down syndrome

Parents of children with DS have many information needs, summarized in a recent review (Bailey & Powell, 2005). Over the past 50 years, we have gone from little available information to mainly negative and deficit-oriented information to a massive amount and variety of information from a tremendous number of sources. An Internet search of the keyword "Down syndrome" produces millions of hits (e.g. 16 million on April 1, 2009). Some of the best information is contained on websites by parent–professional organizations, with a partial listing in Exhibit 2.9.

In contrast to the quotes at the beginning of this chapter, in the present day, expectations are quite different and high. For instance, the optimism expressed in the website for the Down Syndrome Research and Treatment Foundation (DSRTF) (see www/dsrtf.org) is now fairly common:

DSRTF sees a new world coming in which people with Down syndrome are fully included in academic and social environments and where they can live independently as adults, if they choose so.

Treatments … will allow individuals with Down syndrome to participate more fully in school; lead more active and independent lives; and prevent early cognitive decline.

Follow-up studies of adults with Down syndrome

The current optimism about outcomes and long-term functioning of persons with DS may be overly hopeful, however, considering available research data. Few follow-up studies that included adults with DS are available, but those that do exist yielded sobering results. For instance, Hanson (2003) reported about adult outcomes of her sample of 15 children who had participated in an experimental EI program in 1974–1977 in Oregon; they were 24–26 years old in 2000–2001. Hanson found that participation in inclusive educational settings decreased as the children aged. She also found disappointing results with regard to adult outcomes (social, employment, independence). Furthermore, services and supports for these adults were found to be lacking. On a positive note, however, families had strong positive feelings and experiences as a family and fondly remembered EI 25 years later and cited its importance for laying a foundation for the child's and family's long-term adaptation.

In a more recent study of a nationally representative sample of young adults with disabilities in the United States who participated in special education, the National Longitudinal Transition Study 2 (NLTS2), children were followed and data collected four years after they left high school (Wagner et al., 2005). The data are not reported separately for young adults with DS specifically, but the data for the group with mental retardation showed wide variations in outcomes. For instance, overall,

- 72% were high school graduates in 2003 (51% in 1987)
- 25% had participated in some level of postsecondary education
- 30% were employed (compared with 56% for the young adults across all disabilities and 66% for the general population)
- 15% were living independently
- 72% reported that they were seeing friends outside of school or work.

These findings, which undoubtedly reflect many individuals with DS, show that attainment of expected positive adult outcomes is still out of reach of many young adults in this group with mental retardation.

Conclusions and looking to the future

Much progress has been made in the past 50 years in the provision of early intervention for infants and young children with DS and their families. Given the currently available data about adult outcomes, however, it is clear that more progress is required. Continuing research is sorely needed about educational approaches to increase attainment of meaningful and generalizable academic success, social and communication skills, and vocational and recreational skills that will lead to better child and long-term adult outcomes (Spiker et al., 2005). An urgent need exists for long-term follow-up studies of new and contemporary cohorts of children with DS, those who have been the beneficiaries of better educational and rearing opportunities as well as better healthcare, nutrition, and physical fitness than were available to earlier cohorts of children. The continuing advocacy for full participation goals must also be supported by more research about how to implement effective inclusive educational programs. Evidence-based programs, those achieving positive child and adult outcomes, should form the basis of educational policies, funding allocations, and professional development systems. Future research should also include a continuing focus on key functions and developmental processes that support young children's active participation in daily activities and routines and the development of behaviors and skills that enhance the young child's active participation in learning, referred to as learning to learn. Programs also need to use assessment information about key processes for planning interventions to promote the child's emerging skills over the first five years of life. With a continuing synergy between research, advocacy, and policy, current optimism and high expectations for children and adults with DS may be fully realized.

Summary

Fifty years ago, formalized or universal early intervention (EI) for infants and young children with Down syndrome (DS) did not exist . The field of EI for infants and young children with disabilities began with a few experimental programs instigated by the advocacy of parents and the forward thinking of researchers. In this chapter, progress in EI for infants and young children with DS and their families is reviewed by showing how it has been sustained by an accumulation of research studies, by the active and persistent advocacy efforts of parents and professionals, and by major policy developments concerning the treatment of individuals with disabilities. This history of EI includes summaries of: (1) the changing goals of EI for both the children and their families; (2) research on the efficacy and practice of EI; (3) how research in early childhood and early learning has and will affect the practice of EI; and (4) how research and policy developments concerning older children and adults with disabilities are influencing the practice of EI. The review focuses on changes in research, practice, and policy that are having significant impacts on EI for children with disabilities, including those with DS. Conclusions about past research and policy developments are used to discuss implications for future directions of EI.

References

Bailey, D. B., Jr., Bruder, M. B., Hebbeler, K., et al. (2006). Recommended outcomes for families of young children with disabilities. *Journal of Early Intervention*, 28(4), 227–251.

Bailey, D. B., McWilliam, R. A., Darkes, L. A., et al. (1998). Family outcomes in early intervention: a framework for program evaluation and efficacy research. *Exceptional Children*, 64, 313–328.

Bailey, D. B., Jr. & Powell, T. (2005). Assessing the information needs of families in early intervention. In M. J. Guralnick (ed.), *The Developmental Systems Approach to Early Intervention*, pp. 151–183. Baltimore: Brookes.

Bowman, B. T., Donovan, M. S., Burns, M. S. (eds.) (2001). *Eager to Learn: Educating our Preschoolers*. Washington, DC: National Academies Press.

Bricker, D. (2000). Inclusion: how the scene has changed. *Topics in Early Childhood Special Education*, 20(1), 14–19.

Bruder, M. B. & Dunst, C. J. (1999). Expanding learning opportunities for infants and toddlers in natural environments: a chance to reconceptualize early intervention. *Zero To Three*, 20, 34–36.

Buysse, V. & Bailey, D. B. (1993). Behavioral and developmental outcomes in young children with disabilities in integrated and segregated settings: a review of comparative studies. *Journal of Special Education*, 26, 434–461.

Chapman, R. S. (1995). Language development in children and adolescents with Down syndrome. In P. Fletcher & B. MacWhinney (eds.), *Handbook of Child Language*, pp. 641–663. Oxford: Blackwell.

Clibbens, J. (2001). Signing and lexical development in children with Down syndrome. *Down Syndrome Research and Practice*, 7, 101–105.

Cooper, J. O., Heron, T. E., Heward, W. L. (2007). *Applied Behavior Analysis* (2nd edn.). Upper Saddle River: Prentice Hall.

Crnic, K. & Stormshak, E. (1997). The effectiveness of providing social support for families of children at risk. In M. J. Guralnick (ed.), *The Effectiveness of Early Intervention*. Baltimore: Brookes.

DEC/NAEYC. (2009). *Early Childhood Inclusion: A joint position statement of the Division for Early Childhood* (DEC) *and the National Association for the Education of Young Children* (NAEYC). Chapel Hill: The

University of North Carolina, FPG Child Development Institute.

Division for Early Childhood (DEC). (2007). *Promoting Positive Outcomes for Children with Disabilities: Recommendations for Curriculum, Assessment, and Program Evaluation.* Missoula, MT: Author.

Dunst, C. J., Bruder, M. B., Trivette, C. M., Hamby, D. W. (2006). Everyday activity settings, natural learning environments, and early intervention practices. *Journal of Policy and Practice in Intellectual Disabilities,* **3**(1), 3–10.

Dunst, C. J., Trivette, C. M., Jodry, W. (1997). Influences of social support on children with disabilities and their families. In M. J. Guralnick (ed.), *The Effectiveness of Early Intervention.* Baltimore: Brookes.

Fewell, R. R. & Oelwin, P. L. (1991). Effective early intervention: results from the model preschool program for children with Down syndrome and other developmental delays. *Topics in Early Childhood Special Education,* **11**, 56–68.

Fidler, D. J. (2006). The emergence of a syndrome-specific personality profile in young children with Down syndrome. In J. A. Rondal & J. Perera (eds.), *Down Syndrome,* pp. 139–152. West Sussex: Wiley.

Fuchs, D. & Fuchs, L. (1994). Inclusive schools movement and the radicalization of special education reform. *Exceptional Children,* **60**, 294–309.

Gallagher, J. (2000). The beginnings of federal help for young children with disabilities. *Topics in Early Childhood Special Education,* **20**(1), 3–6.

Gardner, W. I. (2006). *Behavior Modification in Mental Retardation.* New York: Aldine De Gruyter.

Gibson, D. & Harris, A. (1988). Aggregated early intervention effects for Down's syndrome persons: patterning and longevity of benefits. *Journal of Mental Deficiency Research,* **32**, 1–17.

Glenn, S., Dayus, B., Cunningham, C., Horgan, M. (2001). Mastery motivation in children with Down syndrome. *Down Syndrome Research and Practice,* **7**, 52–59.

Guralnick, M. J. (ed.) (1997). *The Effectiveness of Early Intervention.* Baltimore: Brookes.

Guralnick, M. J. (ed.) (2001). *Early Childhood Inclusion.* Baltimore: Brookes.

Guralnick, M. J. (2005). Inclusion as a core principle in the early intervention system. In M. J. Guralnick (ed.), *The Developmental Systems Approach to Early Intervention,* pp. 59–69. Baltimore: Brookes.

Guralnick, M. J. & Bricker, D. (1987). The effectiveness of early intervention for children with cognitive and general developmental delays. In M. J.Guralnick & F. C. Bennett (eds.), *The Effectiveness of Early Intervention for At-risk and Handicapped Children,* pp. 115–173. New York: Academic Press.

Guralnick, M. J., Neville, B., Hammond, M. A., Connor, R. T. (2008). Continuity and change from full-inclusion early childhood programs through the early elementary period. *Journal of Early Intervention,* **30**(3), 237–250.

Hanson, M. J. (2003). Twenty-five years after early intervention. *Infants and Young Children,* **16**(4), 354–365.

Hart, B. & Risley, T. (1995). *Meaningful Differences in the Everyday Experience of Young American Children.* Baltimore: Brookes.

Hayden, A. H. & Dmitriev, V. (1975). The multidisciplinary preschool program for Down's syndrome children at the University of Washington model preschool center. In B. Z. Friedlander, G. M. Sterritt, G. E. Kirk (eds.), *Exceptional Infant.* New York: Brunner/Mazel.

Hebbeler, K. & Barton, L. (2007). The need for data on child and family outcomes at the Federal and State levels. *Young Exceptional Children Monograph Series,* **9**, 1–15.

Hebbeler, K., Barton, L., Mallik, S. (2008). Assessment and accountability for programs serving young children with disabilities. *Exceptionality,* **1**(16), 48–63.

Hebbeler, K., Spiker, D., Bailey, D., et al. (2007). *Early intervention for infants and toddlers with disabilities and their families: Participants, services, and outcomes. Final Report of the National Early Intervention Longitudinal Study (NEILS).* Menlo Park: SRI International.

Hebbeler, K., Spiker, D., Morrison, K., Mallik, S. (2008). A national look at the characteristics of Part C early intervention services. *Young Exceptional Children Monograph Series No. 10.*

Hemmeter, M. L. (2000). Classroom-based interventions: evaluating the past and looking toward the future. *Topics in Early Childhood Special Education,* **20**(1), 56–61.

Hepburn, S. L. (2003). Clinical implications of temperamental characteristics of young children with developmental disabilities. *Infants and Young Children,* **16**, 59–76.

Kasari, C., Freeman, S., Mundy, P., Sigman, M. D. (1995). Attention regulation by children with Down syndrome: coordinated joint attention and social referencing looks. *American Journal on Mental Retardation,* **100**, 128–136.

Kelly, J. F., Booth-LaForce, C., Spieker, S. J. (2005). Assessing family characteristics relevant to early intervention. In M. J. Guralnick (ed.), *The Developmental Systems Approach to Early Intervention,* pp. 235–265. Baltimore: Brookes.

Kelly, J. F., Zuckerman, T., Rosenblatt, S. (2008). Promoting first relationships: a relationship-focused early intervention approach. *Infants and Young Children,* **21**, 285–295.

Kim, J. & Mahoney, G. (2004). The effects of mother's style of interaction on children's engagement: Implications for using responsive interventions with parents. *Topics in Early Childhood Special Education,* **24**, 31–38.

Koegel, R. L. & Koegel, L. K. (2006). *Pivotal Response Treatments for Autism.* Baltimore: Brookes.

Landry, S. H., Miller-Loncar, C. L., Swank, P. R. (1998). Goal-directed behavior in children with Down syndrome: the role of joint play situations. *Early Education & Development,* **9**, 264–278.

Linn, M. I., Goodman, J. F., Lender, W. L. (2000). Played out? Passive behavior by children with Down syndrome during unstructured play. *Journal of Early Intervention,* **23**, 264–278.

Mahoney, G., Boyce, G., Fewell, R. R., Spiker, D., Wheeden, C. A. (1998). The relationship of parent-child interaction to the effectiveness of early intervention services for at-risk children and children with disabilities. *Topics in Early Childhood Special Education,* **18**, 5–17.

Mahoney, G. & Perales, F. (2003). Using relationship-focused intervention to enhance the social-emotional functioning of young children with autism spectrum disorders. *Topics in Early Childhood Special Education,* **23**(2), 77–89.

Mahoney, G. & Perales, F. (2005). Relationship-focused intervention with children with pervasive developmental disorders and other disabilities: a comparative study. *Journal of Developmental and Behavioral Pediatrics,* **26**, 77–85.

Markowitz, J., Carlson, E., Frey, W., et al. (2006). *Preschool with Disabilities: Wave 1 Overview Report from the Pre-Elementary Education Longitudinal Study (PEELS).* Washington: Institute for Education Sciences.

McCathren, R. B., Yoder, P. J., Warren, S. F. (1995). The role of directives in early language intervention. *Journal of Early Intervention,* **19**, 91–101.

McLanahan, S. (2005). School readiness: closing racial and ethnic gaps. *The Future of Children,* **15**(1).

McLean, M., Wolery, M., Bailey, D. B., Jr. (2004). *Assessing Infants and Preschoolers with Special Needs* (3rd edn.), Upper Saddle River: Prentice Hall.

McWilliam, R. A. (2005). Assessing the resource needs of families in the context of early intervention. In M. J. Guralnick (ed.), *The Developmental Systems Approach to Early Intervention,* pp. 215–233. Baltimore: Brookes.

National Association for the Education of Young Children (NAEYC) & National Association of Early Childhood Specialists (NAECS) in State Departments of Education. (2003). *Where We Stand on Curriculum, Assessment, and Program Evaluation.* Retrieved from http://www.naeyc.org/about/positions/pdf/StandlCurrAss.pdf.

National Education Goals Panel. (1997). *Special Early Childhood Report 1997.* Washington: Author.

National Research Council and Institute of Medicine. (2000). *From Neurons to Neighborhoods: The Science of Early Childhood Development*. Washington: National Academy Press.

Niccols, A., Atkinson, L., Pepler, D. (2003). Mastery motivation in young children with Down's syndrome: relationship with cognitive and adaptive competence. *Journal of Intellectual Disability Research*, **47**(2), 121–133.

Orsmond, G. I. (2005). Assessing interpersonal and family distress and threats to confident parenting in the context of early intervention. In M. J. Guralnick (ed.), *The Developmental Systems Approach to Early Intervention*, pp. 185–213. Baltimore: Brookes.

Ramruttun, B. & Jenkins, C. (1998). Prelinguistic communication and Down syndrome. *Down Syndrome Research and Practice*, **5**, 53–62.

Roper, N. & Dunst, C. J. (2003). Communication interventions in natural environments: guidelines for practice. *Infants and Young Children*, **16**, 215–226.

Rynders, J. & Horrobin, J. (1975). Project EDGE: a communication stimulation program for Down's syndrome infants. In B. Friedland, G. Steritt, G. Kirk (eds.), *Exceptional Infant: Assessment and Intervention*, pp. 173–192. New York: Brunner/Mazel.

Rynders, J. E. & Horrobin, J. M. (1990). Always trainable? Never educable? Updating educational expectations concerning children with Down syndrome. *American Journal on Mental Retardation*, **95**, 77–83.

Rynders, J. E., Spiker, D., Horrobin, J. (1978). Underestimating the educability of Down's syndrome children: examination of methodological problems in recent literature. *American Journal of Mental Deficiency*, **82**, 440–448.

Scarborough, A. A., Hebbeler, K. M., Spiker, D. (2006). Eligibility characteristics of infants and toddlers entering early intervention in the United States. *Journal of Policy and Practice in Intellectual Disabilities*, **3**(1), 57–64.

Scarborough, A., Spiker, D., Mallik, S., et al. (2004). Who are the children and families receiving early intervention services? *Exceptional Children*, **70**, 469–483.

Smith, G. F. & Berg, J. M. (1976). *Down's Anomaly* (2nd edn.). New York: Longman Group Limited.

Spiker, D. (2006). Off to a good start: early interventions for infants and young children with Down syndrome and their families. In J. A. Rondal & J. Perera (eds.), *Down Syndrome: Neurobehavioral Specificity*, pp. 176–190. West Sussex: Wiley.

Spiker, D., Boyce, G., Boyce, L. (2002). Parent-child interactions when infants and young children have disabilities. In L. Gidden (ed.), *International Review of Research in Mental Retardation*, Vol. 25, pp. 35–70. San Diego: Academic Press.

Spiker, D., Hebbeler, K., Mallik, S. (2005). Developing and implementing early intervention programs for children with established disabilities. In M. J. Guralnick (ed.), *The Developmental Systems Approach to Early Intervention*, pp. 305–349. Baltimore: Brookes.

Spiker, D. & Hopmann, M. R. (1997). The effectiveness of early intervention for children with Down Syndrome. In M. J. Guralnick (ed.), *The Effectiveness of Early Intervention*, pp. 271–306. Baltimore: Brookes.

Turnbull, A. P., Turbiville, V., Turnbull, H. R. (2000). Evolution of family-professional partnerships: collective empowerment as the model for the early twenty-first century. In J. P. Shonkoff & S. J. Meisels (eds.), *Handbook of Early Childhood Intervention* (2nd edn.), pp. 630–650. New York: Cambridge University Press.

Vincent, L. J., Salisbury, C. L., Strain, P., McCormick, C., Tessier, A. (1990). A behavioral-ecological approach to early intervention: focus on cultural diversity. In S. J. Meisels & J. P. Shonkoff (eds.), *Handbook of Early Childhood Intervention*, pp. 173–195. New York: Cambridge University Press.

Wagner, M., Newman, L., Cameto, R., Levine, P. (2005). *Changes Over Time in the Early Postschool Outcomes of Youth with Disabilities*. Menlo Park: SRI International.

Walker, D., Bigelow, K. M., Harjusola-Webb, S. (2008). Increasing communication and language-learning opportunities for infants and toddlers. *Young Exceptional Children Monograph Series No.* **10**, 105–121.

Warren, S. F. (2000). The future of early communication and language intervention. *Topics in Early Childhood Special Education*, **20**, 33–37.

Wishart, J. (1993). The development of learning difficulties in children with Down's syndrome. *Journal of Intellectual Disability Research*, **37**, 389–403.

Wishart, J. (1996). Learning in young children with Down syndrome: developmental trends. In J. A. Rondal & J. Perera (eds.), *Down Syndrome: Psychological, Psychobiological, and Socio-educational Perspectives*, pp. 81–96. London: Whurr.

Wishart, J. (2001). Motivation and learning styles in young children with Down syndrome.

Down Syndrome Research and Practice, **7**, 47–51.

Wolery, M. (2000). Behavioral and educational approaches to early intervention. In J. P. Shonkoff & S. J. Meisels (eds.), *Handbook of Early Childhood Intervention* (2nd edn.), pp. 179–203. New York: Cambridge University Press.

Wolery, M. & Wilbers, J. S. (eds.). (1994). *Including Children with Special Needs in Early Childhood Programs*. Washington: National Association for the Education of Young Children.

Yoder, P. J. & Warren, S. F. (2004). Early predictors of language in children with and without Down syndrome. *American Journal on Mental Retardation*, **109**, 285–300.

Chapter

3

Advances in clinical endpoints for neurocognitive rehabilitation in Down syndrome

Jamie Edgin, Goffredina Spanō, Lynn Nadel

Considerable progress in our understanding of the cognitive profile of Down syndrome (DS) has occurred in the last decade. Complementing this progress has been a series of landmark studies highlighting promise for pharmacological intervention for cognitive deficits in this population (Fernandez et al., 2007; Salehi et al., 2009). Movement forward has also been demonstrated by the development of behavioral cognitive interventions targeting specific aspects of the cognitive profile (e.g. Fidler et al., Chapter 15 of this book). With pharmacological and behavioral clinical trials coming to fruition in the next few years, there is an immediate need for valid and reliable clinical endpoints in DS. These trials will only be meaningful if they include a battery of measurements that are well suited for this population and sensitive enough to detect change. Our group has been involved in the development of such a battery, the Arizona Cognitive Test Battery (ACTB) (Figure 3.1), which serves as a foundation for assessing characteristics of the phenotype of DS.

The history of pharmacological and dietary interventions for the cognitive deficits in humans with DS is largely one of disappointment (Salman, 2002). A number of drugs [e.g. drugs used in Alzheimer's disease, such as donepezil (Prasher et al., 2002)] or dietary supplements currently on the market have been tested for use in individuals with DS, with little effect on the whole. It is unclear if these interventions were unsuccessful because of ineffective drugs aimed at inappropriate targets, methodological shortcomings related to power and outcome measures, or both (see Chapter 7 of this book).

In the past five years, there has been considerable progress in understanding the neuropathological basis of cognitive and memory deficits in DS. Several studies have revealed well-defined neuropathological pathways, modification of which could support enhanced cognitive development in DS. For instance, studies have suggested an imbalance in excitatory and inhibitory inputs at the synaptic level, with excessive inhibition in the dentate gyrus of the hippocampus leading to the dampening of long-term potentiation (LTP) (Kleschevnikov et al., 2004). Some promising treatments have been developed to stabilize this imbalance. Fernandez et al. (2007) found that administration of pentylenetetrazole (PTZ, a gamma-aminobutyric acid [GABA] inverse agonist) eliminated deficits on a test of memory and learning in a mouse model of Down syndrome (Ts65Dn mice), an effect that persisted beyond the administration period. Follow-up studies have solidified the promise of GABA inverse agonists, showing that PTZ was more effective than donepezil in reducing memory impairments in Ts65Dn mice (Rueda et al., 2008).

Neurocognitive Rehabilitation of Down Syndrome, eds. Jean-Adolphe Rondal, Juan Perera, and Donna Spiker. Published by Cambridge University Press. © Cambridge University Press 2011.

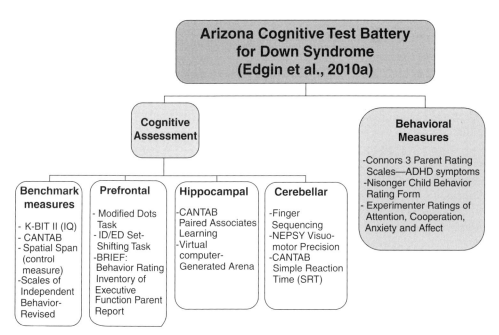

Figure 3.1 Key properties of clinical endpoint assessments: development of the Arizona Cognitive Test Battery for Down syndrome.

In another recent report, Salehi et al. (2009) found that the administration of L-threo-3,4-dihydroxyphenylserine, or xamoterol, a β1-adrenergic receptor partial agonist, normalized deficits in memory and learning in Ts65Dn mice, suggesting that modifications of the adrenergic system may be of additional benefit to cognitive outcomes. While this study detected changes in the hippocampus after drug administration, modification of adrenergic neurotransmitters has the potential to affect multiple brain systems, including the prefrontal cortex.

Other promising treatment pathways target the modification of early neural development, with the aim to counteract the processes contributing to intellectual disability as early as possible. For instance, there is some evidence that the overexpression of specific chromosome 21 genes, such as DYRK1A, may underlie cognitive deficits. Treatments have been developed to counteract these effects in mouse models (Kim et al., 2006). Other treatments may involve the modification of key neurodevelopmental pathways not directly linked to chromosome 21. Roper et al. (2006) found that exposing newborn trisomic mouse pups to an agonist of Sonic Hedgehog, a mitogen influencing neural crest development, reduced cerebellar neuropathology to normal.

Once the safety of each of these protocols is clearly established, the next step is the development of intervention protocols in humans. In order to bring the findings from basic science closer to the clinic, we require clinical endpoint assessments that can accurately detect meaningful changes in individuals with DS. The best trial design will incorporate a range of assessments, with direct consideration of the broader cognitive profile in humans with DS (Heller et al., 2006). Ideally, the tests should be specific enough to tap targeted neural structures so that the mechanisms of drug action may be better understood in humans. The ACTB

(Figure 3.1) is focused on neuropsychological domains specific to deficits in this population and is well suited to achieve these goals.

Key properties of clinical endpoint assessments: development of the Arizona Cognitive Test Battery for Down syndrome

Heller et al. (2006) and Edgin et al. (2010b) described the challenges for outcome assessments in this population. For accurate and sensitive assessment, it is important to take into account floor and ceiling effects (primarily the former) and the effects of confounding factors such as motivation, behavioral problems, and significant difficulties with language. Very few outcome assessments have been validated specifically for this population and sample-specific estimates of test-retest reliability are rare.

Other groups have addressed the general measurement challenges in clinical trials. One prominent group doing so is the OMERACT initiative (Outcome Measures in Rheumatology, http://reuma.rediris.es/omeract/index.html). This initiative served as a model for addressing issues in clinical trials in other medical conditions, and similar initiatives have been developed to provide a foundation for measurement selection for clinical trials in autism [i.e. The Autism Research Units on Pediatric Psychopharmacology (RUPP Autism Network, Arnold et al., 2000)]. For a measure to pass OMERACT's standard it must be feasible, truthful to the measurement construct, and able to discriminate both between typical and atypical populations and within the atypical population over the time intervals involved in the clinical trial. Feasibility involves a set of measures that can be applied easily given the time constraints. The truthfulness of a measure relates to whether or not it measures what it intends to measure and if it is unbiased and relevant. Thus, the truth component addresses issues of face and construct validity. The final component involves the choice of measures that are sensitive indicators of change.

Taking into account these properties and the specific measurement challenges in individuals with DS, we developed the ACTB. The ACTB includes primarily nonverbal tests of prefrontal, hippocampal, and cerebellar function in addition to general cognitive ability and behavior. The tasks were drawn from the Cambridge Neuropsychological Testing Automated Battery (CANTAB) (Lowe & Rabbitt, 1998), Eclipse battery, or based on established paradigms [e.g. NEPSY (Korkman et al., 1998), a computer-generated spatial arena (c-g arena, Thomas et al., 2001), and the Dots task (Davidson et al., 2006)]. Tests from the CANTAB battery have been used in earlier studies of individuals with DS, showing consistent impairments (Pennington et al., 2003; Visu-Petra et al., 2007). Widely used batteries of tests, such as the CANTAB and NEPSY, benefit from the breadth of this use and hence the range of comparable data. For instance, the CANTAB has been used in several neuroimaging studies and with a wide range of patient populations, including individuals with intellectual disability. Many of these tests are error based, helping to limit floor effects, are applicable to children across a wide range of ages, and have alternate forms to decrease practice effects. Another positive aspect of the CANTAB tests chosen for the ACTB is that there is evidence for their effective use across languages and cultures (Luciana & Nelson, 2002).

In the validation study, 74 individuals with DS (ages 7–38 years) and 50 mental age (MA)-matched controls (ages 3–8 years) were tested across three sites. Important for the generation of variables sensitive to change, several ACTB tests yielded low floor performance levels and produced impairments in comparison to a MA-matched sample. Alongside the ACTB, we administered benchmark and parent–report assessments of cognition and behavior.

Battery measures also correlated with these parent reports, including reports of adaptive skills, demonstrating concurrent validity and measure relevance. Preliminary data on test-retest reliability specific to the population were strong.

Many properties of the ACTB overlap with the requirements of ideal assessments for clinical trials as described previously. Measurements were chosen for purity in their constructs, and several have neuroimaging evidence linking them with specific brain regions, albeit in other populations. Limiting floor effects is an essential property for outcome assessments and will directly relate to the measure's sensitivity to detect change. Finally, the ACTB is an excellent set of tests in terms of feasibility. It has been implemented across four sites to date and involves a number of tests with computerized scoring, which limits the burden on the examiner and reduces error. It can be administered during one 2–3-hour session, which aids in reducing participant burden.

In the following sections we review the key cognitive and behavioral endpoints that are important to measure in a clinical trial in DS. We discuss the usefulness of the ACTB in each of these areas, and discuss future goals for the development of clinical endpoints.

The cognitive and behavioral profile of Down syndrome: key clinical endpoints

In the ideal clinical trial, assessment of a broad profile of skills is needed. DS involves a complex constellation of symptoms, including deficits in language, adaptive skills, learning and memory, motor skills, and behavior. Given this constellation of symptoms, the most effective intervention will show an impact on many aspects of cognitive and behavioral function. In the following sections we detail the main domains of function that are important to consider, recent research on the cognitive profile in each of these domains in DS, and approaches to effective measurement of each outcome.

Hippocampal memory

Based on animal models and the human literature, there is a wide body of evidence suggesting episodic memory difficulties in the DS population, particularly on tests of spatial memory and navigation, which tap the functions of the hippocampus (Carlesimo et al., 1997; Hyde et al., 2001; Nadel, 2003; Pennington et al., 2003). In contrast, there is consistent evidence for relatively preserved spatial short-term memory in individuals with DS (Wang & Bellugi, 1994). The ACTB currently incorporates two paradigms with close links to the hippocampus, including the CANTAB Paired Associates Learning (PAL) and the c-g arena task, a virtual version of the Morris Water Maze. The CANTAB PAL is a particularly robust assessment of episodic memory in this population: three separate studies of individuals with DS have demonstrated impairments on this task (Pennington et al., 2003; Visu-Petra et al., 2007; Edgin et al., 2010a). In Edgin et al. (2010a), the CANTAB PAL was found to have very low levels of participant loss and normally distributed outcomes. This task also correlated highly with other assessments, including intelligence quotient (IQ) and parent report of memory on the Behavior Rating Inventory of Executive Function (BRIEF) inventory (Gioia et al., 2000). Two separate studies have found a correlation between the PAL and adaptive scores on the Scales of Independent Behavior-Revised (Edgin et al., 2010a,b). Therefore, the bulk of information on this measure suggests it will be an excellent instrument for the detection of change in a clinical trial. The c-g arena task also provides a direct analog of memory assessment in the mouse model, providing a bridge between intervention trials in animal models and humans.

An important new approach to measurement of episodic memory in this population will involve the use of tasks that are dependent on different regions within the medial temporal lobe, such as the various regions of the hippocampus (dentate gyrus, CA fields, and subiculum), and the entorhinal, perirhinal, and parahippocampal cortices. Vicari & Carlesimo (2006) have begun work in this direction, by assessing dissociations in spatial and object memory in DS and Williams syndrome, another syndrome with hippocampal involvement (Meyer-Lindenberg et al., 2005). This study has suggested greater impairment in object than spatial memory in DS, a finding that could be consistent with impairments in another medial temporal lobe structure, the perirhinal cortex (Murray & Richmond, 2001). It is particularly difficult at present to find assessments for younger children that are targeted at these specific regions. Further development of such early tests that could be used in the context of a clinical trial is a priority.

Verbal short-term memory

One of the most robust cognitive impairments in DS is a deficit in verbal short-term memory. In a recent paper, Edgin et al., (2010b) found that deficits in verbal short-term memory were primary predictors of IQ scores in adolescents and young adults with DS ($r > 0.70$), while hippocampal based memory tasks (i.e. CANTAB PAL) were the primary correlate of adaptive behavior. Verbal short-term memory also correlates with language development (Seung & Chapman, 2000; Chapman et al., 2002). It is important to note that these verbal short-term memory deficits are not a result of peripheral factors, such as impaired audition and speech (Jarrold et al., 2002). More research is needed on the neural basis of these deficits in this population. In the general population, auditory working memory tasks engage a network of posterior and frontal regions (Martin, 2005). Therefore, deficits in verbal short-term memory in the DS population are likely to be linked to dysfunction of a network of brain regions, including the frontal cortex.

The robust nature of this deficit and strong relationship with other outcomes suggest that a verbal short-term memory task could be a useful complement to the ACTB. While not directly validated within the ACTB, there is evidence that these measures can be resistant to floor effects. Edgin (2003) found no issues with floor effects on the forward digit span, as every individual in this sample could complete this task at the level of two digits.

Frontal functions

Recent research has also suggested the importance of frontal functions in DS. While Pennington et al. (2003) found no evidence for frontal dysfunction, several studies since have reported deficits, including deficits in working memory (Rowe et al., 2006; Visu-Petra et al., 2007; Edgin et al., 2010a) and cognitive flexibility (Edgin et al., 2010a). In Figure 3.2 we present data gathered from a sample of 26 individuals with DS, ages 13–26 years (mean = 17.75) on the BRIEF inventory (Gioia et al., 2000), a parent–report assessment of everyday executive skills. Individuals above 18 years of age were given T scores based on the 18-year-old norms. The figure shows elevated mean scores in relation to the general population ($T > 60$) on several scales, including the Global Executive Composite score. Mean Ts on all of the scales were elevated with the exception of inhibition, emotional control, and organization of materials, which fell in the normal range. These findings are consistent with our study of

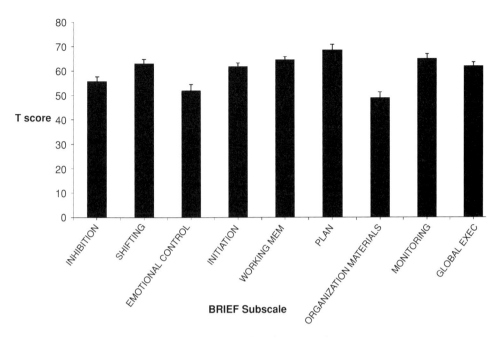

Figure 3.2 BRIEF subscale T score in twenty-six individuals with Down syndrome.

prefrontal function in Edgin et al. (2010a), in which we found deficits in working memory and set-shifting, but not in inhibitory control.

The largest challenge for assessment in this domain is to find assessments that generate a range of scores in the population. The mental age of most individuals with DS falls in a critical age-range for prefrontal development (i.e. between ages 3 years and late childhood). Tests administered to very young children or in late childhood [e.g. A-not-B (Diamond & Goldman-Rakic, 1989) or Wisconsin Card Sorting Test (Heaton et al., 1993)] are not appropriate across the range of ability in DS. Only recently have assessments been developed that can be administered across a broad range of ages (Luciana & Nelson, 2002; Davidson et al., 2006), including one measure in use in the ACTB that clearly dissociates components of inhibitory control and working memory (the Dots task, Davidson et al., 2006). On the ACTB we found deficits in relation to MA controls, excellent inter-task correlations and promising estimates of concurrent validity on the CANTAB IDED (intradimensional–extradimensional) and a modified version of the Dots task.

Cerebellar functions

The cerebellum is one of the most affected neural structures in DS (Pinter et al., 2001), with clear deficits found in this domain in both mouse models and humans (Frith & Frith, 1974; Olson et al., 2004). Given the broad range of cognitive and motor functions involving the cerebellum, pinpointing tasks that tap specific functions of this structure is extremely difficult. Furthermore, measures that are portable and easily implemented across several sites are rare. Eyeblink conditioning is perhaps the purest measure of cerebellar function available. However, eyeblink conditioning has led to inconsistent results in the literature, possibly because of differences in how well tolerated the procedure is (Woodruff-Pak et al., 1994;

Stedron, 2004). In the ACTB we have designed a computerized measure of finger sequencing that is well tolerated by this group (Edgin et al., 2010a). Similar paradigms relate to cerebellar structure and function in other populations, such as autism (Mostofsky et al., 2009). This measure complements measures of visuomotor precision from the NEPSY and the CANTAB simple reaction time task in the ACTB.

Language

While not directly measured on the ACTB, language is an important aspect of the phenotype. Mervis & Robinson (2005) provide an extensive review of measurement issues in phenotype assessment of developmental language disorders, including direct consideration of appropriate measures of language in DS. Language difficulties emerge from a very early age in individuals with DS, including gaps between production and comprehension noticeable in the toddler years (Miller, 1992; Chapman, 1995). Expressive language delays are most evident through delays in syntactic production and articulation. While receptive language is relatively strong, some areas are more impaired than others, including receptive syntax (Rondal & Comblain, 2002; Abbeduto et al., 2003). In past studies of drug intervention in DS, the Clinical Evaluation of Language Fundamentals (third edition) (CELF-3) (Semel et al., 1980) has been used with some success (Heller et al., 2004). Pennington et al. (2003) reported data from the Test for the Reception of Grammar (TROG; Bishop, 1989), CELF-3, and Peabody Picture Vocabulary Test (fourth edition) (Dunn & Dunn, 1997), with few issues in floor performance using raw scores. However, few language measures are able to capture the range of functioning in DS well enough to avoid floor effects with standard scores.

Practice effects are an issue in this domain. While many nonverbal tests, such as the ACTB, include or easily allow for alternate forms, language measures rarely include alternate forms. One exception is the Peabody Picture Vocabulary Test (fourth edition) (PPVT-4) (Dunn & Dunn, 2007), which includes an alternate form and growth scores. The PPVT-4 also has a wide range of standard scores and has been validated across an extensive age-range (floor = 20, 2.5–90 years), allowing it to be a very appropriate measure of receptive vocabulary in this population. The PPVT has consistently been considered an excellent measure of receptive vocabulary in this population and was included in batteries developed for the assessment of dementia in DS (Haxby, 1989; Mervis & Robinson, 2005). The Expressive Vocabulary Test (second edition) (EVT-2; Williams, 2007) was co-normed with the PPVT-4 in individuals 2.5–90 years of age (lowest standard score = 20) and provides growth scores. The combination of these two measures could be quite informative in the context of a clinical trial.

Adaptive behavior

Adaptive behavior is clearly an important aspect of the functional profile of anyone with an intellectual disability (ID). The definition of ID includes a reduction in both IQ and adaptive behavior (standard scores < 70). Any successful intervention will need to be reflected in changes in cognition as well as everyday function. Adaptive behavior itself involves a complex set of skills that most often are assessed through parent report of motor skills, social skills and communication, personal living skills (e.g. self-help skills), and skills in community living (e.g. writing checks, understanding time and money).

There is some evidence that adaptive skills are a relative strength in this population. In the report of Edgin et al. (2010a), we found that children and adults with DS had stronger adaptive skills on average than chronological aged (CA)- and IQ-matched individuals with Williams syndrome as measured on the Scales of Independent Behavior-Revised (SIB-R) (Bruininks et al., 1997). Edgin (2003) reported that the group with DS had higher overall motor and personal living skills standard scores on the SIB-R than did the group with Williams syndrome, while social and communication and community living skills (e.g. daily tasks like work skills) were equivalent. Despite a profile of relative strengths in adaptive skills in comparison to individuals with other types of IDs, adaptive skills have been found to plateau in adolescence in individuals with DS (Dykens et al., 2006).

There are several issues regarding the assessment of adaptive skills for clinical trials. One question is whether adaptive skills may dramatically change across a brief interval of time, often six months to one year for any trial. A clinically significant change on adaptive measures may require the attainment of skills that take some time to acquire, even when there is a drug effect. These measures are often a parent–report only, which can be problematic in terms of reporter bias. Another hurdle with the use of these measures is that many of these tasks are parent motivated (Mervis & Morris, 2007). For instance, take the hypothetical 18-year-old person with DS who scores 50 on the SIB-R (Bruininks et al., 1997), the adaptive measure included alongside the ACTB. To achieve a 10-point increase in the adaptive behavior standard score, he/she would need to have some substantial changes in the everyday level of function, including changes on some items that would require more independent transportation and ability to engage in activities that are often restricted (e.g. cooking independently using the stove). In some instances, change may require a perspective shift in the parent as well as a change in the general skill level of the child. However, this problem may not stand for adaptive behavior alone, but could be an issue in other domains as well (e.g. vocabulary development).

Clearly, assessments are needed that tap everyday skills in a more comprehensive manner, with the ability to detect fine-grained changes. New measurements have been developed for clinical trials in Alzheimer's disease, in which everyday tasks are individually administered across the trial (Loewenstein & Acevedo, 2010). Another option for assessment in this domain is the precise measurement of the component areas of adaptive behavior. For instance, adaptive behavior measures query parents about scholastic achievement, such as progress in reading and numerical ability. Having a direct assessment of these domains could be useful. In summary, the development of a set of tasks that resist practice effects, limit reporter bias, and which could be individually administered across the trial is crucial to the accurate and sensitive measurement of this important domain of function.

Maladaptive behavior

The variety of behavioral problems present in individuals in this population must be addressed in the design of any clinical trial. Fidler and Nadel (2007) reviewed a line of research that suggests that individuals with DS may be more likely to have a personality style including low task persistence and avoidance, a set of problems that could limit learning in multiple domains. Furthermore, Capone et al. (2006) reviewed the literature on the comorbidity of behavioral disorders in DS, reporting that the incidence of various behavioral problems ranges from 18% to 38% in this population. The problems reported included hyperactivity and inattention, conduct problems, depression, and symptoms of autism. A recent population study in Colorado suggested that a diagnosis of autism was found in 10%–15% of individuals with DS (DiGuiseppi et al., 2010).

Addressing these maladaptive behaviors could substantially impact on the quality of life of individuals with DS and their families. In recent work, our group has examined the relationship between maladaptive outcomes and cognition and a parent's level of stress in 19 individuals with DS, 12 years of age on average (Tandyasraya & Mason, 2010). Similar to past research, we found no significant difference between levels of parent stress in the group with DS versus an MA-control sample. Of further interest was the finding that IQ and neuropsychological function showed no relation to parent levels of stress. However, maladaptive behaviors, such as conduct problems, were related. Therefore, an intervention that decreases maladaptive behaviors could have a substantial impact on the quality of life for families and children. The assessments that will be most valid in this domain are ones that have been specifically designed to address the maladaptive behavior profile of those with intellectual disabilities. The Nisonger Child Behavior Report Form (NCBRF) (Aman et al., 1996), which was validated in conjunction with the ACTB, was designed for use in IDs, is suitable across a wide range of ages, and includes both parent and teacher ratings of behavior.

Intelligence quotient

Owing to the diverse nature of the cognitive components of many IQ tests, full IQ standard scores may be less likely to show change in the context of a clinical trial. However, tests that provide a profile, such as the Differential Ability Scales (second edition) (DAS-II) (Elliott, 2007), may be helpful. The main measurement issue in choosing IQ tests in a clinical trial is the selection of a test with appropriately low floor levels on standard scores. The Kaufmann Brief Intelligence Test (second edition) (KBIT-II) (Kaufman & Kaufman, 2004), used in the ACTB, provides a floor standard score of 40, one of the lowest in brief IQ assessments and normative data from 4 to 90 years of age. Of the full IQ scales, the Stanford-Binet (fifth edition) provides normative data in a wide range of ages (2-85 years) and has standard scores extending down to 40 (Roid, 2003). Similarly, the DAS-II (both the early years and school-aged core) provides normative data from early childhood to 18 years of age and a floor level of performance at a standard score of 30. The DAS-II provides one of the most comprehensive profiles of cognitive outcome for any IQ measure appropriate to this population and also includes growth scores that could be useful in a clinical trial.

In summary, in recent years great progress has been made in refining our definition of the phenotype in individuals with DS. The field has offered some assessments, including the ACTB, which could serve as valid indictors of change. We now turn to key issues with the design and interpretation of clinical trials in this population, including: (1) translation between animal models and human trials; (2) the age at which we intervene; and (3) how we might define statistically and clinically significant change on measures.

Key issues in efficacy assessment of neurocognitive intervention in Down syndrome

Translation from rodents to humans

Human drug trials based on successful interventions in animal models are now emerging. Whether these interventions will translate into success in humans rests on two primary assumptions: (1) drug effects will be similar in humans; and (2) the neural systems modified will have a substantial impact on key outcomes in humans, including everyday skills. In recent pharmacological intervention studies in mouse models, hippocampal or cerebellar functions have often been the focus of clinical endpoints. However, as we have illustrated here, the cognitive and behavioral profile of DS has a complexity that cannot always be measured in animal models. Given this disconnect, there is always the possibility that a promising drug in an animal model may not affect cognitive outcome to the same extent in humans. One strategy to counteract this issue is to ensure that the tests administered in humans and mice are as directly comparable as possible. The ACTB provides a bridge between mouse models and humans, particularly with the tasks of hippocampal memory. However, more effort is required to develop animal assessments specific to the cognitive and behavioral phenotype of DS.

Shamloo et al. (2010) report a more comprehensive set of behavioral assays in mice to aid translation between animal models and humans, including measurements of animal hyperactivity. However, language skills and verbal short-term memory are clearly missing endpoints in animal models. While direct measures of productive language are impossible, recent studies have indicated that auditory learning tasks (i.e. oddball discrimination) can be completed in mice (Villers-Sidani et al., 2010). The addition of auditory learning tasks to batteries of rodent measures could allow for the testing of the effects of drugs on multiple neural systems and key aspects of the phenotype prior to trials in humans.

Which age?

Studies show clear possibilities for intervention in both young children and adults with neurodevelopmental disorders (reviewed in Silva & Ehninger, 2009). Given the developmental course of cognitive function in DS, it is also our belief that effective interventions may be executed across the lifespan. However, the preschool and early adulthood periods could be particularly beneficial timepoints on which to focus. During these times, intervention could provide a foundation for later cognitive development or work to counteract cognitive decline. For instance, there is evidence that IQ declines in early childhood in individuals with DS, causing them to lose ground in relation to same-age peers (i.e. decreases in IQ standard score) (Hodapp & Zigler, 1990). Similarly, in late childhood and early adulthood, adaptive behavior has been found to plateau (Dykens et al., 2006). During early adulthood, it will be important to execute treatments to sustain cognitive skills in adults with DS and support independent everyday skills development. Currently, neuropsychological assessments are maximally effective in late childhood (11 years old and on, Edgin et al., 2010a) and adulthood, in which there has been a lot of work on batteries of assessments to detect cognitive decline (Haxby, 1989; Burt & Aylward, 2000). However, for interventions to move forward in preschool-aged children, tests must be developed and validated at this young age.

What constitutes significant change?

The extent that a therapy or drug will be adopted into clinical practice rests on its ability to generate a significant change in an individual's level of function. The therapy must not only generate statistically significant change, but the change must carry some value of clinical relevance. Statistically significant change, beyond the range of measurement error, is calculated through a process of determining a confidence interval for a true score that is generated based on test-retest reliability estimates and adjusted for practice effects (i.e. the reliable change index, Hageman & Arrindell, 1993).

Beyond proving statistical change, an intervention must demonstrate clinically significant change. Unfortunately, there are no set definitions for clinical significance. Past clinical trials have often utilized global assessments of change (GCI) from doctors, parents, or the participants themselves, as these outcomes are clear indicators of the everyday significance of any change. The subjective nature of these assessments can be problematic for drugs targeting cognitive functions.

The best indicator of change would be the movement of an individual's score outside a confidence interval on a norm-referenced test. This finding would indicate that the individual's developmental trajectory had been modified by the intervention. However, two major problems with this approach are that: (1) norm-referenced tests generally have not been validated in a wide enough range of individuals to have norms with variability at the lower end (Hessl et al., 2009); and (2) when tests are able to detect variation at the lower standard scores, they generally do not include measurements of specific cognitive skills (e.g. neuropsychological tests). For instance, measurements such as the KBIT-II and PPVT-4 provide low norms (i.e. standard scores of 40 and 20, respectively), but they may not measure skills that are immediately affected in a clinical trial. Other promising batteries have been developed to measure neuropsychological skills in children [NEPSY (Korkman et al., 1998); the automated working memory assessment (AWMA) (Alloway et al., 2004)]. However, these do not provide standard scores lower than 50–60.

One exception for an adequate standardized measure in children up to 18 years is the newly revised DAS-II (Elliot, 2007). The DAS-II provides standard scores as low as 30 and measures a range of skills, including some measures of verbal and episodic memory. The DAS-II is a clear advance on other IQ batteries, because of the addition of memory measures. However, tests specific to cerebellar and prefrontal function are not included.

In another approach to this problem, Hessl et al. (2009) discuss a strategy for dealing with the lack of variability in standard scores, which involves calculating normalized scores for each participant's raw score using a z-score transformation in relation to the mean and standard deviation of the raw scores generated by the standardization sample. While this procedure allowed for more variability and normally distributed data, it required permission to use the raw data sets from the test company (i.e. Psychological Corporation). Similar approaches could be used to generate meaningful scores with greater variability on batteries such as the NEPSY, AWMA, and CANTAB.

To determine the specific effects of a drug agent or an intervention, the best endpoints will come from targeted neuropsychological tests validated in the population. Given the number of individuals who have completed ACTB assessments in our past work, we can begin to generate sample-specific normative data for individuals between the ages of 11 and 20 years on some measures of the ACTB. The comparison of change in relation to peers within the group of individuals with DS could be particularly useful, with significant change marked by movement outside the confidence interval for the sample-specific normative score. A goal of our future research is to expand these norms to allow for more accurate estimates of the population.

However, without the availability of normative scores, one must call on other approaches to determine clinically significant change. One approach has used clinical anchor points which can help determine cutoffs when normative data are unavailable (Crosby et al., 2003). These methods were originally devised to determine the meaning of changes in quality of life for clinical trials of cancer patients, another set of measurements for which it is particularly difficult to define meaningful change. In short, the process involves choosing a measure and determining the point at which change relates the most to ratings on another scale (i.e. the point at which sensitivity and specificity is maximized). Batteries, such as the ACTB, that include cognitive assessment as well as a range of other outcomes (e.g. parent–teacher report of skills) are better placed to determine significant changes associated with these anchor points.

In summary, more work is needed to allow for measures that detect meaningful change in this population, through the development of normative tests that specifically include this population or individuals of a similar developmental level in the standardization sample. Specific neuropsychological tests should be the target of this development, with tests that are normed across a large age-range.

Discussion

Outcome assessment in individuals with DS has reached a turning point. We can no longer discuss the application of basic science to the clinic simply in hypothetical terms. Tests of the efficacy of neurocognitive rehabilitation have already started and will increase in number in the next few years. Therefore, assessments that are valid, reliable, feasible, and have properties allowing for the sensitivity to detect change are essential. Our development of the ACTB is one step in this process. To move forward, we require a consensus on a battery of tests that captures the complexity of the cognitive profile of DS through direct assessment as well as informant report. These tests must stand up to the measurement demands in this dynamic syndrome, including being aimed at a developmental level at which there is great variability. While we have made a first step through our validation of several neuropsychological measures in the ACTB, this is an area requiring the attention of the community. Researchers examining DS could greatly benefit from a process such as the OMERACT initiative.

Future directions for the field will be the development and validation of assessments of neuropsychological function with even more specific targets (e.g. dissociation of components of the hippocampal formation) and assessments to measure the cognitive and behavioral profile in very young children. While we discussed how interventions may be beneficial throughout life, ideally they will be executed as early as possible in order to maximize benefit. The evaluation of early intervention strategies cannot occur without better assessments of cognitive and behavioral function in early childhood. More work is also needed to support the use of analogous tasks in mouse models of DS and in humans. Studies incorporating neuroimaging are also needed as the neural underpinnings of any test can vary in children and adults (Casey et al., 2000), a pattern that is also likely to be true in individuals with ID versus the typical population. In summary, the development of the ACTB has allowed for several significant advances in measuring cognitive and behavioral changes in individuals with DS in the context of a clinical trial. However, more effort is required to hone these tools and address measurement challenges across the lifespan in DS.

Summary

The last decade has seen significant advances in our understanding of the neurobiological bases of the intellectual disability observed in Down syndrome (DS), generating several potential targets for neurocognitive rehabilitation. To accurately test the efficacy of interventions in DS, reliable and valid assessments of cognitive outcome are needed. In the current chapter, we discuss recent advances in neurobiological targets for treatment and current knowledge of the cognitive and behavioral phenotype. Given these targets, we describe the ideal properties of assessments for these interventions. We describe the Arizona Cognitive Test Battery (Edgin et al., 2010a), a set of primarily nonverbal neuropsychological assessments, and detail additional assessments that could be included in the context of a clinical trial. Significant issues and future directions in the development of clinical endpoints are discussed.

Acknowledgments

Many thanks to Carolyn Mervis who provided comments on the draft of this chapter. We thank the families who made this work possible. This study was supported in part by grants from the Down Syndrome Research and Treatment Foundation, DSRTF (to L.N. and J.O.E.), the Anna and John Sie Foundation (to L.N.), the National Down Syndrome Society Charles Epstein Award (to J.O.E.), the Lejeune Foundation (to J.O.E.), the Arizona Alzheimer's Research Consortium (to L.N.), and the University of Arizona Foundation (to L.N.).

References

Abbeduto, L., Murphy, M. M., Cawthon, S. W., et al. (2003). Receptive language skills of adolescents and young adults with Down syndrome or fragile X syndrome. *American Journal on Mental Retardation*, **108**, 149–160.

Alloway, T. P., Gathercole, S. E., Pickering, S. J. (2004). *The Automated Working Memory Assessment*. Test battery available from authors.

Aman, M. G., Tassé, M. J., Rojahn, J., Hammer, D. (1996). The Nisonger CBRF: a child behavior rating form for children with developmental disabilities. *Research in Developmental Disabilities*, **17**(1), 41–57.

Arnold L. E., Aman M.G., Martin A., et al. (2000). Assessment in multisite randomized clinical trials of patients with autistic disorder: the Autism RUPP Network. *Journal of Autism and Developmental Disorders*, **30**, 99–111.

Bishop, D. V. M. (1989). *Test for Reception of Grammar* (2nd edn.). Manchester: Chapel Press.

Bruininks, R. K., Woodcock, R. W., Weatherman, R. F., Hill, B. K. (1997). *Scales of Independent Behavior-Revised (SIB-R)*. The Rolling Meadows: Riverside.

Burt, D. & Aylward, E. (2000). Test battery for the diagnosis of dementia in individuals with intellectual disability. *Journal of Intellectual Disability Research*, **44**, 262–270.

Capone, G., Goyal, P., Ares, W., Lannigan, E. (2006). Neurobehavioral disorders in children, adolescents, and young adults with Down syndrome. *American Journal of Medical Genetics. Part C, Seminars in Medical Genetics*, **142C**, 158–172.

Carlesimo, G. A., Marotta, L., Vicari, S. (1997). Long-term memory in mental retardation: evidence for a specific impairment in subjects with Down's syndrome. *Neuropsychologia*, **35**, 71–79.

Casey, B. J., Giedd, J. N., Thomas, K. M. (2000). Structural and functional brain development and its relation to cognitive development. *Biological Psychology*, **54**, 241–257.

Chapman, R. S. (1995). Language development in children and adolescents with Down Syndrome. In P. Fletcher & B. MacWhinney (eds.), *The Handbook of Child Language*, pp. 664–689. Oxford: Blackwell.

Chapman, R. S., Hesketh, L. J., Kistler, D. (2002). Predicting longitudinal change in language production and comprehension in individuals with Down syndrome: hierarchical linear modeling. *Journal of Speech, Language, and Hearing Research*, **45**, 902–915.

Crosby, R. D., Kolotkin, R. L., Williams, G. R. (2003). Defining clinically meaningful change in health-related quality of life. *Journal of Clinical Epidemiology*, **56**, 395–407.

Davidson, M. C., Amso, D., Anderson, L. C., Diamond, A. (2006). Development of cognitive control and executive functions from 4 to 13 years: evidence from manipulations of memory, inhibition, and task switching. *Neuropsychologia*, **44**, 2037–2078.

Diamond, A. & Goldman-Rakic, P. S. (1989). Comparison of human infants and rhesus monkeys on Piaget's A-not-B task: evidence for dependence on dorsolateral prefrontal cortex. *Experimental Brain Research*, **74**, 24–40.

DiGuiseppi, C., Hepburn, S., Davis, J. M., et al. (2010). Screening for autism spectrum disorders in children with Down syndrome: population prevalence and screening test characteristics. *Journal of Developmental & Behavioral Pediatrics*, **31**(3), 181–191.

Dunn, L. M. & Dunn, D. M. (2007). *Peabody Picture Vocabulary Test* (4th edn.). Minneapolis: Pearson Assessments.

Dykens, E.M., Hodapp, R.M., Evans, D.W. (2006). Profiles and development of adaptive behavior in children with Down syndrome. *Down Syndrome Research and Practice*, **9**(3), 45–50.

Edgin, J. O. (2003). *A neuropsychological model for the development of the cognitive profiles in mental retardation syndromes: evidence from Down syndrome and Williams syndrome* [doctoral dissertation]. Denver: University of Denver.

Edgin, J. O., Mason, G., Allman, M. J., et al. (2010a). Development and validation of the Arizona Cognitive Test Battery for Down syndrome. *Journal of Neurodevelopmental Disorders*, **2**, 149–164.

Edgin, J. O., Pennington, B. F., Mervis, C. B. (2010b). Neuropsychological components of intellectual disability: the contributions of immediate, working, and associative memory. *Journal of Intellectual Disability Research*, **54**, 406–417.

Elliott, C. D. (2007). *Differential Ability Scales (2nd edn): Introductory and Technical Handbook*. San Antonio: The Psychological Corporation.

Fernandez, F., Morishita, W., Zuniga, E., et al. (2007). Pharmacotherapy for cognitive impairment in a mouse model of Down syndrome. *Nature Neuroscience*, **10**, 411–413.

Fidler, D. J. & Nadel, L. (2007). Education and children with Down Syndrome: neuroscience, development, and intervention. *Mental Retardation and Developmental Disabilities Research Reviews*, **13**, 262–271.

Frith, U. & Frith, C. D. (1974). Specific motor disabilities in Down's syndrome. *Journal of Child Psychology and Psychiatry*, **15**, 293–301.

Gioia, G. A., Isquith, P. K., Guy, S. C., Kenworthy, L. (2000). *Behavior Rating Inventory of Executive Function*. Odessa: Psychological Assessment Resources.

Hageman, W. L. & Arrindell, W. A. (1993). A further refinement of the reliable change index by improving the pre–post difference score: introducing the RCID. *Behaviour Research and Therapy*, **51**, 693–700.

Haxby, J. V. (1989). Neuropsychological evaluation of adults with Down's syndrome: patterns of selective impairment in non-demented old adults. *Journal of Mental Deficiency Research*, **33**, 193–210.

Heaton, R. K., Chelune, G. J., Talley, J. L., Kay, G. G., Curtiss, G. (1993). *Wisconsin Card Sorting Test Manual: Revised and Expanded*. Odessa: Psychological Assessment Resources.

Heller, J. H., Spiridigliozzi, G. A., Crissman, B. G., et al. (2006). Clinical trials in children with Down syndrome: issues from a cognitive research perspective. *American Journal of Medical Genetics. Part C, Seminars in Medical Genetics*, **142C**, 187–195.

Heller, J. H., Spiridigliozzi, G. A., Doraiswamy, P. M., et al. (2004). Donepezil effects on language in children with Down syndrome: results of the first 22-week pilot clinical trial. *American Journal of Medical Genetics. Part A, Seminars in Medical Genetics*, **130A**, 325–326.

Hessl, D., Danh V., Nguyen, C. G., et al. (2009). A solution to limitations of cognitive testing in children with intellectual disabilities: the case of fragile X syndrome. *Journal of Neurodevelopmental Disorders*, **1**, 33–45.

Hodapp, R. M. & Zigler, E. F. (1990). Applying the developmental perspective to individuals with Down syndrome. In D. Cicchetti & M. Beeghly (eds.), *Children with Down Syndrome: A Developmental Perspective*, pp. 1–28. New York: Cambridge University Press.

Hyde, L. A, Frisone, D. F., Crnic, L. S. (2001). Ts65Dn mice, a model for Down syndrome, have deficits in context discrimination learning suggesting impaired hippocampal function. *Behavioural Brain Research*, **118**, 53–60.

Jarrold, C., Baddeley, A., Phillips, C. E. (2002). Verbal short-term memory in Down syndrome: a problem of memory, audition or speech? *Journal of Speech, Language and Hearing Research*, **45**, 531–544.

Kaufman, A. S. & Kaufman, N. L. (2004). *Kaufman Brief Intelligence Test* (2nd edn.). Bloomington: Pearson.

Kim, N. D., Yoon, J., Kim, J. H., et al. (2006). Putative therapeutic agents for the learning and memory deficits of people with Down syndrome. *Bioorganic & Medicinal Chemistry Letters*, **16**, 3772–3776.

Kleschevnikov, A. M., Belichenko, P. V., Villar, A. J., et al. (2004). Hippocampal long-term potentiation suppressed by increased inhibition in the Ts65Dn mouse, a genetic model of Down syndrome. *Journal of Neuroscience*, **24**, 8153–8160.

Korkman, M., Kirk, U., Kemp, S. (1998). *NEPSY: A Developmental Neuropsychological Assessment*. San Antonio: The Psychological Corporation.

Loewenstein, D. & Acevedo, A. (2010). The relationship between instrumental activities of daily living and neuropsychological performance. In T. D. Marcotte & I. Grant (eds.), *Neuropsychology of Everyday Functioning*, pp. 93–112. New York: Guilford.

Lowe, C. & Rabbitt, P. (1998). Test/re-test reliability of the CANTAB and ISPOCD neuropsychological batteries: theoretical and practical issues. Cambridge Neuropsychological Test Automated Battery. International Study of Post-operative Cognitive Function. *Neuropsychologia*, **36**, 915–923.

Luciana, M. & Nelson, C. (2002). Assessment of neuropsychological function through use of the Cambridge Neuropsychological Testing Automated Battery: performance in 4- to 12-year-old children. *Developmental Neuropsychology*, **22**, 595–624.

Martin, R. C. (2005). Components of short-term memory and their relation to language processing: evidence from neuropsychology and neuroimaging. *Current Directions in Psychological Science*, **14**, 204–208.

Mervis, C. B. & Morris, C. A. (2007). Williams syndrome. In M. M. M. Mazzocco & J. L. Ross (eds.), *Neurogenetic Developmental Disorders: Variation of Manifestation in Childhood*, pp. 199–262. Cambridge: MIT Press.

Mervis, C.B. & Robinson, B.F. (2005). Designing measures for profiling and genotype/phenotype studies of individuals with genetic syndromes or developmental language disorders. *Applied Psycholinguistics*, **26**, 41–64.

Meyer-Lindenberg, A., Mervis, C.B., Sarpal, D., et al. (2005). Functional, structural, and metabolic abnormalities of the hippocampal formation in Williams syndrome. *Journal of Clinical Investigation*, **115**, 1888–1895.

Miller, J. F. (1992). Development of speech and language in children with Down Syndrome. In I. T. Lott & E. E. McCoy (eds.), *Down Syndrome: Advances in Medical Care*, pp. 39–50. New York: Wiley-Liss.

Mostofsky, S. H., Powell, S. K., Simmonds, D. J., et al. (2009). Decreased connectivity and cerebellar activity in autism during motor task performance. *Brain*, **132**, 2413–2425.

Murray, E. A. & Richmond, B. J. (2001). Role of perirhinal cortex in object perception, memory, and associations. *Current Opinion in Neuro Biology*, **11**, 188–193.

Nadel, L. (2003). Down's syndrome: a genetic disorder in biobehavioral perspective. *Genes, Brain and Behavior*, **2**(3), 156–166.

Olson, L. E., Roper, R. J., Baxter, L. L., et al. (2004). Down syndrome mouse models Ts65Dn, Ts1Cje, and Ms1Cje/Ts65Dn exhibit variable severity of cerebellar phenotypes. *Developmental Dynamics*, **230**, 581–589.

Pennington, B. F., Moon, J., Edgin, J., Stedron, J., Nadel, L. (2003). The neuropsychology of Down syndrome: evidence for hippocampal dysfunction. *Child Development*, **74**, 75–93.

Pinter, J. D., Eliez, S., Schmitt, J. E., Capone, G. T., Reiss, A. L. (2001). Neuroanatomy of Down's syndrome: a high-resolution MRI study. *The American Journal of Psychiatry*, **158**, 1659–1665.

Prasher, V. P., Huxley, A., Haque, M. S. (2002). The Down syndrome ageing study group, a 24-week, double-blind, placebo-controlled trial of donepezil in patients with Down syndrome and Alzheimer's disease – pilot study. *International Journal of Geriatric Psychiatry*, **17**, 270–278.

Roid, G. H. (2003). *Stanford–Binet Intelligence Scale Manual* (5th edn.). Itasca, IL: Riverside.

Rondal, J. A. & Comblain, A. (2002). Language in ageing persons with Down syndrome. *Down Syndrome Research and Practice*, **8**(1), 1–9.

Roper, R. J., Baxter, L. L., Saran, N. G., et al. (2006). Defective cerebellar response to mitogenic Hedgehog signaling in Down syndrome mice. *Proceedings of the National Academy of Sciences of the United States of America*, **103**, 1452–1456.

Rowe, J., Lavender, A., Turk, V. (2006). Cognitive executive function in Down's syndrome. *British Journal of Clinical Psychology*, **45**, 5–17.

Rueda, N., Florez, J., Martinez-Cue, C. (2008). Chronic pentylenetetrazole but not donepezil treatment rescues spatial cognition in Ts65Dn mice, a model for Down syndrome. *Neuroscience Letters*, **433**, 22–27.

Salehi, A., Faizi, M., Colas, D., et al. (2009). Restoration of norepinephrine modulated contextual memory in a mouse model of Down syndrome. *Science Translational Medicine*, **1**(7), 7–17.

Salman, M. S. (2002). Systematic review of the effect of therapeutic dietary supplements and drugs on cognitive function in subjects with Down syndrome. *European Journal of Paediatric Neurology*, **6**, 213–219.

Semel, E., Wiig, E., Secord, W. (1980). *CELF: Clinical Evaluation of Language Fundamentals*. San Antonio: Psychological Corporation.

Seung, H. K. & Chapman, R. (2000). Digit span in individuals with Down syndrome and in typically developing children: temporal aspects. *Journal of Speech, Language, and Hearing Research*, **43**, 609–620.

Shamloo, M., Belichenko, P. V., Mobley, W. C. (2010). Comprehensive behavioral assays to enhance phenotype to genotype linkages and therapeutic screening in mouse models of Down syndrome. *Future Neurology*, **5**, 467–471.

Silva, A. J. & Ehninger, D. (2009). Adult reversal of cognitive phenotypes in neurodevelopmental disorders. *Journal of Neurodevelopmental Disorders*, **1**, 150–157.

Stedron, J. (2004). *Cerebellar function in Down syndrome.* (doctoral dissertation). Denver: University of Denver.

Tandyasraya, P. & Mason, G. (2010). *Parental stress and child characteristics of children with Down syndrome.* Poster presented at the annual meeting of The American Association for the Advancement of Science (AAAS), San Diego, CA.

Thomas, K. G. F., Hsu, M., Laurance, H. E., Nadel, L., Jacobs, W. W. (2001). Place learning in virtual space III: investigation of spatial navigation training procedures and their application to fMRI and clinical neuropsychology. *Behavior Research Methods, Instruments, & Computers*, **33**(1), 21–37.

Vicari, S. & Carlesimo, G. A. (2006). Short-term memory deficits are not uniform in Down and Williams syndromes. *Neuropsychology Review*, **16**, 87–94.

Villers-Sidani, E., Alzghoul, L., Zhou, X., et al. (2010). Recovery of functional and structural age-related changes in the rat primary auditory cortex with operant training. *Proceedings of the National Academy of Sciences of the United States of America*, **107**(31), 13900–13905.

Visu-Petra, L., Benga, O., Tincas, I., Miclea, M. (2007). Visual-spatial processing in children and adolescents with Down's syndrome: a computerized assessment of memory skills. *Journal of Intellectual Disability Research*, **51**, 942–952.

Wang, P. P. & Bellugi, U. (1994). Evidence from two genetic syndromes for a dissociation between verbal and visual-spatial short-term memory. *Journal of Clinical and Experimental Neuropsychology*, **16**, 317–322.

Williams, K. T. (2007). *Expressive Vocabulary Test* (2nd edn.). Minneapolis: Pearson Assessments.

Woodruff-Pak, D. S., Papka, M., Simon, E. (1994). Eyeblink classical conditioning in Down's Syndrome, Fragile X syndrome and normal adults over and under age 35. *Neuropsychology*, **8**, 14–24.

New perspectives on molecular and genic therapies in Down syndrome

Jean-Maurice Delabar

Down syndrome and phenotypes

Trisomy 21 exerts a powerful downward effect on intelligence quotient (IQ). In contrast to normally developing children, there is a progressive IQ decline in Down syndrome (DS) beginning in the first year of life. The ratio of mental age to chronological age is not constant. By adulthood, IQ is usually in the moderately to severely retarded level (IQ 25–55) with an upper limit on mental age of approximately 7–8 years although a few individuals have IQ in the lower normal range (70–80). The molecular basis and the genes involved in this early decline across development are not known. This low IQ corresponds to an overall mental retardation. The short-term memory development of individuals with DS has been the subject of considerable research. Recent observation of the development of encoding strategies through the ages of 5 to 8 years suggests that this is a complex process involving the maturation of attentional and inhibitory processes (Palmer, 2000). The alterations in the cognition processes have not yet been related to the neuropathological features of DS.

At a gross morphological level, DS brains are smaller than normal. A 15%–20% decrease is generally reported (Jernigan et al., 1993; Pinter et al., 2001). Three brain areas are mainly altered: prefrontal cortex, hippocampus, and cerebellum. Postmortem studies and noninvasive brain imaging have revealed reduced sizes of the brain hemispheres, brainstem, and cerebellum (Kesslak et al., 1994; Raz et al., 1995). In vivo magnetic resonance imaging (MRI) studies have also revealed the relative increase of specific brain regions, such as the subcortical gray matter (Pinter et al., 2001). In addition, regional differences were also reported in a voxel-based MRI study (White et al., 2003). Neuronal number is reduced in distinct regions and abnormal neuronal morphology is observed, especially in the cerebral cortex. In fetuses, brain examination has revealed abnormal cortical lamination patterns (Golden & Hyman, 1994), altered dendritic arborization and spine morphology, reduction of spine number (Becker et al., 1991; Schulz & Scholz, 1992), and altered electrophysiological properties of cell membranes (Becker et al., 1991).

People with DS are much more likely to develop dementia than the general public. The neuropathological changes seen in DS brains (beyond 35 years old) are identical to those seen in sporadic Alzheimer's disease (AD) in terms of pattern of distribution of lesions (plaques and tangles) and immunostaining properties of lesions, although the changes in DS seem more pronounced. These changes are associated with dementia in 30%–50% of the patients beyond 50 years old (Franceschi et al., 1990; Mann et al., 1990). The reasons why DS patients

Neurocognitive Rehabilitation of Down Syndrome, eds. Jean-Adolphe Rondal, Juan Perera, and Donna Spiker. Published by Cambridge University Press. © Cambridge University Press 2011.

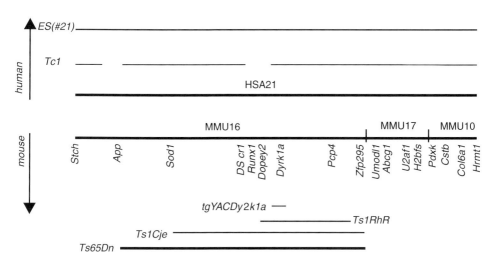

Figure 4.1 Existing mouse models with partial trisomy of regions syntenic to human chromosome 21.

develop these lesions and that they are at increased risk for development of dementia are unknown. The current knowledge of the genes that predispose or participate in the AD of DS does not yet provide a satisfactory explanation of their pathophysiology. AD is characterized by the deposition of senile plaques and neurofibrillary tangles in vulnerable brain regions. One hypothesis to explain the AD phenotype in DS is that triplication of the gene encoding the amyloid precursor protein (APP) would lead to the overproduction of A-beta peptides; however, other HSA21 genes might also be involved in the process.

Murine models

Mouse orthologs of HSA21 genes are located on chromosome 16 (MMU16), chromosome 10 (MMU10), and chromosome 17 (MMU17) (Figure 4.1). Thus, the characterization of mouse models that have an extra copy of all or part of MMU16, MMU10, or MMU17 should be useful for the understanding of DS alterations. Davisson et al. (1990) used radiation-induced translocations to produce Ts65Dn, a mouse trisomic for a long fragment of MMU 16 (more than 20 Mb) syntenic to segment MRPL39-ZNF295 in humans (132 genes). A second partial trisomy 16 model has recently been developed, the Ts1Cje mouse (Sago et al., 1998). This mouse resulted from a reciprocal translocation between the end of chromosome 12 and the distal part of chromosome 16 at the level of the Sod1 gene: the partial trisomy 16 resulting from this event contains functional genes distal to Sod1 (one copy of Sod1 has been knocked out). The region present in three copies is syntenic to a smaller fragment than the syntenic region in Ts65Dn mice, corresponding to only 85 human genes (Figure 4.1). The Ts65Dn mice present some features of DS: craniofacial abnormalities, developmental delay, and impaired performance in various learning tests. In addition, alterations in long-term potentiation (LTP) and long-term depression (LTD) have been reported in young and old Ts65Dn mice (Siarey et al., 1997, 1999).

Kleschevnikov et al. (2004) and stereological morphometric studies have demonstrated reduction in the volume of CA2 and in the mean neuron number in the dentate gyrus (Insausti et al., 1998). Electron microscopy showed that boutons and spines are enlarged and that abnormalities in the internal membranes are present in both models (Holtzmann et al., 1996; Belichenko et al., 2005). Stereological measurements gave evidence of an age-related degeneration of septohippocampal cholinergic neurons and of astrocytic hypertrophy. Finally, high resolution MRI and histological analysis revealed a reduction in cerebellar volume in Ts65Dn mice owing to a reduction of both the internal granule layer and the molecular layer, with a parallel reduction in granule cell number (Baxter et al., 2000). In contrast, the brain, with the exception of the cerebellum, is not significantly smaller in segmentally trisomic mice and, indeed, tends to be larger than that of euploid mice if measurements of area at the midline level are taken into account (9% increase). In addition, Ts1Cje show a cerebellar hypoplasia with a lower decrease in granule cell density (Olson et al., 2004). The Ts1Cje mice perform efficiently in the Morris water maze test when the platform is visible, but they show impairment in the hidden platform and probe tests, and in the reverse platform test (Sago et al., 1998), indicating that learning impairment is less severe than in Ts65Dn mice.

Recently two models of chimeric mice containing a large part of an extra human chromosome 21 with a varying degree of mosaicism have also been constructed (Shinohara et al., 2001; O'Doherty et al., 2005): the first one demonstrated a correlation between phenotype severity (learning impairment and heart defect with a double-outlet right ventricle and riding aorta) and the percentage of cells with an extra HSA21; the second model (Tc1) showed germline transmission resulting in living animals with various mosaicism and phenotypic alterations in behavior, synaptic plasticity, cerebellar neuronal number, and heart development (ventricular septal defect and atrioventricular septal defect).

Smith and colleagues (1997) used smaller human chromosome fragments inserted into yeast artificial chromosomes to create an in vivo library spanning 1.8 Mb of 21q22.2. Two YAC-transgenic mice presented brain abnormalities: tg230E8 (with nine genes) had a high density of cortical neurons and tg152F7 (with five genes including DYRK1A, encoding a serine threonine kinase) had a 15% heavier brain, with larger cortical (layer V) and hippocampal (dentate gyrus) neurons (15%) than euploid mice (Branchi et al., 2004). A smaller human fragment containing only the DYRK1A gene was used by Ahn et al. (2006) to generate a line of transgenic mice with heavier than normal brains (19% heavier).

Other groups have created models for single gene overexpression and the observation of these models, together with other datasets, is intended to identify potential candidate genes.

Candidate genes
Criteria used to define candidate genes
The rational basic assumptions guiding DS research are that: (1) individual chromosome 21 genes will show gene dosage effects that increase expression by 50% at the RNA and protein level; (2) at least some of these increases will result in perturbations of the pathways and cellular processes in which these genes are involved; and (3) these perturbations will result, possibly additively, in the neurodevelopmental and cognitive abnormalities that characterize the mental retardation of DS. These assumptions emphasize that, in comparison with mental retardation as a result of single gene defects, DS presents unique complexities: there is no absent gene function and there is a large number of candidate genes (more than 300) (Gardiner et al., 2004).

Chromosomic localization

The gene must be localized on chromosome 21 which, owing to the sequencing of the human genome, is now an easy-to-answer question. Obviously, genes other than those encoded by HSA21 are involved in DS phenotypes, but the primary cause of their dysregulation is thought to be a result of a triplicated gene on HSA21. However, the question of the regional localization of the genes on the chromosome is also important: genotype–phenotype correlation studies in ten patients with partial trisomy 21 suggested that there is a region of about 2.5 Mb between the genes CBR and ERG that, if triplicated, is associated with numerous features of DS. These include facial dysmorphology (flat nasal bridge, protruding tongue, high arched palate, folded ears), hand and foot features, joint hyperlaxity, muscular hypotonia, short stature, and mental retardation (Delabar et al., 1993). Pooling data from the literature allowed us to compare 40 patients: 30 patients carrying this region in three copies presented a characteristic phenotype that included mental retardation; among nine individuals with a duplication of the proximal HSA21q region, only two presented a weak form of mental retardation, indicating that a second locus (with lower penetrance) may be involved in mental retardation. It was proposed (Korenberg et al., 1997) to name the CBR-ERG region as DSCR1 (DS chromosomal region 1). A gene localized outside this region will have a lower probability to be a strong player in mental retardation. Recently a family carrying duplication of 10 genes only and showing head phenotypes and mental retardation has allowed narrowing down of this region (Ronan et al., 2007).

Functions or potential functions

The protein characteristics must suggest a relevant function and there is still a large number of genes of unknown function. Functional hypotheses might also come from the known target of the gene or from the interacting proteins. The analysis of pathways is a further source of relevant hypotheses (Gardiner et al., 2004; Pellegrini-Calace & Tramontano, 2006). The interrelation between pathways is not yet very well explored; however, gene dosage errors of genes belonging to the transcription factor family or to the kinases family will definitely be good candidates to explain pleiotropic phenotypic actions.

Territories of expression

The gene must be found expressed in relevant body tissues; some expression studies have now been performed either on a large scale to first visualize expression patterns (Gitton et al., 2002; Reymond et al., 2002) or, more accurately, at different developmental stages and in specific brain tissues. Sim2 (single minded): *in situ* hybridization of a probe, derived from one exon of this gene, with human and rat fetuses showed that the corresponding gene is expressed during early fetal life in the central nervous system and in other tissues, including the face, skull, palate, and vertebra primordial tissues (Dahmane et al., 1995); pcp4: PCP4 is expressed in the central nervous system, in the myenteric plexus, and in other ectodermal derivatives, for instance the lens, the hair cells of the cochlea, the enamel organ, and the hair follicles (Thomas et al., 2003); dopey2 (C21orf5): a wide but differential expression was detected in the nervous system during embryogenesis, with a relatively lower level in the forebrain than in the midbrain and hindbrain, and the highest transcription intensity in the future cerebellum (Rachidi et al., 2006); DYRK1A: a high expression is detected in the cerebral cortex, the cerebellum, the hippocampus, and the thalamo-hypothalamus regions (Rahmani et al., 1998).

Level of expression in Down syndrome or in transgenic mice

Transcriptome analyses of these mouse models have shown that most of the genes in three copies are 1.5 times overexpressed. However, some genes are more than 1.5-fold overexpressed and others are submitted to compensatory mechanisms with no change in expression or, more rarely, decreased expression (Lyle et al., 2004; Dauphinot et al., 2005). Studying lymphoblastoid cell lines, Aït Yahya-Graison and colleagues (2007) have shown, using HSA21-oligoarrays combined with a powerful statistical analysis protocol, that it is possible to classify HSA21 genes according to their level of expression in DS lymphoblastoid cell lines: among the expressed transcripts, 29% are sensitive to the gene dosage effect or amplified, 56% are compensated, and 15% are highly variable among individuals. Obviously a gene, expression of which is found compensated, will not be a good candidate for a phenotype found in the studied tissue.

Associated phenotypic changes in murine models

Finally, the best evidence remains the demonstration of a phenotype arising from overexpression in a mouse model and these phenotypes are used as markers of the efficiency of the assessed therapeutic strategies.

Gene-based corrective strategies

Associated with the identification of candidate genes is the possibility of designing corrective strategies directly targeting the gene products or targeting downward pathways. The main caveat to these strategies is that some genes are sensitive to a decreased gene dosage below the normal level; therefore reaching a level of 50% of the normal situation might induce dramatic consequences.

RNA targets

The first consequence of the presence of three copies of HSA21 genes is thought to be, for the largest part of the genes, an increase of the corresponding messenger RNA (mRNA). The use of a new class of small RNAs, the small interfering RNAs (siRNAs), is one of the strategies allowing the decrease of the amount of: first, the targeted RNA and, second, the encoded protein.

RNA interference (RNAi) is an ancient mechanism of gene regulation, which plays a central role in controlling gene expression in all eukaryotes including yeast. Using siRNA molecules, RNAi can selectively silence essentially any gene in the genome. Once in a cell, a short double-stranded RNA (dsRNA) molecule is cleaved by an RNA sequence called Dicer into 21–23 nucleotide-guide RNA duplexes called siRNAs that become bound to the RNA-induced silencing complex (RISC). Within the RISC, one of the two strands of the siRNA is chosen as the antisense strand via cleavage of the passenger strand, so that they can target complementary sequences in mRNAs. After pairing with an siRNA strand, the targeted mRNA is cleaved and undergoes degradation thereby interrupting the synthesis of the disease-causing protein.

One example is an experiment targeting DSCR1, a gene that belongs to a family of conserved proteins, also termed calcipressins; the protein functions as a small cytoplasmic

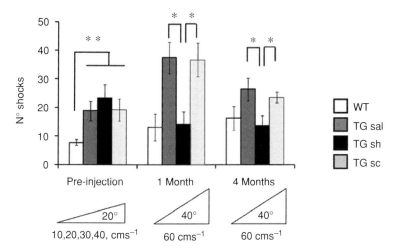

Figure 4.2 Behavioral analysis of motor tasks in TgDYRK1A mice treated with intra-striatal injections of AAVshDYRK1A. Animals were randomly assigned to four treatment groups: wild-type (saline) and TgDYRK1A (saline, AAVshDYRK1A, and AAVscDYRK1A) (sal: saline, sh: short hairpin RNA, sc: scrambled control; WT: wild-type). Treadmill test: the results are expressed as the total number of shocks received. Non-treated mice confirmed the presence of motor coordination alterations in TgDYRK1A mice ($F1.22 = 11.937$, **$P = 0.002$). One month after the intervention, the AAVshDYRK1A TgDYRK1A group received significantly fewer shocks compared to the groups of TgDYRK1A injected with either saline or AAVscDYRK1A, reaching levels similar to those of the control groups (TG sal versus TG sh: $F1.6 = 8.669$, *$P = 0.032$; TG sc versus TG sh: $F1.8 = 9.844$, *$P = 0.016$). This effect was maintained four months after treatment in AAVshDYRK1A TgDYRK1A mice (TG sal versus TG sh: $F1.10 = 5.575$, *$P = 0.043$; TG sc versus TG sh: $F1.10 = 6.094$, *$P = 0.033$), (n = 6 mice/group). (Reproduced with permission from Ortiz-Abalia et al., 2008.)

signaling molecule. Two research groups (Hesser et al., 2004 and Arron et al., 2006) have established a regulatory role for DSCR1 that controls the level of nuclear factor of activated T-cells (NFAT), a transcription factor, in the nucleus. Using an siRNA targeting DSCR1, Hesser and colleagues have shown, in endothelial cells, that they can increase the NFAT activity, which is reduced in DS.

A second example is an experiment targeting DYRK1A, an important kinase localized in the DCR-1 region: viral delivery of small hairpin RNA (shRNA) candidates presents an alternative approach to mouse genetic engineering with which to understand pathophysiology and test potential therapeutic targets. To investigate the effects of inhibiting DYRK1A overexpression in the case of established motor deficits seen in a TgDYRK1A model (a complementary (cDNA) driven by an exogen promoter), Ortiz-Abalia and colleagues (2008) have injected AAVshDYRK1A (a modified viral genome with an siRNA-targeting DYRK1A) into the striatum of two- to three-month-old adult TgDYRK1A mice, and performed behavioral phenotyping at pre-injection and different post-injection timepoints. They demonstrated that intrastriatal injections of AAVshDYRK1A in TgDYRK1A mice normalize DYRK1A gene expression in the striatum and correct established motor alterations, as shown in Figure 4.2 in a treadmill experiment.

Protein targets

The second strategy directly targets the protein product of the candidate gene.

The two following examples illustrate the use of antibodies to decrease the amount of the amyloid-beta (A-beta) peptide. In the amyloid cascade hypothesis, memory deficits in patients with AD are caused by increased brain levels of both soluble and insoluble A-beta peptide(s), which are derived from the larger amyloid precursor protein (APP) by sequential proteolytic processing (Hardy & Selkoe, 2002). Bales et al. (2006) have found that A-beta proteins can directly interact with the high-affinity choline transporter, which may impair acetylcholine release and related neurotransmission. Using an anti-A-beta antibody, they treated mice that overexpress a mutation-associated tone of the mutation, associated with familial AD, by direct hippocampal perfusion and they restored hippocampal acetylcholine release and reduced impaired habituation learning.

In a similar study, Lee and colleagues (2006) designed a monoclonal antibody preferentially targeting the higher order A-beta structures and verified that this antibody is specific for fibrillar A-beta in brain sections of individuals with mild cognitive impairment, DS, or AD. Intraperitoneal injections of this antibody in mice carrying the mutation 2576 found in familial AD induced significant improvements in spatial learning and memory relative to control mice.

These results suggest that pathological A-beta conformers produced in vivo are capable of disrupting neuronal function, and substantiate the therapeutic potential of targeting A-beta oligomers for the treatment of AD in patients with AD or DS.

Protein activities as targets

A third possibility is to use compounds acting to modify the activity of a targeted protein or pathway. These strategies are being focused either on cell cycle or central nervous system functions.

Cell cycle pathways

Sonic hedgehog pathway

Roper and colleagues (2006, 2009) have demonstrated that, in cell culture, developing cerebellar granule cell precursors (GCP) respond to the addition of Sonic hedgehog (Shh) protein by proliferating. This response is reduced in trisomic mice. These results indicate that failure to generate sufficient progeny from GCP is an important component of the GC deficit associated with reduced cerebellar size in adult Ts65Dn mice. On the day of birth, the number of progenitors is identical, but the number of mitotic GCP is significantly reduced in trisomic mice. By P6, the total number of precursor cells has been compromised, such that normal levels of GCP production are not achieved in Ts65Dn mice. The authors show that an intrinsic deficit in the response of trisomic GCP to Shh underlies the reduced generation of GC in Ts65Dn mice. Introduction of a Shh-pathway agonist early in development stimulated mitosis of GCP and corrected this deficit, such that the number of GCP and the rate of mitosis were normal one week after treatment (Figure 4.3).

In a second set of experiments, these authors investigated the involvement of an attenuated response to Shh in neural crest (NC) cells. The NC contributes to the majority of the bone, cartilage, connective tissue, and peripheral nervous tissue in the head. Because NC is a common precursor of many structures affected in DS, it has been hypothesized that trisomy 21 affects the NC. Using crosses between Ts65Dn mice and mice expressing lacZ under control of the Wnt1 promoter, the authors showed a reduction of the first pharyngeal arch (PA1) size. They also showed that concomitant with the reduction of PA1 size, there were significantly fewer NC cells within PA1 of trisomic compared to euploid embryos. To

A

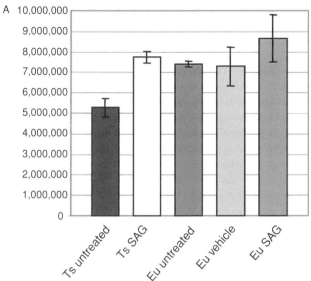

B

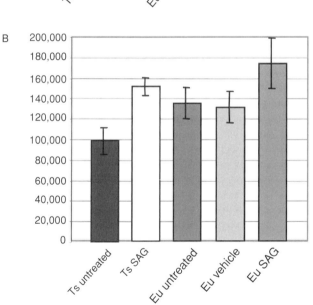

Figure 4.3 Mitotic and granule cell precursor deficits of trisomic mice are reversed by injection of a Sonic hedgehog-pathway agonist. Progeny of Ts65Dn mothers received a spinal cord injection of a Shh-pathway agonist, 20 g SAG 1.1 Shh agonist, on the day of birth. The animals were killed, genotyped, and assessed by stereology at P6. ANOVA with multiple comparisons was used to analyze results. A: for GCP, the trisomic (Ts) agonist, euploid (Eu) vehicle, and euploid untreated groups were not different from each other, but were significantly increased relative to untreated trisomic mice (F = 5.6, P = 0.009, $\alpha = 0.05$). B: for mitotic cells, the trisomic agonist group was significantly different from trisomic untreated mice (F = 3.06, P = 0.06, $\alpha = 0.05$), but not different from euploid or euploid vehicle groups. (Reproduced with permission from Roper et al., 2006.)

examine the Shh response in a controlled condition, they isolated cells from PA1 of trisomic or euploid T14 embryos and cultured them for 12 h in media containing 2, 4, or 8 μg/mL of Shh. Trisomic cells showed a smaller increase in cell number than euploid cells at all concentrations of Shh, but the addition of 4 μg/mL of Shh increased the cell number of trisomic PA1 cells to the same level as untreated euploid cells (Figure 4.4). This response was concentration dependent, because addition of 2 or 8 μg/mL of Shh did not increase the cell number of either trisomic or euploid PA1 cells. These results suggest that the NC proliferative response in PA1 responds to specific concentrations of Shh, and that stimulation of the Shh pathway can overcome the mitogenic deficit in trisomic cells.

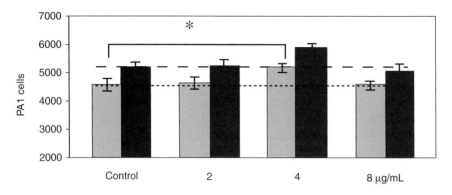

Figure 4.4 Effect of Sonic hedgehog protein on proliferation of first pharyngeal arch cells. 2500 PA1 cells from each of nine Ts65Dn and five euploid T14 embryos were plated in culture dishes, incubated with or without Shh, and the total cell number was determined after 12 h. Trisomic (gray bars) PA1 cells proliferated significantly less than euploid (black bars) at all concentrations of Shh after 12 h in culture ($P < 0.05$ for the control, 4 and 8 μg/mL; $P < 0.08$ for 2 μg/mL Shh). Addition of 4 μg/mL Shh to trisomic cells (third group) caused a significant increase in proliferation of trisomic cells, returning it to the level of proliferation seen in untreated euploid PA1 cells. *Statistically significant with Student's t-test ($P = 0.02$). (Reproduced with permission from Roper et al., 2009.)

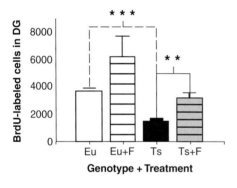

Figure 4.5 Fluoxetine increases adult hippocampal neurogenesis in Ts65Dn mice. Stereological analysis indicates that the total estimated population of BrdU-labeled cells in euploid (3642.25±257.4 1) and fluoxetine-treated Ts65Dn (3134.37±483.04) is significantly greater than for untreated Ts65Dn (1506.5±168.51, n = 8, ***$P < 0.001$, **$P < 0.01$) mice. Fluoxetine treatment (F) in euploid mice (Eu) resulted in an increase in neurogenesis. (Reproduced with permission from Clark et al., 2006.)

Prozac and neurogenesis

In seeking mechanisms underlying memory and learning deficits in Ts65Dn mice, Clark et al. (2006) assessed adult neurogenesis in the dentate gyrus of these animals. They found that the Ts65Dn dentate gyrus showed less neurogenesis than that in euploid animals. Chronic use of antidepressants (like Prozac or fluoxetine) has been shown to counter the behavioral aspects of stress and depression by increasing neurogenesis. To determine whether antidepressant-induced neurogenesis is also efficient in Ts65Dn mice, they chronically treated young Ts65Dn mice (2.5 months) with fluoxetine for 24 days with bromodeoxyuridine (BrdU) given for the last nine days, which resulted in significant increases in neurogenesis in Ts65Dn hippocampi. Stereological analysis revealed a significant increase in total neurogenesis (Figure 4.5).

Synaptic plasticity and memory pathways

Gamma-aminobutyric acid pathways

Previous research suggested that cognitive deficits are not a result of gross abnormalities in Ts65Dn neuroanatomy, but rather derive from selective decreases in the number of

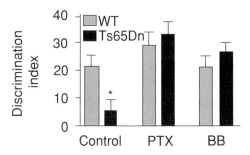

Figure 4.6 Picrotoxin and bilobalide rescue Ts65Dn performance in the novel object recognition task. Compilation of wild-type (WT) and Ts65Dn mouse novelty dicrimination indices (DIs) with no treatment or treatment with saline, picrotoxin (PTX), or bilobalide (BB), showing that PTX and BB normalized Ts65Dn object recognition memory ($F_{5,187}$ = 5.204, P < 0.0002; all post hoc comparisons with Ts65Dn control, P < 0.05; all other post hoc comparisons, P > 0.05). Control observations were pooled from untreated and saline-treated (PTX-naive) mice, and PTX observations from mice given PTX in either the first or second two weeks. (Reproduced with permission from Fernandez et al., 2007.)

excitatory synapses in the brain and corresponding changes in synaptic connectivity. These findings are supported by in vitro studies showing that excessive gamma-aminobutyric acid (GABA)-mediated inhibition impairs induction of LTP. Assuming that triplicated genes found in Ts65Dn mice shift the optimal balance of excitation and inhibition in the dentate gyrus (and perhaps other brain regions) to a state in which excessive inhibition obscures otherwise normal learning and memory, Fernandez and colleagues (2007) theorized that reducing the inhibitory load in the Ts65Dn brain with GABA$_A$-receptor antagonists might rescue defective cognition. They assessed whether a non-epileptic dose of the noncompetitive GABA$_A$ antagonist picrotoxin [PTX; via intraperitoneal (i.p.) injection] could improve Ts65Dn object recognition memory. Ts65Dn mice treated with PTX for two weeks showed normalized object recognition performance, as did those that received bilobalide (BB) throughout the study (Figure 4.6). To extend these findings, they next evaluated the effects of pentylenetetrazole (PTZ; via voluntary oral feeding), a noncompetitive GABA$_A$ antagonist, on declarative memory in the novel object recognition test. PTZ-treated Ts65Dn mice showed discrimination indices (DIs) on a par with those of wild-type mice.

Another study by Rueda et al. (2008) has used the Morris water maze to evaluate spatial learning after a treatment with PTZ. They showed an improvement of the performances (latency to reach the platform) after the treatment.

N-methyl-D-aspartate receptor antagonist memantine

Recently, Arron et al. (2006) suggested that the 50% increased dosages of DSCR1 and DYRK1A (which encode for a nuclear serine–threonine kinase) cooperatively lead to reduced activity of calcineurin-dependent transcriptional activity of NFAT. N-methyl-D-aspartate receptors (NMDARs) are among the targets of calcineurin (CaN). The pharmacological inhibition of CaN activity leads to increased NMDAR mean open-time and opening probability. Because the uncompetitive NMDAR antagonist memantine produces changes in NMDAR kinetics that at least qualitatively mimic the actions of CaN at the single channel level, this drug may partially restore the physiological function of NMDAR and potentially improve learning and memory in these animals. Costa and colleagues (2008) used a simple fear conditioning protocol to test the capacity for contextual memory of four- to six-month-old Ts65Dn

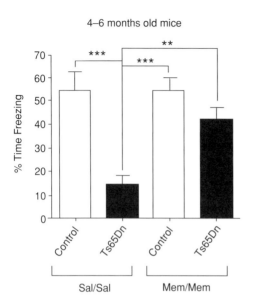

4–6 months old mice

Figure 4.7 Memantine rescues performance deficits of four- to six-month-old Ts65Dn mice on a fear conditioning test. Bar graphs represent mean percentage freezing (7 SEM) during the context test. In a context-shock protocol, saline-injected euploid control mice (n = 10) displayed freezing for about 50% of the total time, whereas saline-injected Ts65Dn mice (n = 10) displayed freezing behavior for only about 15% of the total time. In contrast, memantine-treated Ts65Dn mice (n = 10) displayed freezing at a comparable percentage to both saline-injected and memantine-treated control animals (n = 10). (Reproduced with permission from Costa et al., 2008.)

mice compared to euploid control mice of the same age. During the context test, saline-injected control mice displayed a larger percentage of freezing compared to saline-injected Ts65Dn mice (Figure 4.7). They found that memantine-treated Ts65Dn mice displayed freezing at a comparable percentage to both saline-injected and memantine-treated control animals.

DYRK1A pathway

Minibrain kinase or dual-specificity tyrosine phosphorylation-regulated kinase (Mnb; DYRK1A) is a proline-directed serine–threonine kinase (Kentrup et al., 1996; Himpel et al., 2000) encoded by a gene located within the DSCR1 involved in mental retardation in DS (Delabar et al., 1993; Korenberg et al., 1997). Its expression is elevated in DS brain fetuses (unpublished results) and in individuals with DS (Guimera et al., 1999). Several endogenous substrates for this kinase have been identified, such as transcription factor FKHR (Woods et al., 2001b), microtubule-associated protein tau (Woods et al., 2001a), and proteins engaged in endocytosis such as dynamin (Chen-Hwang et al., 2002) and synaptojanin (Adayev et al., 2006). It is thought to be involved in the control of neurogenesis and of neuronal plasticity. YAC-transgenic mice carrying an extra copy of this gene present alterations of brain morphology and of cognitive functions (Branchi et al., 2004; Chabert et al., 2004). This gene is also overexpressed in specific neurons of patients with AD (Ferrer et al., 2005).

MRI was used to characterize brain morphology alterations during development: total brain volume of transgenic animals is found increased by 14%–15% in comparison with controls, and this difference is seen as early as two days postnatally.

The regional assessment of the volumes allowed the identification of a region, the thalamus–hypothalamus area, which is specifically increased (30%) in transgenic mice (Sebrié et al., 2008).

Kinases catalyze the addition of a phosphate group to various substrates. The main class of inhibitors of kinases are molecules taking the place of the donor molecule, ATP, or modifying

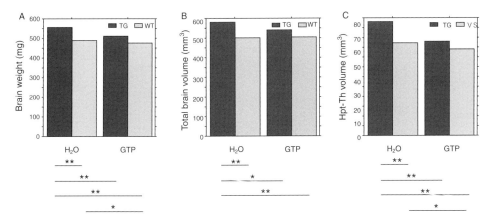

Figure 4.8 Effect of green tea polyphenol (GTP) treatment on DYRK1A-induced brain alterations. A: weight of total brain (mg) in wild-type (WT, n = 26), YACtg152F7 (TG, n = 13) water-fed (H_2O), and in wild-type (WT, n = 13), YACtg152F7 transgenic (TG, n = 18) green tea-fed GTP; B: in vivo MRI assessment of total brain volume (mm^3) in wild-type (n = 10) and YACtg152F7 transgenic (n = 10) water-fed (H_2O) and in wild-type (n = 9) and YACtg152F7 transgenic (n = 11) green tea-fed GTP; C: in vivo MRI assessment of hypothalamus–thalamus volume (mm^3) in wild-type (n = 6) and YACtg152F7 transgenic (n = 6) water-fed (H_2O) and in wild-type (n = 5) and YACtg152F7 transgenic (n = 7) green tea-fed GTP. (Details of the MRI experiments in supplementary data). ** for $p < 0.01$; * for $p < 0.05$. (Reproduced with permission from Guedj et al., 2009.)

the active site. Bain and colleagues (2003) have shown in vitro that DYRK1A is specifically inhibited by epigallocatechin gallate (EGCG), a natural molecule that is the main component of the polyphenols from green tea (PGT).

These observations were used to design a diet given to the gestating mothers and continued postnatally until the MRI analysis. It was found that PGT corrected alterations of morphogenesis. Guedj et al. (2009) also demonstrated that chronic administration of PGT can have a similar (although less efficient than normalizing the gene copy number) corrective effect on brain alterations indicating that the diet brings the level of active DYRK1A to a value between those produced in the transgenic and wild-type situations (Figure 4.8).

The effect of the polyphenols is also visible when comparing water-fed and green tea-fed wild-type animals: the diet induces a significant reduction of brain weight and thalamus–hypothalamus volume, suggesting that the diet-induced reduction of active DYRK1A is equivalent to a genic content below two copies. Polyphenol treatment had no effect on the results of the spontaneous alternation paradigm: transgenic animals do not show any impairment of this task and behave similarly to the control animals. Using a novel object recognition paradigm to assess long-term memory, transgenic mice with three copies of DYRK1A were clearly impaired: polyphenol treatment ameliorates cognitive deficits in YACtg152F7 mice (Figure 4.9).

Other groups have shown an effect of polyphenols on brain functions: in a study designed to determine whether cognition could be influenced by a flavanol rich diet. Van Praag et al. (2007) found that memory, hippocampal vascularization, and neuronal spine density were enhanced in mice fed an (-)epicatechin-containing diet compared with controls. The polyphenol treatment does not modify the amount of DYRK1A mRNA. These results suggest either a direct effect of EGCG on the activity of DYRK1A or an indirect effect, acting via

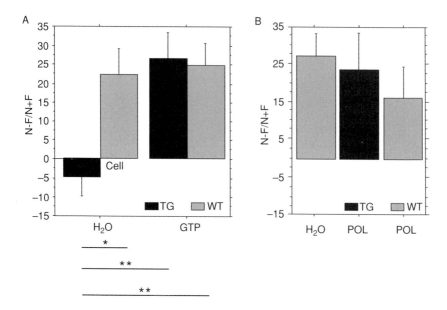

Figure 4.9 Effect of green tea polyphenol (GTP) treatment on short- and long-term memory. In wild-type (WT, n = 10) and YACtg152F7 transgenic (TG, n = 10) water-fed (H_2O) and in wild-type (WT, n = 10) and YACtg152F7 transgenic (TG, n = 10) green tea-fed (GTP, n = 10 mice). A: object recognition test: difference in exploration time between the new and familiar objects, in percentage of total time spent exploring the two objects; 1006 (N-F/N+F). ** for P < 0.01, * for P < 0.05. (According to Wilcoxon test results [two-way ANOVA] in supplementary data.) B: object recognition test on WT H_2O-fed (n = 10), WT polyphenol-fed (n = 10) and TG polyphenol-fed (n = 6) (no significant differences between the three groups). (Reproduced with permission from Guedj et al., 2009.)

a downstream target in the DYRK1A pathway. DYRK1A phosphorylation of trafficking proteins has been observed in cell cultures. Modulation of these trafficking proteins is generally thought to influence synaptic plasticity. LTP and its opposing process, LTD, are widely considered the major cellular mechanisms that underlie learning and memory. LTP was reduced and LTD was augmented in comparison to diploid controls in the isolated hippocampus of Ts65Dn and Ts1Cje, two DS murine models carrying a partial trisomy 16 encompassing the DYRK1A gene. LTP levels can be rescued in hippocampal slices from Ts65Dn mice by EGCG treatment (Xie et al., 2008). This is consistent with observations of long-term memory impairment rescue. These results suggest a central role for DYRK1A in central nervous system functioning and highlight a potential clinical benefit of DYRK1A inhibitors, particularly of natural polyphenol extracts; similar extracts are already used as dietary supplements for the treatment of other disorders and have been shown to be well tolerated at doses similar to those used in the study described here.

Future prospects

Targeting specific genes in animal models is now possible by using one of the strategies presented in this review. These corrective interventions might create side effects, as has been the case with antibody technology used in AD. To avoid the possible negative effects in humans and to choose the best targets or the best combination of targets (those which will allow corrections as close as possible to a normal level), it will be necessary to develop numerous single gene models in mice. The piracetam assay was unfortunately performed only after

Table 4.1 Assessment of therapeutic strategies in mice models

Drugs	Mice models			Teams	Neurogenesis	Morphogenesis	Motor function	Fear conditioning	Learning
	ts65Dn	APP-AD	DYRK1A						
folates									
piracetam									
piracetam	X			Moran et al. 2002					negative effect
SAG1.1	X			Roper et al. 2006	rescue				
fluoxetine	X			Clark et al. 2006	rescue				rescue
memantine		X		Scholtzova et al. 2008					
memantine	X			Costa et al. 2008			rescue	rescue	rescue
donepezil	X			Rueda et al. 2008			no effect		no effect
PTZ	X			Rueda et al.			negative effect		rescue
PTZ	X			Fernandez et al.					rescue
PGT			X	Guedj et al.		rescue	rescue		
AAVshRNA			X	Ortiz-Abalia et al.			rescue		

■ : total or partial rescue; ■ : no effect; ■ : negative effect; □ : not yet done clinical trials in humans; this experiment has demonstrated that this compound was not efficient in rescuing the learning defect in mice (Moran et al., 2002, and Table 4.1).

Unique gene models together with models of partial trisomy will have to be assessed for the efficiency of the corrective strategies at different levels: Table 4.1 shows clearly that many experiments have still to be performed in order to compare the various strategies and eventually to associate different compounds or different strategies. Nevertheless, it is remarkable that strategies targeting specific genes or specific pathways are already giving promising results. One can hope that similar strategies or the development of the strategies reported in this chapter will render it possible to decrease the burden on DS patients.

Summary

Aneuploidies, that is, copy number disorders of functional genomic elements, are common genomic disorders with profound impact on the health of human populations. The phenotypic consequences of aneuploidies are numerous and range from mental retardation, developmental abnormalities, susceptibility to common phenotypes, and to various neoplasms. Trisomy 21 is the most frequent aneuploidy (1 in 700 births and 500,000 patients in Europe) and it is still, even after the improvements of prenatal diagnosis, far outside the range of rare diseases ($<$1 in 2000). This is one of the main genetic causes of mental retardation. This review focuses on new strategies that might allow countering some of the adverse effects of the phenotype.

References

Adayev, T., Chen-Hwang, M. C., Murakami, N., Wang, R., Hwang, Y. W. (2006). MNB/DYRK1A phosphorylation regulates the interactions of synaptojanin 1 with endocytic accessory proteins. *Biochemical and Biophysical Research Communications*, **351**(4), 1060–1065.

Ahn, K. J., Jeong, H. K., Choi, H. S., et al. (2006). DYRK1A BAC transgenic mice show altered synaptic plasticity with learning and memory defects. *Neurobiology of Disease*, **22**(3), 463–472.

Aït Yahya-Graison, E., Aubert, J., Dauphinot, L., et al. (2007). Classification of human chromosome 21 gene-expression variations in Down syndrome: impact on disease phenotypes. *American Journal of Human Genetics*, **81**(3), 475–491.

Arron, J. R., Winslow, M. M., Polleri, A., et al. (2006). NFAT dysregulation by increased dosage of DSCR1 and DYRK1A on chromosome 21. *Nature*, **441**(7093), 595–600.

Bain, J., McLauchlan, H., Elliott, M., Cohen, P. (2003). The specificities of protein kinase inhibitors: an update. *Biochemical Journal*, **371**(1), 199–204.

Bales, K. R., Tzavara, E. T., Wu, S., et al. (2006). Cholinergic dysfunction in a mouse model of Alzheimer disease is reversed by an anti-A beta antibody. *Journal of Clinical Investigation*, **116**(3), 825–832.

Baxter, L. L., Moran, T. H., Richtsmeier, J. T., Troncoso, J., Reeves, R. H. (2000). Discovery and genetic localization of Down syndrome cerebellar phenotypes using the Ts65Dn mouse. *Human Molecular Genetics*, **9**, 195–202.

Becker, L. E., Mito, T., Takashima, S., Onodera, K. (1991). Growth and development of the brain in Down syndrome. In C. J. Epstein (ed.), *The Morphogenesis of Down Syndrome*, pp.133–152. New York: Wiley-Liss.

Belichenko, P. V., Masliah, E., Kleschevnikov, A. M., et al. (2005). Synaptic structural abnormalities in the Ts65Dn mouse model of Down Syndrome. *Journal of Comparative Neurology*, **480**(3), 281–298.

Branchi, I., Bichler, Z., Minghetti, L., et al. (2004). Transgenic mouse in vivo library of human Down syndrome critical region 1: association between DYRK1A overexpression, brain development abnormalities, and cell cycle protein alteration. *Journal of Neuropathology and Experimental Neurology*, **63**(5), 429–440.

Chabert, C., Jamon, M., Cherfouh, A., et al. (2004). Functional analysis of genes implicated in Down syndrome: 1. Cognitive abilities in mice transpolygenic for Down Syndrome Chromosomal Region-1 (DCR-1). *Behavior Genetics*, **34**(6), 559–569.

Chen-Hwang, M. C., Chen, H. R., Elzinga, M., Hwang, Y. W. (2002). Dynamin is a minibrain kinase/dual specificity Yak1 related kinase 1A substrate. *Journal of Biological Chemistry*, **277**(20), 17597–17604.

Clark, S., Schwalbe, J., Stasko, M. R., Yarowsky, P. J., Costa, A. C. (2006). Fluoxetine rescues deficient neurogenesis in hippocampus of the Ts65Dn mouse model for Down syndrome. *Experimental Neurology*, **200**(1), 256–261.

Costa, A. C., Scott-McKean, J. J., Stasko, M. R. (2008). Acute injections of the NMDA receptor antagonist memantine rescue performance deficits of the Ts65Dn mouse model of Down syndrome on a fear conditioning test. *Neuropsychopharmacology*, **33**(7), 1624–1632.

Dahmane, N., Charron, G., Lopes, C., et al. (1995). Down syndrome-critical region contains a gene homologous to Drosophila sim expressed during rat and human central nervous system development. *Proceedings of the National Academy of Sciences of the United States of America*, **92**(20), 9191–9195.

Dauphinot, L., Lyle, R., Rivals, I., et al. (2005). The cerebellar transcriptome during postnatal development of the Ts1Cje mouse, a segmental trisomy model for Down syndrome. *Human Molecular Genetics*, **14**(3), 373–384.

Davisson, M. T., Schmidt, C., Akeson, E. C. (1990). Segmental trisomy of murine chromosome 16: a new model system for studying Down syndrome. *Progress in Clinical and Biological Research*, **360**, 263–280.

Delabar, J. M., Theophile, D., Rahmani, Z., et al. (1993). Molecular mapping of twenty-four features of Down syndrome on chromosome 21. *European Journal of Human Genetics*, **1**(2), 114–124.

Fernandez, F., Morishita, W., Zuniga, E., et al. (2007). Pharmacotherapy for cognitive impairment in a mouse model of Down syndrome. *Nature Neuroscience*, **10**(4), 411–413.

Ferrer, I., Barrachina, M., Puig, B., et al. (2005). Constitutive Dyrk1A is abnormally expressed in Alzheimer disease, Down syndrome, Pick disease, and related transgenic models. *Neurobiology of Disease*, **20**(2), 392–400.

Franceschi, M., Comola, M., Piattoni, F., Gualandri, W., Canal, N. (1990). Prevalence of dementia in adult patients with trisomy 21. *American Journal of Medical Genetics*, **Suppl. 7**, 306–308.

Gardiner, K., Davisson, M. T., Crnic, L. S. (2004). Building protein interaction maps for Down syndrome. *Briefings in Functional Genomics & Proteomics*, **3**(2), 142–156.

Gitton, Y., Dahmane, N., Baik, S., et al. (2002). HSA21 expression map initiative. A gene expression map of human chromosome 21 orthologues in the mouse. *Nature*, **420** (6915), 586–590.

Golden, J. A. and Hyman, B. T. (1994). Development of the superior temporal neocortex is anomalous in trisomy 21. *Journal of Neuropathology and Experimental Neurology*, **53**, 513–520.

Guedj, F., Sébrié, C., Rivals, I., et al. (2009). Green tea polyphenols rescue of brain defects induced by overexpression of DYRK1A. *PLoS ONE*, **4**(2), e4606.

Guimera, J., Casas, C., Estivill, X., Pritchard, M. (1999). Human minibrain homologue (MNBH/DYRK1): characterization, alternative splicing, differential tissue expression, and overexpression in Down syndrome. *Genomics*, **57**(3), 407–418.

Hardy, J. & Selkoe, D. J. (2002). The amyloid hypothesis of Alzheimer's disease: progress and problems on the road to therapeutics. *Science*, **297**, 353–356.

Hesser, B. A., Liang, X. H., Camenisch, G., et al. (2004). Down syndrome critical region protein 1 (DSCR1), a novel VEGF target gene that regulates expression of inflammatory markers on activated endothelial cells. *Blood*, **104**(1), 149–158.

Himpel, S., Tegge, W., Frank, R., et al. (2000).
Specificity determinants of substrate
recognition by the protein kinase DYRK1A.
Journal of Biological Chemistry, **275**(4),
2431–2438.

Holtzman, D. M., Santucci, D., Kilbridge, J., et al.
(1996). Developmental abnormalities and
age-related neurodegeneration in a mouse
model of Down syndrome. *Proceedings of the
National Academy of Sciences of the United
States of America*, **93**, 13333–13338.

Insausti, A. M., Megias, M., Crespo, D., et al.
(1998). Hippocampal volume and neuronal
number in Ts65Dn mice: a murine model of
Down syndrome. *Neuroscience Letters*, **253**,
175–178.

Jernigan, T. L. A., Sowell, E., Doherty, S.,
Hesselink, J. R. (1993). Cerebral morphologic
distinctions between Williams and Down
syndromes. *Archives of Neurology*, **50**,
186–191.

Kentrup, H., Becker, W., Heukelbach, J., et al.
(1996). Dyrk, a dual specificity protein kinase
with unique structural features whose activity
is dependent on tyrosine residues between
subdomains VII and VIII. *Journal of
Biological Chemistry*, **271**(7), 3488–3495.

Kesslak, J. P., Nagata, S. F., Lott, I., Nalcioglu, O.
(1994). Magnetic resonance imaging analysis
of age-related changes in the brains of
individuals with Down's syndrome.
Neurology, **44**, 1039–1045.

Kleschevnikov, A. M., Belichenko, P. V., Villar,
A. J., et al. (2004). Hippocampal long-term
potentiation suppressed by increased
inhibition in the Ts65Dn mouse, a genetic
model of Down syndrome. *Journal of
Neuroscience*, **24** (37), 8153–8160.

Korenberg, J. R., Aaltonen, J., Brahe, C., et al.
(1997). Report and abstracts of the Sixth
International Workshop on Human
Chromosome 21 Mapping 1996. Cold Spring
Harbor, New York, USA. May 6–8, 1996.
Cytogenetics and Cell Genetics, **79**(1–2),
21–52.

Lee, E. B., Leng, L. Z., Zhang, B., et al. (2006).
Targeting amyloid-beta peptide (Abeta)
oligomers by passive immunization with a
conformation-selective monoclonal antibody
improves learning and memory in Abeta

precursor protein (APP) transgenic mice.
Journal of Biological Chemistry, **281**(7),
4292–4299.

Lyle, R., Gehrig, C., Neergaard-Henrichsen, C.,
Deutsch, S., Antonarakis, S. E. (2004). Gene
expression from the aneuploid chromosome
in a trisomy mouse model of Down
syndrome. *Genome Research*, **14**(7),
1268–1274.

Mann, D. M., Royston, M. C., Ravindra, C. R.
(1990). Some morphometric observations on
the brains of patients with Down's syndrome:
their relationship to age and dementia.
Journal of the Neurological Sciences **99**,
153–164.

Moran, T. H., Capone, G. T., Knipp, S., et al.
(2002). The effects of piracetam on cognitive
performance in a mouse model of Down's
syndrome. *Physiology & Behavior*, **77**(2–3),
403–409.

O'Doherty, A., Ruf, S., Mulligan, C., et al. (2005).
An aneuploid mouse strain carrying human
chromosome 21 with Down syndrome
phenotypes. *Science*, **309**(5743), 2033–2037.

Olson, L. E., Roper, R. J., Baxter, L. L., et al.
(2004). Down syndrome mouse models
Ts65Dn, Ts1Cje, and Ms1Cje/Ts65Dn exhibit
variable severity of cerebellar phenotypes.
Developmental Dynamics, **230**(3), 581–589.

Ortiz-Abalia, J., Sahún, I., Altafaj, X., et al.
(2008). Targeting Dyrk1A with AAVshRNA
attenuates motor alterations in TgDyrk1A, a
mouse model of Down syndrome. *American
Journal of Human Genetics*, **83**(4), 479–488.

Palmer, S. (2000). Working memory: a
developmental study of phonological
recoding. *Memory*, **8**, 179–193.

Pellegrini-Calace, M. & Tramontano, A. (2006).
Identification of a novel putative
mitogen-activated kinase cascade on human
chromosome 21 by computational
approaches. *Bioinformatics*, **22**(7), 775–778.

Pinter, J. D., Eliez, S., Schmitt, J. E., Capone,
G. T., Reiss, A. L. (2001). Neuroanatomy of
Down's syndrome: a high-resolution MRI
study. *American Journal of Psychiatry*, **158**,
1659–1665.

Rachidi, M., Lopes, C., Delezoide, A. L., Delabar,
J. M. (2006). C21orf5, a human candidate
gene for brain abnormalities and mental

retardation in Down syndrome. *Cytogenetic and Genome Research*, **112**(1–2), 16–22.

Rahmani, Z., Lopes, C., Rachidi, M., Delabar, J. M. (1998). Expression of the mnb (dyrk) protein in adult and embryonic mouse tissues. *Biochemical and Biophysical Research Communications*, **253**(2), 514–518.

Raz, N., Torres, I. J., Briggs, S. D., et al. (1995). Selective neuroanatomic abnormalities in Down's syndrome and their cognitive correlates: evidence from MRI morphometry. *Neurology*, **45**, 356–366.

Reymond, A., Marigo, V., Yaylaoglu, M. B., et al. (2002). Human chromosome 21 gene expression atlas in the mouse. *Nature*, **420**(6915), 582–586.

Ronan, A., Fagan, K., Christie, L., et al. (2007). Familial 4.3 Mb duplication of 21q22 sheds new light on the Down syndrome critical region. *Journal of Medical Genetics*, **44**(7), 448–451.

Roper, R. J., Baxter, L. L., Saran, N. G., et al. (2006). Defective cerebellar response to mitogenic Hedgehog signaling in Down [corrected] syndrome mice. *Proceedings of the National Academy of Sciences of the United States of America*, **103**(5), 1452–1456.

Roper, R. J., VanHorn, J. F., Cain, C. C., Reeves, R. H. (2009). A neural crest deficit in Down syndrome mice is associated with deficient mitotic response to Sonic hedgehog. *Mechanisms of Development*, **126**(3–4), 212–219.

Rueda, N., Flórez, J., Martínez-Cué, C. (2008). Chronic pentylenetetrazole but not donepezil treatment rescues spatial cognition in Ts65Dn mice, a model for Down syndrome. *Neuroscience Letters*, **433**(1), 22–27.

Sago, H., Carlson, E. J., Smith, D. J., et al. (1998). Ts1Cje, a partial trisomy 16 mouse model for Down syndrome, exhibits learning and behavioral abnormalities. *Proceedings of the National Academy of Sciences of the United States of America*, **95**, 6256–6261.

Scholtzova, H., Wadghiri, Y. Z., Douadi, M., et al. (2008). Memantine leads to behavioral improvement and amyloid reduction in Alzheimer's-disease-model transgenic mice shown as by micromagnetic resonance imaging. *Journal of Neuroscience Research*, **86**(12), 2784–2791.

Schulz, E. & Scholz, B. (1992). [Neurohistological findings in the parietal cortex of children with chromosome aberrations.] *Journal für Hirnforschung*, **33**(1), 37–62.

Sebrié, C., Chabert, C., Ledru, A., et al. (2008). In vivo MRI study of brain volumetric alterations in a transgenic YAC model of partial trisomy 21. *Anatomical Record*, **291**(3), 254–262.

Shinohara, T., Tomizuka, K., Miyabara, S., et al. (2001). Mice containing a human chromosome 21 model behavioral impairment and cardiac anomalies of Down's syndrome. *Human Molecular Genetics*, **10**(11), 1163–1175.

Siarey, R. J., Carlson, E. J., Epstein, C. J., et al. (1999). Increased synaptic depression in the Ts65Dn mouse, a model for mental retardation in Down syndrome. *Neuropharmacology*, **38**(12), 1917–1920.

Siarey, R. J., Stoll, J., Rapoport, S. I., Galdzicki, Z. (1997). Altered long-term potentiation in the young and old Ts65Dn mouse, a model for Down Syndrome. *Neuropharmacology*, **36**, 1549–1554.

Smith, D. J., Stevens, M. E., Sudanagunta, S. P., et al. (1997). Functional screening of 2 Mb of human chromosome 21q22.2 in transgenic mice implicates minibrain in learning defects associated with Down syndrome. *Nature Genetics*, **16**(1), 28–36.

Thomas, S., Thiery, E., Aflalo, R., et al. (2003). PCP4 is highly expressed in ectoderm and particularly in neuroectoderm derivatives during mouse embryogenesis. *Gene Expression Patterns*, **3**(1), 93–97.

Van Praag, H., Lucero, M. J., Yeo, G. W., et al. (2007). Plant-derived flavanol (-)epicatechin enhances angiogenesis and retention of spatial memory in mice. *Journal of Neuroscience*, **27**(22): 5869–5878.

White, N. S., Alkire, M. T., Haier, R. J. (2003). A voxel-based morphometric study of nondemented adults with Down Syndrome. *NeuroImage*, **20**, 393–403.

Woods, Y. L., Cohen, P., Becker, W., et al. (2001a). The kinase DYRK phosphorylates protein-synthesis initiation factor eIF2Bepsilon at Ser539 and the microtubule-associated protein tau at Thr212: potential role for DYRK as a glycogen synthase kinase 3-priming kinase. *Biochemistry Journal*, **355**(3), 609–615.

Woods, Y. L., Rena, G., Morrice, N., et al. (2001b). The kinase DYRK1A phosphorylates the transcription factor FKHR at Ser329 in vitro, a novel in vivo phosphorylation site. *Biochemistry Journal*, **355**(3), 597–607.

Xie, W., Ramakrishna, N., Wieraszko, A., Hwang, Y. W. (2008). Promotion of neuronal plasticity by (-)-epigallocatechin-3-gallate. *Neurochemical Research*, **33**(5): 776–783.

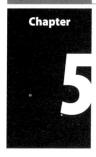

Chapter

5

Brain plasticity and environmental enrichment in Ts65Dn mice, an animal model for Down syndrome

Adam Golabek, Katarzyna Jarząbek, Sonia Palminiello,
Marius Walus, Ausma Rabe, Giorgio Albertini,
Elizabeth Kida

The concept of neuronal plasticity and enriched environment

With an occurrence of ~1 in 800 live births, Down syndrome (DS), a chromosome 21 (HSA21) trisomy, is the most common genetic cause of mental retardation (Epstein, 1986). Although the somatic phenotype of DS affects nearly every organ in the body, the predominant and most consistent feature of DS is subnormal intellectual functioning, ranging from mild to severe (Chapman & Hesketh, 2000), resulting from abnormal cognitive and language development, learning and memory impairments, and significant behavioral alterations (Pennington et al., 2003). Underlying the complex neurological phenotype of DS are a number of different central nervous system abnormalities such as hypocellularity (already observed in the fetus), delayed myelination, altered cortical lamination, dendritic and synaptic alterations, and abnormal neurogenesis (Wisniewski et al., 2006). Despite enormous scientific efforts, the cause of the subnormal intellectual functioning of DS patients on the molecular level remains unanswered. It is also unknown whether, which, and to what extent the developmental abnormalities caused by the triplicated chromosome 21 can be mitigated by environmental factors and behavioral therapies (Guralnick, 2005).

Although sophisticated genetic and epigenetic programs predetermine the structural integrity and basal functionality of the mammalian brain at the time of birth, further brain development and refinement of neuronal circuitry are determined through interaction with the surrounding environment. Only with the development of the concepts of neuronal (brain) plasticity and enriched environment has it been possible to more rigorously study the effect of environment on the development and functioning of the mammalian brain in adulthood, under normal and various pathological conditions, both genetic and acquired.

The concepts of neuronal plasticity and environmental enrichment were first formulated by Hebb in the late 1940s (van Praag et al., 2000). On the basis of observations that rats kept at home as pets showed behavioral improvements over their littermates kept in laboratories (Hebb, 1947), Hebb introduced a notion of neuronal plasticity in the adult brain, defined

Neurocognitive Rehabilitation of Down Syndrome, eds. Jean-Adolphe Rondal, Juan Perera, and Donna Spiker. Published by Cambridge University Press. © Cambridge University Press 2011.

as changes taking place in cells that were repeatedly excited, leading to a more efficient firing on successive stimulation (Hebb, 1949). Since then, the ideas of neuronal plasticity and enriched environment have been extended and refined following the accumulation of extensive experimental data. The standard definition of an enriched environment is a combination of complex inanimate and social stimulation (Rosenzweig et al., 1978). In laboratory settings, an enriched environment usually refers to housing conditions that facilitate enhanced sensory, cognitive, and motor stimulation. Enhanced stimulation is achieved by housing multiple animals in larger-than-standard cages, equipped with multiple objects (toys) varying in size, shape, color, texture, and often location within the cage. The cage may be outfitted with a running wheel, allowing for physical activity (Nithianantharajah & Hannan, 2006).

Currently, no single cognitive theory explaining the mechanism by which an enriched environment affects the brain is widely accepted, even though most investigators favor the learning-and-memory hypothesis in which the mediators of the observed morphological changes are the molecular mechanisms underlying the memory process (van Praag et al., 2000). Nevertheless, it is well documented that an enriched environment may promote neuronal activation, signaling, and plasticity in the somatosensory, visual, and motor cortices, hippocampus, and cerebellum. Numerous behavioral, morphological, and molecular studies have revealed significant effects of an enriched environment on the brains of rodents and other mammalian species and provided new insights into the mechanisms of experience-dependent plasticity.

Earlier experiments in rodents showed that environmental enrichment increases hippocampal thickness, increases dendritic arborization, and increases the number of glial cells in the hippocampus (Rosenzweig, 1966; Walsh et al., 1969; Fiala et al., 1978). More recent studies demonstrated that an enriched environment also enhances adult neurogenesis, a prominent form of structural plasticity leading to continuous generation of new neurons in the mature mammalian brain (Kempermann et al., 1997). In addition, environmental enrichment has a survival-promoting effect on the progeny of neuronal precursor cells in the hippocampus of mice (van Praag et al., 1999).

An enriched environment is also beneficial for the brain exposed to various pathological conditions, stress, and ageing. Thus, an enriched environment was shown to protect dopaminergic neurons in an MPTP-induced mouse model of Parkinson's disease (Bezard et al., 2003), to rescue protein deficits in a mouse model of Huntington's disease (Spires et al., 2004), to reduce amyloid-beta (A-beta) levels and amyloid deposition in amyloid precursor protein (APP)-transgenic mice, to increase the expression of genes associated with neurogenesis, cell survival, learning, and memory (Lazarov et al., 2005), and to promote behavioral and morphological recovery in a mouse model of the fragile-X syndrome (Restivo et al., 2005). Amyotrophic lateral sclerosis, epilepsy, stroke, and traumatic brain injury animal models also benefited from enriched environmental conditions (Nithianantharajah & Hannan, 2006).

Mouse models of Down syndrome

Mouse models of neurological disorders provide the opportunity to define the abnormal molecular and cellular mechanisms underlying the particular disease and allow for experimental manipulation of those mechanisms, which is not possible in humans. To date, a number of mouse models of HSA21 have been generated. HSA21 genes are conserved in the orthologous regions of mouse chromosomes 16, 17, and 10 (MMU16, MMU17, and MMU10). Because of this multi-chromosomal distribution of HSA21 genes in the mouse, the development of a mouse model that is trisomic for all orthologous genes of HSA21 was difficult, and mostly partial trisomies have been generated.

The first mouse model of HSA21 was labeled Ts16 and was created by using spontaneous Robertsonian translocations. The main features of Ts16 mice included moderate general hypoplasia, slight developmental retardation, and cardiovascular anomalies (Miyabara et al., 1982). However, given the presence of syntenies between MMU16 and HSA3, HSA8, HSA16, and HSA21 and the nonviability of the trisomic fetuses beyond term, the value of mouse Ts16 as a model for human Ts21 is limited. The second model, Ts65Dn mice, represented a partial (segmental) trisomy of MMU16 encompassing genes from Mrp139 to Znf259 (Davisson et al., 1990). Some behavioral, cellular, and molecular abnormalities demonstrated in these animals indeed replicate human disease. Importantly, Ts65Dn mice are viable, have cognitive impairments that center on hippocampal function (Reeves et al., 1995), and are impaired in tasks that require spatial and working memory (Lorenzi & Reeves, 2006; Sérégaza et al., 2006; Gardiner, 2010).

Two other DS mouse models carry triplication of smaller fragments of MMU16. The triplicated fragment of MMU16 includes genes from SOD1 to Znf295 in Ts1Cje mice (Sago et al., 1998), and from App to SOD1 (a centromeric part) in Ms1Ts65 (Sago et al., 2000). Ts1Cje mice are trisomic for ~78% of the genes triplicated in Ts65Dn mice and show milder learning deficits than Ts65Dn mice as well as abnormal short- and long-term synaptic plasticity (Siarey et al., 2005). In contrast to Ts65Dn mice, degeneration of basal forebrain cholinergic neurons is absent in Ts1Cje (Sago et al., 1998). Interestingly, Ms1Ts65 mice also demonstrate poor performance in the Morris water maze, although less severely than in Ts65Dn mice, which suggests that not only triplication of the region from SOD1 to Znf295 but also imbalance of the region from App to SOD1 may contribute to the DS phenotype (Sago et al., 2000).

Earlier studies proposed that a small region of HSA21 spanning 3.8–6.5 Mb and containing ~25–50 genes, the so-called DS critical region (DSCR), may play a major role in DS phenotypes (Korenberg et al., 1992; Delabar et al., 1993; Antonarakis et al., 2004). To test the hypothesis implying that the DSCR contains a gene or genes sufficient to cause impairment in learning and memory tasks involving the hippocampus, Ts1Rhr and Ms1Rhr mice that are either trisomic or monosomic, respectively, for the region extending from Cbr3 to Mx2 have been generated (Olson et al., 2004, 2007). Trisomy for the DSCR alone was not sufficient to produce the characteristic facial phenotype as well as structural and functional features of hippocampal impairment that are seen in the Ts65Dn mouse and DS. However, when the critical region is returned to normal dosage in trisomic Ms1Rhr/Ts65Dn mice, performance in the Morris water maze is identical to that in euploid mice, demonstrating that this region is necessary for the phenotype. That important neurobiological phenotypes characteristic of DS are conserved in Ts1Rhr mice was also documented in another study (Belichenko et al., 2009). Nevertheless, two recent genotype–phenotype mapping analyses in DS subjects with partial trisomy (Korbel et al., 2009) and partial trisomy and partial monosomy (Lyle et al., 2009) excluded the existence of a single DSCR being responsible for all or most aspects of the DS phenotype, providing evidence for a contribution to the overall DS phenotype of many genes along HSA21. As a consequence, it was proposed that the DSCR represents a susceptibility region (SR) modified by other loci on HSA21 and elsewhere in the genome (Lyle et al., 2009).

In agreement with this assumption, TsYah mice that are trisomic for the Abcg1-U2af1 interval, located on MMU17 that contains only 12 genes present in the HSA21 sub-telomeric region, show defects in novel object recognition and open-field and Y-maze tests, similar to other DS models, which also implicates the Abcg1-U2af1 orthologous region in the DS phenotype (Pereira et al., 2009). Interestingly, in contrast to other DS model animals, TsYah mice demonstrate an unexpected gain of cognitive function in spatial memory.

Recently, two new DS mouse models have been generated: Tc1 mice and Dp(10)1Yey/+; Dp(16)1Yey/+; Dp(17)1Yey/+ mice. Tc1 mice, a transchromosomic strain, carry almost complete HSA21 with two small deletions eliminating only ~8% of HSA21 genes. These mice manifest alterations in behavior, synaptic plasticity, cerebellar neuronal number, heart development, and mandible size that relate to human DS (O'Doherty et al., 2005). However, while Tc1 mice show short-term memory impairments, their long-term memory and synaptic plasticity are preserved (Morice et al., 2008). Both mosaicism and/or internal deletions in HSA21q, leaving some genes disomic, could contribute to the apparently milder phenotype of the Tc1 model (Gardiner, 2010). Dp(10)1Yey/+; Dp(16)1Yey/+; Dp(17)1Yey/+ mice are trisomic for all of the HSA21 syntenic regions by carrying duplications spanning the entire HSA21 syntenic regions on all three mouse chromosomes (Yu et al., 2010). These mutant animals are impaired in spatial learning and memory and in context-associated learning, and have significant defects in hippocampal long-term potentiation (LTP). Approximately 6.5% of Dp(10)1Yey/+; Dp(16)1Yey/+; Dp(17)1Yey/+ mice exhibit hydrocephalus with aqueductal stenosis at ~6–8 weeks of age and die usually at ~8–10 weeks of age.

Of all DS mouse models created to date, the most widely utilized and best characterized is the Ts65Dn mouse strain. Nevertheless, only a very few studies have analyzed the effect of an enriched environment on the phenotype of Ts65Dn mice. When applied to Ts65Dn pups for seven weeks after weaning, an enriched environment induced significant behavioral and learning changes in a battery of tests. However, improvement of spatial memory in the Morris water maze and improved performance in the acquisition trials was demonstrated only in females, indicating that gender significantly modifies the effect of environmental enrichment in Ts65Dn mice (Martínez-Cué et al., 2002). It was also reported that wild-type (wt) mice housed under enriched conditions demonstrated significantly more branched and more spinous pyramidal cells in the frontal cortex than non-enriched animals, but this effect was very small in Ts65Dn animals (Dierssen et al., 2003).

The effect of an enriched environment on Ts65Dn mice

Thus, it is still uncertain which structural and molecular abnormalities manifested by Ts65Dn mice can be improved by an enriched environment. Furthermore, it is unclear which molecular mechanisms may underlie the cognitive and behavioral improvement that was observed in Ts65Dn mice in an enriched environment. To address these issues, we initiated studies aimed at characterizing whether and how an environmental enrichment affects: (1) synaptic vesicles trafficking proteins, (2) dentate gyrus neurogenesis/cell divisions, and (3) levels of selected proteins encoded by the triplicated genes.

Synaptic plasticity

Synapses are specialized sites of information exchange between neurons and their target cells, where an arriving electrical signal is transformed rapidly and efficiently into a chemical signal through the regulated exocytosis of neurotransmitter-filled synaptic vesicles (SVs) (Sudhof, 2004). Abnormalities in the structure and development of synapses have been documented in humans with DS (Wisniewski et al., 1986, 2006). A lasting decrease in synaptic development beginning in the first postnatal week has been reported recently in Ts65Dn animals

(Chakrabarti et al., 2007). Already at postnatal day 21, enlargement of presynaptic (boutons) and postsynaptic (spines) elements, decreased spine density on the dendrites of dentate granule cells, a decrease in input to dendritic shafts, and an increase in input to the necks of spines were also found (Belichenko et al., 2004). In older Ts65Dn mice, fewer asymmetric synapses in the dentate gyrus and CA3/CA1 hippocampal sectors, a deficit in symmetric synapses in the dentate gyrus, and greater apposition zone lengths of asymmetric synapses were detected (Kurt et al., 2004). These structural synaptic changes are associated in Ts65Dn mice with functional alterations. An in vitro synaptic plasticity of brain slices measured as LTP is an experimental correlate of the cellular and molecular changes observed in learning and memory processes in vivo. Unlike for wt littermates, LTP could not be elicited in the dentate gyrus of Ts65Dn mice (Kleschevnikov et al., 2004) as a result of inadequate synaptic activation of N-methyl-D-aspartate (NMDA) receptors, similar to what was observed in the CA1 region (Siarey et al., 1999). Suppression of gamma-aminobutyric acid (GABA) receptor-mediated inhibition with picrotoxin restored the LTP induction in these animals, suggesting that enhanced inhibitory synaptic transmission is the underlying cause of the LTP induction failure (Kleschevnikov et al., 2004).

Fusion of SVs with the presynaptic plasma membrane is a tightly controlled process, both spatially and temporally (Brodsky et al., 2001; Sudhof, 2004). Vesicles cluster, dock, fuse, and release neurotransmitter at a restricted and highly specialized plasma membrane called the active zone. The release of SVs is followed by their recycling, which is crucial for the continuation of synaptic transmission, because the number of quanta released during a short burst of intense nerve activity is much greater than the total number of synaptic vesicles present in the nerve terminal. Slight differences in SV trafficking may directly or indirectly contribute to the pathophysiology associated with some neurodevelopmental disorders through frequency-dependent changes in chemical neurotransmission. Pathological expression of a presynaptic protein could affect both pre- and postsynaptic long-term plasticity. Thus, analysis of the presynaptic function might reveal a cause for the cognitive deficits in neurodevelopmental disorders and a potential therapeutic target.

In this regard, Pollonini et al. (2008) reported on reduced levels of synaptophysin in the homogenates from the hippocampus of a four-month-old Ts65Dn mouse, but normal levels of this protein were found in the whole brain extracts of newborn animals. However, Fernandez and colleagues (2009) were unable to detect significant changes in synaptophysin levels in synaptosomal fractions prepared from the brains of three-month-old Ts65Dn mice in comparison with wt littermates. In addition, the levels of several other proteins associated with synaptic junctions studied by these authors, such as RIM1/2, Munc-13, synapsin I, Munc-18, synaptotagmin, and SNAP-25, were not altered except for increased levels of synaptojanin, encoded on triplicated chromosome, and modest decreases in the levels of the presynaptic protein ERC1/CAST2/ELKS, postsynaptic PSD-95 and CAMKIIα, and the α1 subunit of the GABA$_A$ receptor.

We have investigated the effect of an enriched environment on the levels of 10 SV proteins involved in either SV integrity like synaptophysin, or SV trafficking such as amphiphysin 1, BRAMP2 (amphiphysin 2), Munc-18, rab3, Rim, sec8, SNAP-25, synapsin IIa, and synaptotagmin. Only female mice were used for these experiments because both control and Ts65Dn males displayed an overly aggressive behavior when housed in larger groups. Two sets of animals were studied. The first group consisted of 12 younger females reared from the age of 16–25 days in an enriched cage and their 10 littermates housed 4–5 in a smaller cage. The second group consisted of eight older females maintained in an enriched cage and their six littermates housed in two standard cages from the age of four months. The animals were maintained either under an enriched environmental or under standard conditions (controls) for the same period of 3.5 months. Each enriched cage contained many different objects of various textures and sizes and two activity wheels, exposing the mice to social interactions and learning and physical activities. The levels of SV proteins in the brain homogenates prepared from the cerebral hemispheres were examined by immunoblotting.

To determine whether changes in SV proteins' levels in Ts65Dn mice correlate with those in the brain tissue of DS subjects, we also analyzed the levels of SV proteins in the frontal cortices of four DS subjects and four normal control subjects at 8–23 years of age. The levels of synaptophysin, Munc-18, and SNAP-25 were similar in both groups. The levels of rab3 and RIM were lower in DS than in controls, but the difference was not statistically significant. The levels of amphiphysin1 and 2 as well as synapsin IIa were significantly lower in DS subjects than in controls (up to 50%). Sec8 and synaptotagmin levels were higher in DS subjects than in controls (up to 20%), but these differences were not statistically significant.

The differences in the levels of SV proteins in brain tissue homogenates of Ts65Dn mice and controls were similar to those we observed in human samples; however, they were distinctly milder in the mouse than in the human brain. The levels of synaptophysin were similar in brain homogenates of Ts65Dn and control mice housed under normal conditions, thus confirming the observations of Fernandez and colleagues (2009). An enriched environment led to a significant increase in synaptophysin levels in both young and older disomic animals (not shown), in agreement with earlier studies (Lambert et al., 2005). However, only the older group of Ts65Dn mice housed under enriched conditions showed significantly higher levels of synaptophysin than their trisomic littermates maintained in regular cages.

Amphiphysin is one of the proteins involved in SV endocytosis. It recruits the dynamin to the membrane and maintains it in a dissociated state as well as binds to AP-2 and synaptojanin (Wigge & McMahon, 1998). Amphiphysin 2 is a brain-specific ampiphysin with several splicing variants. Owing to alternative splicing, BRAMP2 appears on immunoblots of mouse tissue as a doublet of ~96 and 89 kDa, and as a single band in human tissues. According to our data, the levels of both amphiphysin 1 (not shown) and BRAMP2 (Figure 5.1B) are lower in the brains of Ts65Dn mice in comparison with wt littermates, similar to what we found in the brains of DS subjects (Figure 5.1A). Interestingly, although BRAMP2 levels in young Ts65Dn mice were normalized by an enriched environment (Figure 5.1B), they were not significantly changed in older Ts65Dn mice (not shown). The levels of synapsin IIa and RIM increased mildly whereas the levels of sec8 decreased in younger and older groups of Ts65Dn mice exposed to an enriched environment.

These observations revealed mild abnormalities in the levels of some SV proteins implicated in SV trafficking in Ts65Dn mice, which may contribute to the cognitive deficit in these animals, and demonstrate that some of these deficiencies respond to an enriched environment, suggesting that environmental stimulation may improve, at least to a certain degree, altered synaptic plasticity in these animals.

Neurogenesis

Altered neurogenesis represents another molecular abnormality that may bring about the cognitive dysfunction observed in individuals with DS and in model animals. Neurogenesis has long been believed only to occur during brain development. In the 1960s, pioneering studies by Altman and Das (1965) provided the first evidence that new neurons can be generated also in the adult mammalian brain. Neurogenic regions in the adult mammalian brain

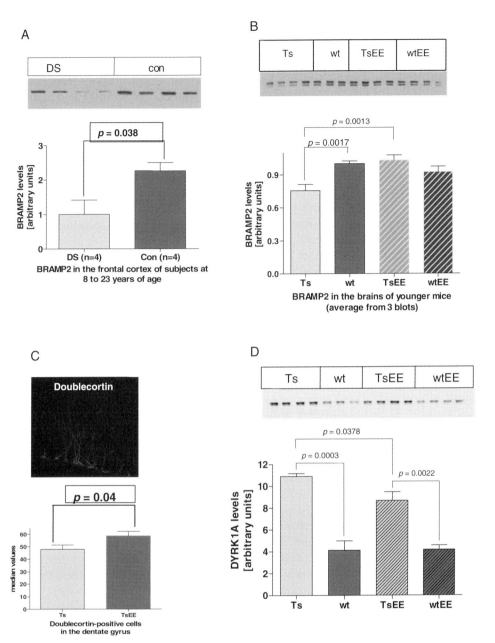

Figure 5.1 The effect of an enriched environment on the brain plasticity of Ts65Dn mice.
A, **B**: the level of BRAMP2 is decreased in the frontal cortices of DS subjects (**A**) and in the cerebral hemispheres of young Ts65Dn mice in comparison with controls (**B**). As shown in (**B**), Ts65Dn mice housed under enriched conditions demonstrate a significant increase in the level of BRAMP2 in comparison with animals kept under standard conditions.
C: the number of doublecortin-positive cells in the hippocampal dentate gyrus (lower panel), as quantitated on 40 μm-thick vibratome sections (upper panel) by using a laser-scanning confocal microscope, is slightly but significantly higher in Ts65Dn mice housed in enriched cages than in mice kept under standard conditions.
D: the levels of DYRK1A non-phosphorylated at Tyr-145 visualized in homogenates of cerebral hemispheres on immunoblots with mAb 8D9 (upper panel) are significantly lower in Ts65Dn mice housed in enriched cages in comparison to Ts65Dn mice housed under standard conditions (lower panel).
DS: Down syndrome; con: control; wt: wild-type; Ts: trisomic; EE: enriched environment. Statistical analyses were performed by using Student's t-test.

include the subventricular zone, the source of new neurons for the olfactory bulb, and the dentate gyrus of the hippocampus (von Bohlen Und Halbach, 2007). In the hippocampal dentate gyrus, neurogenesis is limited to the subgranular zone. The newly formed cells integrate into the granular layer of the dentate gyrus and start to extend axons and dendrites into their target areas. Although it was proposed that adult-generated hippocampal neurons are potentially involved in associative memory formation (Gould et al., 1999), the physiological role of neurogenesis in the adult hippocampus is still a matter of debate.

Abnormal neurogenesis, both prenatally and postnatally, was reported in both DS subjects and mouse models of DS (Clark et al. 2006; Chakrabarti et al., 2007; Contestabile et al., 2007, 2009; Ishihara et al., 2010). In Ts65Dn mice, longer cell cycle duration and reduced neurogenesis from the ventricular zone, leading to delays in prenatal growth of the cerebral cortex and hippocampus, have been described recently, suggesting that postnatal disabilities in Ts65Dn mice and probably in individuals with DS as well, may stem from specific abnormalities in embryonic forebrain precursor cells (Chakrabarti et al., 2007). In addition, elongation of the cell cycle (G2 and G1 phases) was described in the cerebella of neonatal Ts65Dn mice (Contestabile et al., 2009), whereas at P6, an 18% reduction in mitotic cells in the granule cell layer and the hilus was found (Lorenzi & Reeves, 2006). Reduced cell proliferation and density of surviving cells were reported earlier in Ts65Dn mice at 13–15 months of age, but not in young mice at 3–5 months of age, in comparison to controls (Rueda et al., 2005). However, young (2–5 months old) Ts65Dn mice demonstrated markedly fewer 5-bromo-2′deoxyuridine (BrdU)-labeled cells in the hippocampal dentate gyrus than did euploid animals according to another study (Clark et al., 2006). The number of proliferating cells is reduced also in DS fetuses studied at 18–21 weeks' gestation in both the hippocampal dentate gyrus and the cortical germinal zone (Contestabile et al., 2007).

In the adult dentate gyrus, five different stages of neurogenesis spanning ∼2–3 weeks can be distinguished: proliferation, differentiation, migration, axonal and dendritic targeting, and synaptic integration (Kempermann et al., 2003). To assess the effect of an enriched environment on cell divisions in the hippocampal dentate gyrus, we administered two intraperitoneal injections of BrdU at 100 mg/kg of weight within a four-hour interval to Ts65Dn females (aged 3.5–5 months), which after weaning were maintained either in standard or enriched cages. The animals were sacrificed two hours after the second injection. As revealed by quantitative analyses, the number of BrdU-positive cells in the hippocampal dentate gyrus was higher in Ts65Dn mice kept under enriched environmental conditions than in animals maintained in regular cages, but the differences were not statistically significant, partly because of marked differences among animals within the enriched group (not shown).

Proteins encoded by triplicated genes

One of the immunohistochemical markers used to label newly generated neuronal cells is doublecortin. The expression of doublecortin starts at the stage of differentiation and continues through axonal and dendritic targeting (Kempermann et al., 2003). Doublecortin promotes microtubule polymerization, and thus plays a fundamental role in the migration of newly generated neurons. We investigated the number of doublecortin-positive cells in the hippocampal dentate gyri of young Ts65Dn female mice (3.5–5 months of age), maintained after weaning for three months either in regular or enriched cages, as described previously. The expression of doublecortin appeared early in newly born neurons, during the S phase of the cell cycle, as judged from its presence in cells co-labeled with BrdU injected into these animals twice. However, at that early time, immunoreactivity to doublecortin was localized to the cell cytoplasm and usually one, unbranched cell process (not shown), while numerous, abundantly branched processes were visualized by anti-doublecortin antibodies in more mature neurons (Figure 5.1C, upper panel). The number of immunopositive cells was slightly but significantly higher in the dentate gyrus in Ts65Dn mice exposed to an enriched environment than in Ts65Dn mice maintained under standard conditions (Figure 5.1C, lower panel). These results demonstrate that an enriched environment enhances adult neurogenesis in Ts65Dn mice.

Given that an enriched environment improves learning and memory in Ts65Dn female mice (Martínez-Cué et al., 2002), pointing to the preservation of the brain plasticity potential in these genetically compromised animals, we also investigated the possibility that behavioral improvement might be paralleled by normalization/reduction of the increased levels of those proteins encoded by genes located in the triplicated chromosome that are engaged in learning/memory processes. Such a candidate protein is DYRK1A, a protein kinase encoded in humans by a gene mapped to the 21q22.2 locus of HSA21 (Guimerá et al., 1996) and to the triplicated segment of MMU16 in Ts65Dn mice (Song et al., 1996). Overexpression of DYRK1A in mice causes neurodevelopmental delay with motor abnormalities and cognitive deficits (Altafaj et al., 2001), whereas its haplo-insufficiency is associated with developmental delay and abnormal brain morphology (Fotaki et al., 2002).

DYRK1A phosphorylates *in vitro* a wide range of proteins localized in the nucleus and cell cytoplasm; for example, protein-synthesis initiation factor eIF2Bε, the microtubule-associated protein tau, the cAMP-response element-binding protein, the splicing factor SF3b1, dynamin 1, and amphiphysin 1 (Wiseman et al., 2009), suggesting that DYRK1A might function in cell nuclei and extra-nuclear cell compartments (Hämmerle et al., 2003; Wegiel et al., 2008). DYRK1A overexpression in the embryonic mouse neocortex, obtained by using an *in utero* electroporation technique, inhibits neural cell proliferation and promotes premature neuronal differentiation in the developing cerebral cortex without affecting cell fate and layer positioning (Yabut et al., 2010). In the brain tissue of DS subjects, the levels of DYRK1A are increased around 1.5-fold (Dowjat et al., 2007).

We examined the levels of DYRK1A in the brain hemispheres of female Ts65Dn mice and wt animals kept under both an enriched environment and standard conditions, as before. We studied the levels of DYRK1A on immunoblots by using two monoclonal antibodies. One of them, mAb 7D10, is commercially available (Abnova, Taipei, Taiwan) and recognizes both phosphorylated and non-phosphorylated forms of DYRK1A. The second monoclonal antibody, mAb 8D9, was produced at IBR by Dr. Y. Huang. According to our data (unpublished) this mAb is phospho-specific, as it recognizes only a form of DYRK1A that does not carry phosphate at Tyr-145. Western blotting of homogenates from mouse hemispheres revealed up to a 2.2-fold increase in the level of DYRK1A in Ts65Dn mice with both 8D9 and 7D10 in comparison with age-matched wt animals; thus, an even higher increase than that reported in the brains of DS individuals. Enriched housing conditions did not significantly affect the levels of DYRK1A in wt animals. However, they significantly reduced the amounts of DYRK1A non-phosphorylated at Tyr-145 in the hemispheres of both younger (Figure 5.1D) and older (not shown) Ts65Dn animals by up to 30%, not significantly affecting the levels of total DYRK1A (as detected by mAb 7D10). These observations indicate that housing of Ts65Dn mice in enriched environmental conditions affects the phosphorylation level of DYRK1A. Thus, a simple behavioral manipulation owing to environmental enrichment can alleviate genetically determined defects in these animals.

The normalization of some SV protein levels, increased neurogenesis, and changes in phosphorylation levels of DYRK1A we observed in Ts65Dn mice exposed to an enriched environment suggest that environmental conditions can modify the seemingly predetermined biological fate of genetic syndromes and offer additional hope for individuals with DS.

Summary

Brain plasticity is determined by both genetic and environmental factors. Prior experiments in laboratory animals documented that an enriched environment alleviates behavioral abnormalities; improves spatial memory; increases neurotrophic support, the neural stem/progenitor cell pool, and neurogenesis; reduces synaptic alterations; and activates glutamatergic signaling. Encouraging data have also been obtained in some animal models for human disorders. Thus, to address the issue of whether environmental enrichment might have significant implications for the prevention and/or treatment of intellectual disabilities in individuals with Down syndrome (DS), we are using the most popular and best-characterized animal model for DS, Ts65Dn mice. Our studies focus on the effect of an enriched environment on the molecular aspects of synaptic plasticity and on analysis of proteins associated with chemical synaptic transmission, some features of neurogenesis in the adult brain, and the potential to normalize or reduce increased levels of proteins encoded by triplicated genes, which are potentially associated with cognitive dysfunction in subjects with DS (DYRK1A). Our data suggest that environmental enrichment can substantially alleviate some of the molecular abnormalities found in Ts65Dn mice, suggesting that it might also have therapeutic potential in humans with DS.

References

Altafaj, X., Dierssen, M., Baamonde, C., et al. (2001). Neurodevelopmental delay, motor abnormalities and cognitive deficits in transgenic mice overexpressing Dyrk1A (minibrain), a murine model of Down's syndrome. *Human Molecular Genetics*, **10**, 1915–1923.

Altman, J. & Das, G. D. (1965). Autoradiographic and histological evidence of postnatal hippocampal neurogenesis in rats. *Journal of Comparative Neurology*, **124**, 319–335.

Antonarakis, S. E., Lyle, R., Dermitzakis, E. T., Reymond, A., Deutsch, S. (2004). Chromosome 21 and Down syndrome: from genomics to pathophysiology. *National Reviews Genetics*, **5**, 725–738.

Belichenko, N. P., Belichenko, P. V., Kleschevnikov, A. M., et al. (2009). The "Down syndrome critical region" is sufficient in the mouse model to confer behavioral, neurophysiological, and synaptic phenotypes characteristic of Down syndrome. *Journal of Neuroscience*, **29**, 5938–5948.

Belichenko, P. V., Masliah, E., Kleschevnikov, A. M., et al. (2004). Synaptic structural abnormalities in the Ts65Dn mouse model of Down Syndrome. *Journal of Comparative Neurology*, **480**, 281–298.

Bezard, E., Dovero, S., Belin, D., et al. (2003). Enriched environment confers resistance to 1-methyl-4-phenyl-1,2,3,6-tetrahydropyridine and cocaine: involvement of dopamine transporter and trophic factors. *Journal of Neuroscience*, **23**, 10999–101007.

Brodsky, F. M., Chen, C. Y., Knuehl, C., Towler, M. C., Wakeham, D. E. (2001). Biological basket weaving: formation and function of clathrin-coated vesicles *Annual Review of Cell and Developmental Biology*, **17**, 517–568.

Chakrabarti, L., Galdzicki, Z., Haydar, T. F. (2007). Defects in embryonic neurogenesis and initial synapse formation in the forebrain of the Ts65Dn mouse model of Down syndrome. *Journal of Neuroscience*, **27**, 1483–1495.

Chapman, R. S. & Hesketh, L. J. (2000). Behavioral phenotype of individuals with

Down syndrome. *Mental Retardation and Developmental Disabilities Research Reviews*, **6**, 84–95.

Clark, S., Schwalbe, J., Stasko, M. R., Yarowsky, P. J., Costa, A. C. (2006). Fluoxetine rescues deficient neurogenesis in hippocampus of the Ts65Dn mouse model for Down syndrome. *Experimental Neurology*, **200**, 256–261.

Contestabile, A., Fila, T., Bartesaghi, R., Ciani, E. (2009). Cell cycle elongation impairs proliferation of cerebellar granule cell precursors in the Ts65Dn mouse, an animal model for Down syndrome. *Brain Pathology*, **19**, 224–237.

Contestabile, A., Fila, T., Ceccarelli, C., et al. (2007). Cell cycle alteration and decreased cell proliferation in the hippocampal dentate gyrus and in the neocortical germinal matrix of fetuses with Down syndrome and in Ts65Dn mice. *Hippocampus*, **17**, 665–678.

Davisson, M. T., Schmidt, C., Akeson, E. C. (1990). Segmental trisomy of murine chromosome 16: a new model system for studying Down syndrome. *Progress in Clinical and Biological Research*, **360**, 263–280.

Delabar, J. M., Theophile, D., Rahmani, Z., et al. (1993). Molecular mapping of twenty-four features of Down syndrome on chromosome 21. *European Journal of Human Genetics*, **1**, 114–124.

Dierssen, M., Benavides-Piccione, R., Martínez-Cué, C., et al. (2003). Alterations of neocortical pyramidal cell phenotype in the Ts65Dn mouse model of Down syndrome: effects of environmental enrichment. *Cerebral Cortex*, **13**, 758–764.

Dowjat, W. K., Adayev, T., Kuchna, I., et al. (2007). Trisomy-driven overexpression of DYRK1A kinase in the brain of subjects with Down syndrome. *Neuroscience Letters*, **413**, 77–81.

Epstein, C. J. (1986). Developmental genetics. *Experientia*, **42**, 1117–1128.

Fernandez, F., Trinidad, J. C., Blank, M., et al. (2009). Normal protein composition of synapses in Ts65Dn mice: a mouse model of Down syndrome. *Journal of Neurochemistry*, **110**, 157–169.

Fiala, B. A., Joyce, J. N., Greenough, W. T. (1978). Environmental complexity modulates growth of granule cell dendrites in developing but not adult hippocampus of rats. *Experimental Neurology*, **59**, 372–383.

Fotaki, V., Dierssen, M., Alcántara, S., et al. (2002). Dyrk1A haploinsufficiency affects viability and causes developmental delay and abnormal brain morphology in mice. *Molecular and Cellular Biology*, **22**, 6636–6647.

Gardiner, K. J. (2010). Molecular basis of pharmacotherapies for cognition in Down syndrome. *Trends in Pharmacological Sciences*, **31**, 66–73.

Gould, E., Tanapat, P., Hastings, N. B., Shors, T. J. (1999). Neurogenesis in adulthood: a possible role in learning. *Trends in Cognitive Sciences*, **3**, 186–192.

Guimerá, J., Casas, C., Pucharcòs, C., et al. (1996). A human homologue of Drosophila minibrain (MNB) is expressed in the neuronal regions affected in Down syndrome and maps to the critical region. *Human Molecular Genetics*, **5**, 1305–1310.

Guralnik, M. J. (ed.) (2005). *Developmental Systems Approach to Early Intervention*. Baltimore: Brookes.

Hämmerle, B., Carnicero, A., Elizalde, C., et al. (2003). Expression patterns and subcellular localization of the Down syndrome candidate protein MNB/DYRK1A suggest a role in late neuronal differentiation. *European Journal of Neuroscience*, **17**, 2277–2286.

Hebb, D. O. (1947). The effects of early experience on problem solving at maturity. *The American Psychologist*, **2**, 306–307.

Hebb, D. O. (1949). *The Organization of Behavior*. Wiley: New York.

Ishihara, K., Amano, K., Takaki, E., et al. (2010). Enlarged brain ventricles and impaired neurogenesis in the Ts1Cje and Ts2Cje mouse models of Down syndrome. *Cerebral Cortex*, **20**, 1131–1143.

Kempermann, G., Gast, D., Kronenberg, G., Yamaguchi, M., Gage, F. H. (2003). Early determination and long-term persistence of adult-generated new neurons in the hippocampus of mice. *Development*, **130**, 391–399.

Kempermann, G., Kuhn, H. G., Gage, F. H. (1997). More hippocampal neurons in adult mice living in an enriched environment. *Nature*, **386**, 493–495.

Kleschevnikov, A. M., Belichenko, P. V., Villar, A. J., et al. (2004). Hippocampal long-term potentiation suppressed by increased inhibition in the Ts65Dn mouse, a genetic model of Down syndrome. *Journal of Neuroscience*, 24, 8153–8160.

Korbel, J. O., Tirosh-Wagner, T., Urban, A. E., et al. (2009). The genetic architecture of Down syndrome phenotypes revealed by high-resolution analysis of human segmental trisomies. *Proceedings of the National Academy of Sciences of the United States of America*, **106**, 12031–12036.

Korenberg, J. R., Bradley, C., Disteche, C. M. (1992). Down syndrome: molecular mapping of the congenital heart disease and duodenal stenosis. *American Journal of Human Genetics*, **50**, 294–302.

Kurt, M. A., Kafa, M. I., Dierssen, M., Davies, D. C. (2004). Deficits of neuronal density in CA1 and synaptic density in the dentate gyrus, CA3 and CA1, in a mouse model of Down syndrome. *Brain Research*, **1022**, 101–109.

Lambert, T. J., Fernandez, S. M., Frick, K. M. (2005). Different types of environmental enrichment have discrepant effects on spatial memory and synaptophysin levels in female mice. *Neurobiology of Learning and Memory*, **83**, 206–216.

Lazarov, O., Robinson, J., Tang, Y. P., et al. (2005). Environmental enrichment reduces Ab levels and amyloid deposition in transgenic mice. *Cell*, **120**, 701–713.

Lorenzi, H. A. & Reeves, R. H. (2006). Hippocampal hypocellularity in the Ts65Dn mouse originates early in development. *Brain Research*, **1104**, 153–159.

Lyle, R., Béna, F., Gagos, S., et al. (2009). Genotype-phenotype correlations in Down syndrome identified by array CGH in 30 cases of partial trisomy and partial monosomy chromosome 21. *European Journal of Human Genetics*, **17**, 454–466.

Martínez-Cué, C., Baamonde, C., Lumbreras, M., et al. (2002). Differential effects of environmental enrichment on behavior and learning of male and female Ts65Dn mice, a model for Down syndrome. *Behavioral Brain Research*, **134**, 185–200.

Miyabara, S., Gropp, A., Winking, H. (1982). Trisomy 16 in the mouse fetus associated with generalized edema and cardiovascular and urinary tract anomalies. *Teratology* 25, 369–80.

Morice, E., Andreae, L. C., Cooke, S. F., et al. (2008). Preservation of long-term memory and synaptic plasticity despite short-term impairments in the Tc1 mouse model of Down syndrome. *Learning and Memory*, 15, 492–500.

Nithiananantharajah, J. & Hannan, A. J. (2006). Enriched environments, experience-dependent plasticity and disorders of the nervous system. *National Reviews Neuroscience*, 7, 697–709.

O'Doherty, A., Ruf, S., Mulligan, C., et al. (2005). An aneuploid mouse strain carrying human chromosome 21 with Down syndrome phenotypes. *Science*, 23, 2033–2037.

Olson, L. E., Richtsmeier, J. T., Leszl, J., Reeves, R. H. (2004). A chromosome 21 critical region does not cause specific Down syndrome phenotypes. *Science*, **306**, 687–690.

Olson, L. E., Roper, R. J., Sengstaken, C. L., et al. (2007). Trisomy for the Down syndrome 'critical region' is necessary but not sufficient for brain phenotypes of trisomic mice. *Human Molecular Genetics*, **16**, 774–782.

Pennington, B. F., Moon, J., Edgin, J., Stedron, J., Nadel, L. (2003). The neuropsychology of Down syndrome: evidence for hippocampal dysfunction. *Child Development*, **74**, 75–93.

Pereira, P. L., Magnol, L., Sahún, I., et al. (2009). A new mouse model for the trisomy of the Abcg1-U2af1 region reveals the complexity of the combinatorial genetic code of Down syndrome. *Human Molecular Genetics*, **18**, 4756–4769.

Pollonini, G., Gao, V., Rabe, A., et al. (2008). Abnormal expression of synaptic proteins and neurotrophin-3 in the Down syndrome mouse model Ts65Dn. *Neuroscience*, **156**, 99–106.

Reeves, R. H., Irving, N. G., Moran, T. H., et al. (1995). A mouse model for Down syndrome exhibits learning and behaviour deficits. *Nature Genetics*, **11**, 177–184.

Restivo, L., Ferrari, F., Passino, E., et al. (2005). Enriched environment promotes behavioral and morphological recovery in a mouse model for the fragile X syndrome. *Proceedings of the National Academy of Sciences of the United States of America*, **102**, 11557–11562.

Rosenzweig, M. R. (1966). Environmental complexity, cerebral change, and behavior. *The American Psychologist*, **21**, 321–332.

Rosenzweig, M. R., Bennett, E. L., Hebert, M., Morimoto, H. (1978). Social grouping cannot account for cerebral effects of enriched environments. *Brain Research*, **153**, 563–576.

Rueda, N., Mostany, R., Pazos, A., Flórez, J., Martínez-Cué, C. (2005). Cell proliferation is reduced in the dentate gyrus of aged but not young Ts65Dn mice, a model of Down syndrome. *Neuroscience Letters*, **380**, 197–201.

Sago, H., Carlson, E. J., Smith, D. J., et al. (1998). Ts1Cje, a partial trisomy 16 mouse model for Down syndrome, exhibits learning and behavioral abnormalities. *Proceedings of the National Academy of Science of the United States of America*, **95**, 6256–6261.

Sago, H., Carlson, E. J., Smith, D. J., et al. (2000). Genetic dissection of region associated with behavioral abnormalities in mouse models for Down syndrome. *Pediatric Research*, **48**, 606–613.

Sérégaza, Z., Roubertoux, P. L., Jamon, M., Soumireu-Mourat, B. (2006). Mouse models of cognitive disorders in trisomy 21: a review. *Behavior Genetics*, **36**, 387–404.

Siarey, R. J., Carlson, E. J., Epstein, C. J., et al. (1999). Increased synaptic depression in the Ts65Dn mouse, a model for mental retardation in Down syndrome. *Neuropharmacology*, **38**, 1917–1920.

Siarey, R. J., Villar, A. J., Epstein, C. J., Galdzicki, Z. (2005). Abnormal synaptic plasticity in the Ts1Cje segmental trisomy 16 mouse model of Down syndrome. *Neuropharmacology*, **49**, 122–128.

Song, W. J., Sternberg, L. R., Kasten-Sportès, C., et al. (1996). Isolation of human and murine homologues of the Drosophila minibrain gene: human homologue maps to 21q22.2 in the Down syndrome "critical region". *Genomics*, **15**, 331–339.

Spires, T. L., Grote, H. E., Varshney, N. K., et al. (2004). Environmental enrichment rescues protein deficits in a mouse model of Huntington's disease, indicating a possible disease mechanism. *Journal of Neuroscience*, **24**, 2270–2276.

Sudhof, T. C. (2004). The synaptic vesicle cycle. *Annual Review of Neuroscience*, **27**, 509–547.

van Praag, H., Kempermann, G., Gage, F. H. (1999). Running increases cell proliferation and neurogenesis in the adult mouse dentate gyrus. *Nature Neuroscience*, **2**, 266–270.

van Praag, H., Kempermann, G., Gage, F. H. (2000). Neural consequences of environmental enrichment. *Nature Reviews Neuroscience*, **1**, 191–198.

von Bohlen Und Halbach, O. (2007). Immunohistological markers for staging neurogenesis in adult hippocampus. *Cell and Tissue Research*, **329**, 409–420.

Walsh, R. N., Budtz-Olsen, O. E., Penny, J. E., Cummins, R. A. (1969). The effects of environmental complexity on the histology of the rat hippocampus. *Journal of Comparative Neurology*, **137**, 361–366.

Wegiel, J., Dowjat, K., Kaczmarski, W., et al. (2008). The role of overexpressed DYRK1A protein in the early onset of neurofibrillary degeneration in Down syndrome. *Acta Neuropathologica*, **116**, 391–407.

Wigge, P. & McMahon, H. T. (1998). The amphiphysin family of proteins and their role in endocytosis at the synapse. *Trends in Neurosciences*, **21**, 339–344.

Wiseman, F. K., Alford, K. A., Tybulewicz, V. L. J., Fisher, E. M. C. (2009). Down syndrome – recent progress and future prospects. *Human Molecular Genetics*, **18**, R75–R83.

Wisniewski, K. E., Kida, E., Golabek, A. A., et al. (2006). Down syndrome: from pathology to pathogenesis. In J. A. Rondal & J. Perera (eds.), *Down Syndrome: Neurobehavioral Specificity*. Down syndrome series, pp. 17–33. London: Wiley.

Wisniewski, K. E., Laure-Kamnionowska, M., Connell, F., Wen, G. Y. (1986). Neuronal density and synaptogenesis in the postnatal stage of brain maturation in Down syndrome. In C. J. Epstein (ed.), *The Neurobiology of Down Syndrome*, pp. 29–44. New York: Raven Press.

Yabut, O., Domogauer, J., D'Arcangelo, G. (2010). Dyrk1A overexpression inhibits proliferation and induces premature neuronal differentiation of neural progenitor cells. *Journal of Neuroscience*, **30**, 4004–4014.

Yu, T., Li, Z., Jia, Z., et al. (2010). A mouse model of Down syndrome trisomic for all human chromosome 21 syntenic regions. *Human Molecular Genetics*, **5**, 2780–2791.

Development of the brain and metabolism

David Patterson

Introduction

Down syndrome (DS) is the most common genetic cause of significant intellectual disability, affecting roughly 1 in 733 live births in the United States (Centers for Disease Control and Prevention, 2006). It is caused by trisomy of human chromosome 21 (HSA21) and was the first autosomal trisomy identified, a seminal contribution to human genetics (Lejeune et al., 1959). Over 220,000 babies will be born with DS this year worldwide. The features of DS have been described in detail in the past (Roizen & Patterson, 2003; other chapters in this book). Here we focus on the effects of metabolism on brain development. As discussed in the following sections, the effects of nutritional status and levels of particular nutrients that alter metabolism early in development can have profound effects on brain function later in life, at least in animals like the mouse and rat. This topic is of great importance in the context of DS as many attempts to ameliorate the intellectual and other disabilities confronted by individuals with DS have been tried over the years. To date, none of these proposed interventions has been based on validated scientific evidence. Some have been based, at least in part, on limited data regarding biochemical differences observed between people with and without DS, and some have been based on hypotheses derived from the gene content of HSA21 (Salman, 2002; Roizen, 2005).

The effects of metabolism on human brain development are difficult to assess experimentally for a number of reasons. The effects of some nutrients are likely to take many years to manifest themselves. In some cases, it appears that there is a critical, relatively short time in development during which a particular nutrient may be required at a particular level. It is difficult or impossible to define these time periods experimentally in humans, although clinical observations and imaging studies offer considerable insight (Georgieff, 2007). It is very difficult to ascertain the nutritional status of a large number of individuals over long periods of time, and this is particularly true for individuals with DS. There are ethical considerations as well. If one hypothesizes that a particular nutritional regimen will be beneficial, then it may be hard to justify withholding this treatment from some individuals, especially if the hypothesized benefit might be permanent and if there are no known side effects.

One way to overcome some of these concerns is through the study of the effects of alterations in metabolic status in experimental animals. Generally, mice or rats have been the models of choice for these studies. With regard to DS, there have been many mouse models with features reminiscent of DS that have been produced in the laboratory in recent years,

Neurocognitive Rehabilitation of Down Syndrome, eds. Jean-Adolphe Rondal, Juan Perera, and Donna Spiker. Published by Cambridge University Press. © Cambridge University Press 2011.

and these offer particularly robust systems to study metabolic, primarily nutritional, intervention. Studies of these models will be described in some depth as they are useful guides for possible interventions in humans.

Early studies of nutrition in Down syndrome and attempts to improve brain development and ameliorate intellectual disability in Down syndrome

The hypothesis that DS is accompanied by metabolic alterations and that these may be related to the development of the phenotype has existed for decades and was a hypothesis favored by Lejeune, who hypothesized as early as 1979 that there must be perturbations of oxygen metabolism, amino acid metabolism, and one-carbon metabolism (Lejeune, 1981; Lejeune et al., 1986). Because of this idea, attempts to treat DS with nutritional and other supplements have been undertaken at least since the 1960s. An excellent review of these studies has been published (Roizen, 2005). A few important points from this review need to be emphasized here. To date, no nutritional or drug intervention has been shown to ameliorate the intellectual disabilities of DS (also see Salman, 2002). To detect a six-point improvement in intelligence quotient (IQ), 170 individuals with DS would need to be evaluated. However, this does not mean that successful interventions will not be found in the future.

Genes on HSA21 relevant to metabolism and nutrition

With the complete sequencing of the long (q) arm of (HSA21), it is now possible to develop hypotheses regarding the role of particular metabolic pathways that may respond to nutritional intervention on the basis of the gene content of the chromosome. At least 26 genes likely to be directly involved in cellular metabolism are located on HSA21. This is considered to be a minimal list, as it is highly likely that the functioning of many cell pathways respond to altered metabolic status. These 26 genes can be grouped into various metabolic systems. For example, three genes (ATP5J, ATP5O, and NDUFV3) are involved directly in mitochondrial energy generation. At least seven genes (HemK2, GART, CBS, DNMT3L, RFC, FTCD, and PRMT2) are important for one-carbon/folate/transsulfuration metabolism and methylation reactions. Three genes (LIPI, ABCG1, and LSS) are involved in cholesterol/lipid metabolism. At least six genes (NRF2, APP, SOD1, RCAN1, CBR1, and CBR3) are involved in oxidative stress or xenobiotic metabolism. Individual genes are involved in inositol metabolism (SLC5A3), biotin metabolism (HLCS), and pyridoxal metabolism (PDXK). In many cases, these pathways are very likely interrelated. For example, mitochondrial energy generation genes are almost certainly related to oxidative stress genes. In several cases, mutations in these metabolic genes lead to serious developmental disorders, including intellectual disability. A particularly useful source of information on the genes on HSA21 and the equivalent mouse chromosomes is: http://chr21.egr.vcu.edu:8888/.

Interestingly, the localization of these genes on HSA21 was presaged by phenotypic aspects of DS that were discovered prior to the localization of the genes on HSA21. Thus, it has been known for years that individuals with DS have abnormal inositol metabolism, prior to the demonstration that the gene encoding the inositol transporter, SLC5A3, is located on HSA21 (Brooksbank & Martinez, 1989; Fruen & Lester, 1990; Berry et al., 1995). The observation that purine levels are elevated in individuals with DS was made many years before the localization of the GART gene, which encodes a trifunctional protein critical for *de novo* purine synthesis, was localized to HSA21 (Pant et al., 1968; Moore et al., 1977). The unusual sensitivity of persons with DS and leukemia to methotrexate was known long before the gene for the reduced folate carrier (Slc19A1 or RFC) was mapped to HSA21 (Lejeune et al., 1986; Peeters et al., 1986; Yang-Feng et al., 1995).

Mouse models and the study of metabolism, brain development, and Down syndrome

Much has been learned about the role of metabolism in brain development by the study of mouse models. Mice can be subjected to rigorously controlled diets and drug treatments and examined for effects of these on brain development. Several of these studies will be discussed in the following sections. Mice that are models of DS have been produced recently. By this we mean that these mice have phenotypic, neurological, developmental, or biochemical features reminiscent of those we see in individuals with DS and that they bear genetic alterations that can be related to HSA21. These mice are in general of two types. Transgenic mouse models containing one or more human genes located on HSA21 have been produced and characterized for features associated with DS. Some of these have been used to examine metabolism and brain development. An excellent example of the use of transgenic mice for the study of nutritional supplements is presented by Delabar (Chapter 4 in this book; also see Guedj et al., 2009). A second type of mouse model is trisomic for large regions of HSA21 or, more commonly, of regions of the mouse chromosomes that are homologous to HSA21, primarily regions of mouse chromosome 16 (Mmu16). The most widely studied and characterized model is the Ts65Dn mouse (Davisson et al., 1990). Additional models contain larger or smaller regions of Mmu16 (Sago et al., 1998; Olson et al., 2004, 2007; Li et al., 2007). Recently, a transchromosomal mouse model has been described that contains a freely segregating, almost complete HSA21 (O'Doherty et al., 2005). These mice have been widely used to study brain development, including fetal brain development (Chakrabarti et al., 2007; Salehi et al., 2007).

Methyl group metabolism and Down syndrome

The hypothesis that methyl group (one-carbon units) metabolism might be altered in DS was put forward by Lejeune, who hypothesized that the one-carbon cycle might play a central role (Lejeune, 1981; Lejeune et al., 1986). It is still an active area of investigation. Rodents can also be examined for the effects of metabolism on brain development directly by manipulation of the mouse diet before conception and during pregnancy. This can be done either with presumably normal mice or rats or with mice carrying relevant genetic alterations. The example of choline/folate metabolism is particularly relevant to brain development in DS. Folate is a water-soluble vitamin that cannot be synthesized by mammals and so must be obtained from the diet. Choline can be synthesized by mammals in small amounts, but dietary sources are still required for health and development. The role of folate metabolism itself in DS is still controversial because polymorphisms in folate metabolizing enzymes may be related to an increased incidence of births of individuals with DS and because abnormalities in folate metabolism have been reported in individuals with DS or their mothers. However, these findings remain contentious (Patterson, 2008). Choline is the precursor of acetylcholine, a neurotransmitter important for brain function and hypothesized to play a role in DS and in Alzheimer's disease. Folate and choline metabolism are related because they both can supply methyl groups for methionine synthesis, which then leads to S-adenosylmethionine synthesis, which is the essentially universal methyl group donor in biological reactions. In particular for this discussion, it is the methyl donor for DNA and protein methylation. Thus, in rats, deficiency of choline during days 12–17 of fetal development can lead to life-long deficits in learning and memory. Moreover, choline supplementation during this period can ameliorate age-related decline in learning and memory in rats. Recently, it has been found that maternal supplementation with choline can improve the anatomical and behavioral symptoms of offspring with the mouse equivalent of Rett syndrome; hence, the concept of supplementation during fetal development to improve the development of fetuses with DS is not unreasonable (Nag et al., 2008; Ward et al., 2009). Choline deprivation also leads to abnormalities in brain structure that are life-long. Similar abnormalities in brain development can be observed in mice subjected to folate deficiency (Craciunescu et al., 2004). Interestingly, elevations in methyl groups in the diet in pregnant mice can affect DNA methylation patterns in offspring, and these can have permanent effects on gene expression and phenotype. Particularly good reviews of this subject have been published recently (Zeisel, 2009a, b).

It is important in this context to ask what the hypothesized consequences of trisomy of the HSA21 genes relevant to methylation might be. In some cases, there are reasonably straightforward hypotheses that have some experimental support. Thus, trisomy of the RFC gene would be expected to lead to increased intracellular levels of folate compounds since RFC is quantitatively the most significant importer of reduced folate groups (Patterson et al., 2008; Zhao et al., 2009). Some evidence exists for this conclusion. For example, RFC is important for uptake of the antifolate methotrexate, commonly used to treat a wide variety of cancers including leukemia, and individuals with DS show an increased sensitivity to methotrexate (Peeters et al., 1986, 1995). However, other HSA21 genes are hypothesized to increase demand for folates. The GART gene encodes a protein required for *de novo* purine synthesis that uses folate-carried one-carbon units. CBS converts homocysteine to cystathionine, thus potentially decreasing the synthesis of methionine and the availability of methyl groups. Three genes on HSA21 encode proteins for which it is somewhat more difficult to generate hypotheses. The DNMT3L gene, which is homologous to DNA methyltransferase genes but has no DNA methyltransferase activity itself, influences both DNA and histone methylation (Ooi et al., 2007) and methylation of promoters of genes, including its own promoter (Hu et al., 2008). Generally, promoter methylation is associated with decreased gene activity. Mice in which the DNMT3L gene has been inactivated by targeted mutagenesis cannot carry out appropriate DNA methylation during embryogenesis (Hata et al., 2006). These experiments strongly implicate DNMT3L in regulation of gene expression during early mammalian development, but they do not provide evidence of the consequences of overexpression of DNMT3L. Such evidence has now been obtained. Takashima et al. (2009) have demonstrated that overexpression of DNMT3L prevents normal spermatogenesis. It is not clear what other consequences this overexpression might have or whether this is related to the sterility seen in men with DS.

Two genes on chromosome 21 are important for protein methylation: PRMT2 and HemK2, previously known as N6AMT1 or PRED28. PRMT2 is a coactivator of the androgen receptor and the estrogen receptor alpha (Qi et al., 2002; Meyer et al., 2007), both transcription factors. Conversely, PRMT2 appears to repress E2F1 transcription activity and to inhibit NF–KB-dependent transcription (Ganesh et al., 2006; Yoshimoto et al., 2006). PMRT2 is a member of the protein arginine methyltransferase family of proteins by sequence analysis, but may not have endogenous methylation activity, a situation reminiscent of DNMT3L (Ganesh et al., 2006). In some cases, the activity of PMRT2 appears to be inhibited by inhibitors of methylation, but this is not always the case. It could be that the substrate for methylation by PMRT2 has not yet been found. Ganesh et al. (2006) hypothesize that PMRT2 may actually inhibit protein methylation by other PMRT proteins. Thus, it is unclear whether overexpression of PRMT2 in DS would increase or decrease the need for methyl groups during development. Considering that it appears to affect expression of transcription factors, both positively and negatively, it seems reasonable to hypothesize that trisomy of PRMT2 would have consequences for embryonic development that might well be life-long and influence brain development.

The N6AMT1 gene, also known as PRED28, was putatively identified as an N6-adenine DNA-methylation enzyme-encoding gene on HSA21 on the basis of homology to bacterial proteins known to methylate adenine at the N6 position in DNA. However, little or no N6 adenine can be found in mouse DNA, and no N6A methylation activity could be detected for N6AMT1 (Ratel et al., 2006). It turns out that N6AMT1 is actually a glutamine protein methyltransferase, HemK2 (Figaro et al., 2008). HemK2 methylates the translation termination factor eRF1. Methylation of eRF1 appears necessary for appropriate translation termination. This finding has a number of implications. First, it extends the possible effects of trisomy 21 to translation termination, which may have effects on the proteome that cannot be predicted from messenger-RNA (mRNA)-based gene expression studies. Second, it reinforces the importance of methyl group metabolism in mammals. Trisomy of HemK2 might be expected to increase the demand for methyl groups, but perhaps more importantly, would influence levels of proteins on whose mRNA it acts.

Oxidative stress and Down syndrome

The hypothesis that oxidative stress plays a major role in DS has considerable experimental support. Important studies strongly indicate that altered oxidative stress may play a role in embryonic and fetal development of the brain and nervous system in DS. Evidence for oxidative stress during fetal development has been presented and the suggestion put forward that antioxidant supplementation during the prenatal period should be attempted (Perrone et al., 2007). Busciglio and Yankner (1995) reported that cortical neurons from 16- to 19-week fetuses with DS had a three- to four-fold increase in reactive oxygen species compared to euploid fetal neurons. Bahn et al. (2002) produced neurospheres from 8- to 18-week fetuses and found altered gene expression in the DS neurospheres as well as a decreased number of neurons (also see Bhattacharyya & Svendsen, 2003). Reduced neurogenesis has also been found in cortical and hippocampal regions of early embryos of Ts65Dn mice (Chakrabarti et al., 2007). It is not yet known whether oxidative stress is involved in these abnormalities.

Until recently, evidence for elevated oxidative stress was limited in Ts65Dn mice. However, this has now been demonstrated (Lockrow et al., 2009). Of particular interest, long-term dietary supplementation with vitamin E was reported to reduce markers of oxidative stress, protect from cholinergic neuron degeneration, and improve performance on a spatial learning memory task. These studies suggest that it may be worthwhile to consider such supplementation during pregnancy of Ts65Dn mice to see whether this improves the brain and learning and memory development in these mice.

Inositol metabolism and Down syndrome and brain development

As mentioned previously, individuals with DS have high levels of inositol in their brains. This seems likely to be related to trisomy of the SLC5A3 gene, which encodes the major inositol transporter. Inositol levels are unusually high in the brain, and expression of the SLC5A3 gene seems particularly high in the brain in fetal life. Inositol-containing molecules are critical for many cellular signaling pathways. The Ts65Dn mice also have high brain inositol levels and are trisomic for the SLC5A3 gene. To define the role of SLC5A3, mice in which this gene has been inactivated by targeted mutagenesis have been produced. Homozygous knockout mice die *in utero* but addition of 1% inositol to the drinking water of the dam can prevent this. After weaning, the homozygous knockout mice no longer require inositol supplementation. Interestingly, the levels of inositol in the brains of the pups from dams with supplemented inositol levels show very modest increases in brain inositol levels. Later in life, the pups from these dams have behavioral abnormalities (Bersudky et al., 2008; Buccafusca et al., 2008). Thus, it is not clear how the inositol supplementation rescues these pups. The only SLC5A3 transgenic mice overexpress the SLC5A3 gene from a cDNA under the control of a promoter that restricts its expression to eye tissue. These mice develop cataracts (Jiang et al., 2000), a relatively common feature of DS.

Treatment with lithium lowers inositol levels in humans being treated for bipolar disorder, and it has been hypothesized that this lowering of inositol levels may be related to treatment success, although this is by no means firmly established. Lithium has been shown to reduce inositol levels in the brains of Ts65Dn mice (Huang et al., 2000). More recently, treatment of Ts65Dn mice with lithium has been shown to increase neurogenesis in the Ts65Dn mouse brain (Bianchi et al., 2010). These studies were done with adult mice; therefore, no information is available on the effects of lithium supplementation during fetal brain development.

Ts65Dn mice were reported to pass on the extra chromosome to only about 30% of offspring and to have small litters. Moreover, males are sterile, and the mice carry a retinal degeneration gene. These characteristics initially limited the study of fetal development of Ts65Dn mice. However, it appears that the situation may not be as difficult as originally thought. Thus, during fetal life, the fraction of trisomic fetuses does approach the expected 50% (Moore, 2006). A number of trisomic mice die shortly after birth. Thus, these features of this mouse strain may actually be an advantage. That is, it may be that dietary supplementation during fetal development would enhance survival of pups. Moreover, for this type of analysis, the blindness as a result of retinal degeneration is likely to be irrelevant.

Another possible solution to this situation is that a new mouse strain derived from Ts65Dn has been reported, in which the trisomic chromosome appears to have undergone a centric fusion with mouse chromosome 12. These mice then segregate the trisomy in a Mendelian manner. In addition, males appear to be fertile, although it is not clear that their fertility approaches euploid levels (Villar et al., 2005).

"Omics" studies of fetal development in Down syndrome and future directions

Numerous studies have been carried out examining alterations in gene expression on fetal DS material and on material from mouse models (Patterson, 2007). These studies have revealed significant information regarding alterations in gene expression owing to trisomy. Some conclusions appear to be that many genes encoded on chromosomes other than the trisomic chromosome have altered expression. Moreover, decreased expression of some genes is observed. This should not be surprising given some of the previous discussion and the likely impact of transcription factors or methylation alterations on gene expression. A number of studies attempting proteomic analysis have also been attempted on samples from fetal DS material. Thus far, only one study on the proteome of Ts65Dn mouse brain has been published and this was not on fetal material. Again, it is difficult to draw global conclusions from these experiments regarding what might be done to influence fetal brain development.

The relevance of proteomic studies to metabolism is that it may be that alterations in proteins in particular metabolic pathways might lead to new approaches to understanding metabolism in DS. These studies are all exceedingly important. However, it should be remembered that alterations in gene expression do not necessarily translate directly to similar alterations in cognate protein levels. Indeed, it has been difficult to correlate transcriptomic and proteomic studies. Moreover, proteomic studies have other limitations. While it is possible to interrogate essentially the entire transcriptome, it is not possible to interrogate the entire proteome. At present, perhaps only the most abundant one or two percent of proteins can be reliably identified and quantitated. In addition, many mRNAs encode a large number of different proteins, and many protein levels are influenced by post-transcriptional mechanisms. Many proteins are post-translationally modified, and most proteomic studies do not detect these. Even if a protein shows a statistically significant alteration in amount, it is not at all clear that this alteration will be biologically significant. The activities of proteins are often under stringent regulation. For example, feedback inhibition, substrate and cofactor availability, the possible role of multimer formation or multiprotein complexes, and other factors all play a role in the effects alterations in amounts of proteins may have on biological processes. In the case of metabolic pathways, a protein may or may not be rate limiting in the pathway involved. Its activity could be tightly regulated by substrates, products, and cofactors and by interactions with other proteins. In summary, changes at the genome, transcriptome, or proteome level may have no effect unless they change some metabolic, physiological, or biological system.

Conclusions and future directions

As can be seen from this discussion, a critical remaining issue is the accurate determination of the function of the genes on HSA21. It will be important to keep an open mind in this regard. For example, for decades SOD1 was called erythrocuprein or hemocuprein and had no known enzyme activity (McCord & Fridovich, 1969). It may well be that even proteins for which we believe we know the function may have additional or alternative functions. Identification of the functions of the proteins encoded by genes on HSA21 will lead to new hypotheses regarding metabolic influences in DS.

Production of new mouse models will be exceedingly important. To date, trisomic mouse models involve regions of Mmu16. There are important HSA21 genes located on Mmu17 and Mmu10. It should be possible, using chromosome engineering methods, to create mice trisomic for each of these regions, provided that they are viable. Even these mice will not be ideal, as interactions between genes in the various regions, which may be important for DS, will likely be missed. Additional knockout mice hold great promise for aiding in identification of gene function, but also for selectively returning individual trisomic genes in mice like the Ts65Dn mouse to the diploid state. This approach has already been quite fruitful. Fortunately, efforts are underway to make knockout mice for every mouse gene.

Proteomic analysis of DS and mouse models should also be pursued. However, significant technical obstacles need to be overcome to allow a larger fraction of the proteome to be analyzed. In addition, it is important to consider that the proteome is not likely to be static. It likely will change with age and certainly from tissue to tissue.

It seems apparent that there will be significant metabolic changes associated with DS and that these metabolic changes will be important determinants of brain development. Moreover, in principle, it is these metabolic changes that can be most easily influenced by dietary and nutritional alterations. Thus, an important next step in understanding the role of metabolism in brain development will be the analysis of the metabolome of appropriate samples. Metabolomics is the systematic identification, quantification, and mathematical analysis of as many small molecules (metabolites) in a biological sample as possible (Houten, 2009). The endogenous metabolome can be defined as the total of all small molecules an organism is capable of producing endogenously. There may be fewer than 3000 endogenous metabolites in humans. Analysis of the metabolome, while complex, is based on decades of biochemistry, including human biochemistry and the biochemistry of human disease states (Houten, 2009). This area of analysis is in a period of rapid development (Blow, 2008). Several complementary technologies are being explored and the application of these to brain disorders is underway (Kaddurah-Daouk & Krishnan, 2009; Nicholson & Linden, 2008).

Indeed, metabolomics may offer a unique and powerful, and perhaps the most direct way to understand the role of metabolism in brain development. As Acworth and Bowers (1997) point out, "After all, this [metabolome] is just a working expression of an organism's genome." (p. 42).

Summary

Appropriate metabolism of the mother and fetus is essential for proper brain and nervous system development. Deficiencies of nutrients like folic acid and choline can lead to abnormal brain structure and function that can last throughout life. Genes on chromosome 21 are involved in folate, one-carbon, inositol, reactive oxygen species, and energy metabolism. Comprehensive studies of how Down syndrome (DS) affects global metabolism have not been undertaken, although studies of individual metabolic pathways have provided some information. New methods of high throughput analysis of metabolism allow new approaches to assess the metabolic consequences of DS that may be more immediately relevant to the phenotypes of interest than studies of alterations in gene or protein expression, and may lead to new approaches to ameliorate the alterations in brain function and the intellectual disabilities that are features of DS.

Acknowledgments

This work was supported by generous grants from the Lowe Fund of the Denver Foundation, the Bonfils-Stanton Foundation, and the Towne Foundation.

References

Acworth, I. N. & Bowers, M. (1997). An introduction to HPLC-based electrochemical detection: from single electrode to multi-electrode arrays. *Progress in HPLD-HPCE*, **6**, 3–50.

Bahn, S., Mimmack, M., Ryan, M., et al. (2002). Neuronal target genes of the neuron-restrictive silencer factor in neurospheres derived from fetuses with Down's syndrome: a gene expression study. *Lancet*, **359**, 310–315.

Bersudsky, Y., Shaldubina, A., Agam, G., Berry, G. T., Belmaker, R. H. (2008). Homozygote inositol transporter knockout mice show a lithium-like phenotype. *Bipolar Disorders*, 10, 453–459.

Berry, G. T., Mallee, J. J., Kwon, H. M., et al. (1995). The human osmoregulatory Na+/myo-inositol cotransporter gene (SLC5A3): molecular cloning and localization to chromosome 21. *Genomics*, 25, 507–513.

Bhattacharyya, A. & Svendsen, C. N. (2003). Human neural stem cells: a new tool for studying cortical development in Down's syndrome. *Genes, Brain and Behavior*, 2, 179–186.

Bianchi, P., Ciani, E., Contestabile, A., Guidi, S., Bartesaghi, R. (2010). Lithium restores neurogenesis in the subventricular zone of the Ts65Dn mouse, a model for Down syndrome. *Brain Pathology*, 20(1), 106–118.

Blow, N. (2008). Biochemistry's new look. *Nature*, 455, 697–700.

Brooksbank, B. W. & Martinez, M. (1989). Lipid abnormalities in the brain in adult Down's syndrome and Alzheimer's disease. *Molecular and Chemical Neuropathology*, 11, 157–185.

Buccafusca, R., Venditti, C. P., Kenyon, L. C., et al. (2008). Characterization of the null murine sodium/myo-inositol cotransporter 1 (Smit1 or Slc5a3) phenotype: myo-inositol rescue is independent of expression of its cognate mitochondrial ribosomal protein subunit 6 (Mrps6) gene and of phosphatidylinositol levels in neonatal brain. *Molecular Genetics and Metabolism*, 95, 81–95.

Busciglio, J. & Yankner, B. A. (1995). Apoptosis and increased generation of reactive oxygen species in Down's syndrome neurons in vitro. *Nature*, 378, 776–779.

Centers for Disease Control and Prevention. (2006). Improved national prevalence estimates for 18 selected major birth defects – United States, 1999–2001. *Morbidity and Mortality Weekly Report*, 54, 1301–1305.

Chakrabarti, L., Galdzicki, Z., Haydar, T. F. (2007). Defects in embryonic neurogenesis and initial synapse formation in the forebrain of the Ts65Dn mouse model of Down syndrome. *Journal of Neuroscience*, 27, 11483–11495.

Craciunescu, C. N., Brown, E. C., Mar, M. H., et al. (2004). Folic acid deficiency during late gestation decreases progenitor cell proliferation and increases apoptosis in fetal mouse brain. *Journal of Nutrition*, 134, 162–166.

Davisson, M. T., Schmidt, C., Akeson, E. C. (1990). Segmental trisomy of murine Chromosome 16: a new model system for studying Down Syndrome. In D. Patterson & C. J. Epstein (eds.), *Molecular Genetics of Chromosome 21 and Down Syndrome*, pp. 263–280. New York: Wiley-Liss.

Figaro, S., Scrima, N., Buckingham, R. H., Heurgue-Hamard, V. (2008). HemK2 protein, encoded on human chromosome 21, methylates translation termination factor eRF1. *FEBS Letters*, 582, 2352–2356.

Fruen, B. R. & Lester, B. R. (1990). Down's syndrome fibroblasts exhibit enhanced inositol uptake. *Biochemical Journal*, 270, 119–123.

Ganesh, L., Yoshimoto, T., Moorthy, N. C., et al. (2006). Protein methyltransferase 2 inhibits NF-kappaB function and promotes apoptosis. *Molecular and Cellular Biology*, 26, 3864–3874.

Georgieff, M. K. (2007). Nutrition and the developing brain: nutrient priorities and measurement. *American Journal of Clinical Nutrition*, 85, 614S–620S.

Guedj, F., Sébrié, C., Rivals, I., et al. (2009). Green tea polyphenols rescue of brain defects induced by overexpression of DYRK1A. *PLoS ONE*, 4, e4606.

Hata, K., Kusumi, M., Yokomine, T., Li, E., Sasaki, H. (2006). Meiotic and epigenetic aberrations in Dnmt3L-deficient male germ cells. *Molecular and Reproductive Development*, 73, 116–122.

Houten, S. M. (2009). Metabolomics: Unraveling the chemical individuality of common human diseases. *Annals of Medicine*, 3, 1–6.

Hu, Y. G., Hirasawa, R., Hu, J. L., et al. (2008). Regulation of DNA methylation activity through Dnmt3L promoter methylation by Dnmt3 enzymes in embryonic development. *Human Molecular Genetics*, 17, 2654–2664.

Huang, W., Galdzicki, Z., van Gelderen, P., et al. (2000). Brain myo-inositol level is elevated in Ts65Dn mouse and reduced after lithium treatment. *Neuroreport*, **11**, 445–448.

Jiang, Z., Chung, S. K., Zhou, C., Cammarata, P. R., Chung, S. S. (2000). Overexpression of Na(+)-dependent myo-inositol transporter gene in mouse lens led to congenital cataract. *Investigative Ophthalmology and Visual Science*, **41**, 1467–1472.

Kaddurah-Daouk, R. & Krishnan K. R. R. (2009). Metabolomics: a global biochemical approach to the study of central nervous system diseases. *Neuropsychopharmacology*, **34**, 173–186.

Lejeune, J. (1981). Vingt ans apres. In G. R. Burgio, M. Fraccaro, L. Tiepolo, U. Wolf (eds.), *Trisomy 21, an International Symposium*, Convento dele Clarisse, Rapallo, Italy, 1979, pp. 91–102. Berlin: Springer Verlag.

Lejeune, J., Rethore, M. O., de Blois, M. C., et al. (1986). Metabolism of monocarbons and trisomy 21: sensitivity to methotrexate. *Annals of Genetics*, **29**, 16–19.

Lejeune, J., Turpin, R., Gautier, M. (1959). Etudes des chromosomes somatiques de neuf enfants mongoliens. *Comptes Rendus Hebdomadaires des Seances de l'Academie des Sciences*, **248**, 1721–1722.

Li, Z., Yu, T., Morishima, M., et al. (2007). Duplication of the entire 22.9 Mb human chromosome 21 syntenic region on mouse chromosome 16 causes cardiovascular and gastrointestinal abnormalities. *Human Molecular Genetics*, **16**, 1359–1366.

Lockrow, J., Prakasam, A., Huang, P., et al. (2009). Cholinergic degeneration and memory loss delayed by vitamin E in a Down syndrome mouse model. *Experimental Neurology*, **216**, 278–289.

McCord, J. M. & Fridovich, I. (1969). Superoxide dismutase. An enzymatic function for erythrocuprein (hemocuprein). *Journal of Biological Chemistry*, **244**, 6049-6055.

Meyer, R., Wolf, S. S., Obendorf, M. (2007). PRMT2, a member of the protein arginine methyltransferase family, is a coactivator of the androgen receptor. *Journal of Steroid Biochemistry and Molecular Biology*, **107**, 1–14.

Moore, C. S. (2006). Postnatal lethality and cardiac anomalies in the Ts65Dn Down syndrome mouse model. *Mammalian Genome*, **17**, 1005–1012.

Moore, E. E., Jones, C., Kao, F. T., Oates, D. C. (1977). Synteny between glycinamide ribonucleotide synthetase and superoxide dismutase (soluble). *American Journal of Human Genetics*, **29**, 389–396.

Nag, N., Mellott, T. J., Berger-Sweeney, J. E. (2008). Effects of postnatal dietary choline supplementation on motor regional brain volume and growth factor expression in a mouse model of Rett syndrome. *Brain Research*, **1237**, 101–109.

Nicholson, J. K. & Lindon, J. C. (2008). Metabonomics. *Nature*, **455**, 1054–1056.

O'Doherty, A., Ruf, S., Mulligan, C., et al. (2005). An aneuploid mouse strain carrying human chromosome 21 with Down syndrome phenotypes. *Science*, **309**, 2033–2037.

Olson, L. E., Richtsmeier, J. T., Leszl, J., Reeves, R. H. (2004). A chromosome 21 critical region does not cause specific Down syndrome phenotypes. *Science*, **306**, 687–690.

Olson, L. E., Roper, R. J., Sengstaken, C. L., et al. (2007). Trisomy for the Down syndrome 'critical region' is necessary but not sufficient for brain phenotypes of trisomic mice. *Human Molecular Genetics*, **16**, 774–782.

Ooi, S. K. T., Qiu, C., Bernstein, E., et al. (2007). DNMT3L connects unmethylated lysine 4 of histone H3 to de novo methylation of DNA. *Nature*, **448**, 714–717.

Pant, S., Moser, H. W., Krane, S. M. (1968). Hyperuricemia in Down's syndrome. *Journal of Clinical Endocrinology and Metabolism*, **28**, 472–478.

Patterson, D. (2007). Genetic mechanisms involved in the phenotype of Down syndrome. *Mental Retardation and Developmental Disabilities Research Reviews*, **13**, 199–206.

Patterson, D. (2008). Folate metabolism and the risk of Down syndrome. *Down Syndrome Research and Practice*, **12**, 93–97.

Patterson, D., Graham, C., Cherian, C., Matherly, L. H. (2008). A humanized mouse model for the reduced folate carrier. *Molecular Genetics and Metabolism*, **93**, 95–103.

Peeters, M. A., Poon, A., Zipursky, A., Lejeune, J. (1986). Toxicity of leukemia therapy in children with Down syndrome. *Lancet*, **2**(8512), 1279.

Peeters, M. A., Rethore, M. O., Lejeune, J. (1995). In vivo folic acid supplementation partially corrects in vitro methotrexate toxicity in patients with Down syndrome. *British Journal of Haematology*, **89**, 678–680.

Perrone, S., Longini, M., Bellieni, C. V., et al. (2007). Early oxidative stress in amniotic fluid of pregnancies with Down syndrome. *Clinical Biochemistry*, **40**, 177–180.

Qi, C., Chang, J., Zhu, Y., et al. (2002). Identification of protein arginine methyltransferase 2 as a coactivator of estrogen receptor alpha. *Journal of Biological Chemistry*, **277**, 28624–28630.

Ratel, D., Ravanat, J. L., Charles, M. P., et al. (2006). Undetectable levels of N6-methyl adenine in mouse DNA: cloning and analysis of PRED28, a gene coding for a putative mammalian DNA adenine methyltransferase. *FEBS Letters*, **580**, 3179–3184.

Roizen, N. J. (2005). Complementary and alternative therapies for Down syndrome. *Mental Retardation and Developmental Disabilities Research Reviews*, **11**, 149–155.

Roizen, N. J. & Patterson, D. (2003). Down's syndrome. *Lancet*, **361**(9365), 1281–1289.

Sago, H., Carlson, E. J., Smith, D. J., et al. (1998). Ts1Cje, a partial trisomy 16 mouse model for Down syndrome, exhibits learning and behavioral abnormalities. *Proceedings of the National Academy of Sciences of the United States of America*, **95**, 6256–6261.

Salehi, A., Faizi, M., Belichenko, P. V., Mobley, W. C. (2007). Using mouse models to explore genotype–phenotype relationship in Down syndrome. *Mental Retardation and Developmental Disabilities Research Reviews*, **13**, 207–214.

Salman, M. (2002). Systematic review of the effect of therapeutic dietary supplements and drugs on cognitive function in subjects with Down syndrome. *European Journal of Paediatric Neurology*, **6**, 213–219.

Takashima, S., Takehashi, M., Lee, J., et al. (2009). Abnormal DNA methyltransferase expression in mouse germline stem cells results in sperm-togenic defects. *Biology of Reproduction*, **81**(1), 155–164.

Villar, A. J., Belichenko, P. V., Gillespie, A. M., et al. (2005). Identification and characterization of a new Down syndrome model, Ts[Rb(12.1716)]2Cje, resulting from a spontaneous Robertsonian fusion between T(171)65Dn and mouse chromosome 12. *Mammalian Genome*, **16**, 79–90.

Ward, B. C., Kolodny, N. H., Nag, N., Berger-Sweeney, J. E. (2009). Neurochemical changes in a mouse model of Rett syndrome: changes over time and in response to perinatal choline nutritional supplementation. *Journal of Neurochemistry*, **108**, 361–371.

Yang-Feng T. L., Ma, Y. Y., Liang, R., et al. (1995). Assignment of the human folate transporter gene to chromosome 21q22.3 by somatic cell hybrid analysis and in situ hybridization. *Biochemical and Biophysical Research Communications*, **210**, 874–879.

Yoshimoto, T., Boehm, M., Olive, M., et al. (2006). The arginine methyltransferase PRMT2 binds RB and regulates E2F function. *Experimental Cell Research*, **312**, 2040–2053.

Zeisel, S. H. (2009a). Importance of methyl donors during reproduction. *American Journal of Clinical Nutrition*, **89**, 673S–677S.

Zeisel, S. H. (2009b). Epigenetic mechanisms for nutrition determinants of later health outcomes. *American Journal of Clinical Nutrition*, **89**(5), 1488S–1493S.

Zhao, R., Matherly, L. H., Goldman, I. D. (2009). Membrane transporters and folate homeostasis: intestinal absorption and transport into systemic compartments and tissues. *Expert Reviews in Molecular Medicine*, **11**, e4.

Pharmacological and medical management
and treatment

Pharmacotherapy for children with Down syndrome

George Capone

Introduction

The field of cognitive pharmacology for children with intellectual disability (ID) does not actually exist. As defined by the level of support for clinical trials, or FDA-sanctioned indications, most physicians would be hard pressed to name a single medication used for such a purpose in children. There are few clinical paradigms and little informed consensus about how to navigate these uncharted waters. Despite our advance into the era of genome-based medicine, the mechanisms that support cognition and its neurobiological organization in the brain are still very much in a discovery phase. New appreciation for the biochemical and physiological mechanisms of synaptic dysfunction in neurogenetic disorders holds promise for developing novel therapeutic approaches to ID (Johnston, 2006). Recent advancements using animal models have led to clinical trials for fragile-X syndrome, which is leading the effort to develop therapies for ID based on mechanistic principles (Hagerman et al., 2009).

While scientific investigators may be well equipped to grapple with questions of how to achieve a measureable degree of cognitive enhancement in children with Down syndrome (DS) and ID, they are perhaps less inclined to consider their own motives for doing so. Concerns about biologically informed treatments for persons with DS/ID have a long and colored history, which should not be ignored (Rynders, 1987). Hence, as the scientific pursuit of enhancing cognitive function and related outcomes continues, it remains necessary for clinicians and families to contemplate: why do this; for what purpose, and under what circumstances? It is unlikely that biologically based treatments will render current educational and behavioral interventions obsolete. Rather, the more compelling task will be how to prioritize and combine from among other rationally based therapies so as to gain greater benefit for a particular child with DS.

Intelligence: cognition, memory, and learning

Intelligence is no monolithic phenotype, but a rather complex series of brain strategies that confer developmental and evolutionary advantage by potentiating adaptation across diverse and rapidly changing environmental settings. Through some astonishing miracle of nature and nurture, intelligence emerges during childhood, commensurate with experience, learning, rehearsed motor schemes, and social interactions in parallel with advancing neuromaturation (Barsalou et al., 2007). Intelligent behavior may include up to 60 discrete abilities (Carroll, 1993). Not surprisingly, the neural systems supporting cognition are not readily

Neurocognitive Rehabilitation of Down Syndrome, eds. Jean-Adolphe Rondal, Juan Perera, and Donna Spiker. Published by Cambridge University Press. © Cambridge University Press 2011.

localizable, but are widely distributed across frontal, parietal and temporal–limbic brain regions in typical adults (Jung & Haier, 2007). How cognitive abilities mature from being undifferentiated and imprecise to become the domain-specific, modularized processes we measure in adults is unknown (Karmiloff-Smith, 2006). The emergence of any specific functional skill is linked only tenuously to the particular neurobiological events that unfold during postnatal life (Levitt, 2003), and the events underlying cognitive and language skill acquisition are the most elusive of all (Scerif & Karmiloff-Smith, 2005). Intellectual disability as seen in complex neurogenetic syndromes is not simply an absence of, or diminution in intelligent behavior as defined in typical individuals. It is inherently different; which is why attempts to measure ID as phenotype presents such significant challenges, as cognitive profiles differ in unexpected ways according to etiology and across genetic disorders (Vicari, 2004; Edgin et al., 2010).

It is clear to investigators struggling with the potential enhancement of cognitive function by pharmacological means that it is necessary to utilize neuroscience informed models, with explanatory and predictive power that extends well beyond the themes of development delay and intelligence quotients (IQs). If the goal is informed understanding, then phenomenological constructs alone, in the absence of mechanisms, are inadequate for testing hypotheses about cognition or cognitive enhancement. Those involved in designing newer models of assessment and intervention need to remain informed about genetically influenced biological and physiological processes and their functional manifestation in specific conditions (Dykens & Hodapp, 2007; Beauchaine et al., 2008). How these processes proceed in children with DS gives cause for consternation, because in a subset of vulnerable individuals, cognitive growth can decelerate or falter (Castillo et al., 2008). In others, cognitive function can appear to fluctuate across time and circumstances in children with DS, and may even slow during the first decade (Carr, 1988; Sigman & Ruskin, 1999); however, this phenomenon needs to be better studied, in individual cohorts followed longitudinally. Despite such concerns, identification of a neurobiological substrate for cognitive regression or slowing in children with DS would give scientific investigators a distinct advantage in determining the best research strategies for going forward.

Molecular pharmacology

Neurobiological themes commonly held in the study of cognition and learning often emphasize synaptic neurotransmission, its effects on spine plasticity, nuclear gene expression, and how this changes throughout development and across the lifespan (Johnston, 2009; Johnston et al., 2009). There exists a remarkable evolutionarily conserved yet highly diverse network of chemical neurotransmitters, signaling molecules, and neurotrophic factors, which carry out these functions in different regions of the mammalian brain (Woo & Lu, 2006; Calabrese et al., 2009). For example, the identical neurotransmitter molecule is capable of having multiple effects on target neurons depending on the expression of receptor subtypes, linkage to membrane-bound ion channels or second messenger systems, and their ability to induce DNA, RNA, and protein synthesis (Worley et al., 1987; Lauder, 1993; Heuss & Gerber, 2000). Signaling networks and their nodes of intersection permit cross-talk, which enables neurons to encode long-term changes through induction of nuclear gene expression and synaptic protein synthesis in response to patterned signaling (Johnston, 2009; Bito, 2010). Timing, after all, is everything. A pharmacological challenge given too early or too late in maturation may not result in a robust response; whereas one that is strategically delivered during a sensitive period in development could be maximally advantageous. A more detailed understanding of cellular signaling systems in trisomy 21 will be pivotal in attempting to leverage new or existing pharmacological compounds for therapeutic advantage for children with DS (Ma'ayan et al., 2006; Gardiner, 2009; Wetmore & Garner, 2010).

Neurobiology

A cognitive enhancement strategy that augments synaptic signal while simultaneously reducing background noise has been proposed as a general pharmacological strategy. The neurobiological consequences of trisomy 21 result in reductions in synaptic density, plasticity, and spine dysgenesis, all critical determinants of intellectual impairment in DS (Wisniewski, 1990). Given that pharmacological agents require binding to external cell surface receptors that are linked to a network of signaling mechanisms in order to produce a deliberate cellular response, it becomes critical to determine which children with DS achieve the requisite level of maturation necessary to experience a pharmacological response when challenged. As the Merovingian tells it, "There is only one constant in the Universe. The only one real choice [we have] is 'causality.' Action, reaction, cause and effect." (Merovingian 2003). To which some [Morpheus] would plead that, "everything" begins with choice. "No, wrong!" Merovingian retorts. "Choice is an illusion, created between those with power, and those without. We are all victims of causality." Suffice it to say then, that we will always struggle in our attempts to understand causality or predict the biological reaction sequence for any particular child with trisomy 21.

Thinking about clinical trials

Previous strategies

Until very recently, there has been little interest in designing pharmacological trials for persons with DS because efficacious cognitive enhancing drugs simply have not existed, and biomedical researchers have had little incentive to pursue clinical studies founded on anecdotal reports of benefit. Indeed, the motivation for many previous trials had been to challenge uber-testimonials surrounding the use of certain nutritional supplements, which predictably caused quite a stir among willing believers. Many such compounds are vitamin preparations, metabolic precursors, or hormones that were advocated by parents, manufacturers, and healthcare providers to improve developmental outcomes including intelligence. Because most of these compounds lack any known mechanism of action classifying them as pro-cognitive according to the standards of contemporary neuroscience, they are not included in this review. These studies have been well reviewed in detail elsewhere (Salman, 2002; Roizen, 2005).

Recent strategies

In recent years, the motivation for clinical trials has been to test the efficacy and tolerability of medications having a putative memory-enhancing or cognitive benefit in adult human subjects with dementia or organic brain syndromes. What have evolved are small exploratory clinical trials of psychoactive compounds based on their perceived safety–benefit profile, mechanism of action, and supportive evidence for measurable cognitive-enhancement in humans. A recent review discusses the wide variety of drugs and their target mechanisms being developed for Alzheimer's dementia that could be advantageous for persons with DS (Sabbagh, 2009). Medications with an FDA-approved indication for Alzheimer's dementia have been the most actively studied compounds in persons with DS during the last decade (Prasher et al., 2002; Prasher, 2004; Kishnani et al., 2009). Typically, exploratory clinical trials are initiated with adult subjects and move into the pediatric age group pending the outcome of safety, tolerability, and efficacy data. Heller et al. (2006a) have recently reviewed the essential considerations of clinical trial design in children with DS/ID, and provide insight for many of the conceptual and practical barriers which challenge investigation in this field.

How clinical trials are designed presently

Experimental design and subject selection is critical in any clinical trial. The selection of young subjects expected to benefit from a particular pharmacological intervention has proved challenging. An egalitarian approach of enhancement-for-all seems scientifically naive. A less problematic and more practicable approach has been to select out subjects with a low probability of exhibiting a measureable cognitive response, deemed high-risk candidates. In order to obtain homogeneous study samples, it becomes necessary to exclude subjects according to preexisting cognitive, linguistic, and neurobehavioral criteria. Some minimal level of cognitive–linguistic–behavioral function is necessary to provide informative data in accordance with test protocols; the irony being that many of the excluded candidates are those children most in need of a cognitive advantage. In this imperfect manner, established functional skills serve as proxy in estimating whether requisite levels of neural organization and synaptic maturation have been established.

Measuring outcomes

The selection of outcome measures sensitive enough to detect subtle changes in brain signal against the background noise of individual variability, and developmental change continues to be one of the biggest challenges to experimental design. In the few studies completed, language or adaptive function are the preferred targeted outcomes. In contrast, cognitive drug trials utilizing the Ts65Dn model of trisomy can only emphasize visual and spatial memory outcomes, given the limitation of this model. In young children with DS, desired outcomes should not simply strive for improved memory as learning, but rather the enhancement of central–executive control and the capacity for behavioral self-regulation, under the control of prefrontal cortex (Fuster, 2000; Bell & Deater-Deckard, 2007), potentially setting the stage for improvement in pro-cognitive adaptive function throughout early development. The hierarchical organization of intelligence involves refinement in prefrontal connections, which undergo extensive maturation and reorganization during childhood and adolescence, making these circuits an important target for pharmacological intervention during the first decade of life (Benes et al., 2000; Andersen, 2003).

Meaningful candidate outcomes, applicable to typically developing children with DS include: (1) the capacity for sustained attention, set shifting, and planning; (2) increased capacity of auditory working memory (Vicari et al., 2004; Baddeley & Jarrold, 2007; Edgin et al., 2010); (3) improved sensory–motor processing required for speech production (Vicari et al., 2000; Fidler, 2005); and (4) any neuroimaging marker or characteristic physiological signature that correlates with these functions. Additionally, measures that capture subtle changes in the trajectory of cognitive growth, during the first decade of life, would be valuable. Depending on the specific skill(s) measured, a 10%–15% improvement above baseline function could translate into an adaptive advantage for young children with DS; or perhaps a 5%–10% improvement in multiple domains could result in similar benefit. Such conjectures are speculative, but not unrealistic.

Overlooked physiological variables

Any carefully designed therapeutic trial will require a thorough accounting of secondary physiological impairments (i.e. peripheral auditory impairment, hypothyroidism, sleep fragmentation, or sleep apnea) prior to randomization to ensure the best possible setting for a therapeutic response. Failure to account for these potential saboteurs of brain function will confound data collection and interpretation or, worse, mask any real treatment response. To date, no clinical trials in DS have screened participants for the presence of all known secondary impairments. Auditory function and thyroid status are straightforward enough, but the insidious nature of sleep disturbance needs to be brought to the fore and addressed explicitly.

Cognitive medication trials

Neuroscience informed enhancement of cognition generally involves sensory experience enrichment paradigms or the use of pharmacological agents that target synaptic mechanisms of experience-dependent information coding. The anatomy of memory function emphasizes connections between the thalamus, sensory cortices, and amygdala–hippocampus; structures critical for memory consolidation, storage, and retrieval (Mishkin & Appenzeller, 1987; Wang et al., 2006; Deng et al., 2010).

Acetylcholine and the cholinergic system

Acetylcholine (ACh)-synthesizing neurons are located in the basal forebrain complex, which provides diffuse input to the cerebral cortex, hippocampus, and limbic system. In primates, most cortically projecting ACh fibers arise from the nucleus basalis of Meynert (NbM) and to a lesser extent from the diagonal band of Broca (Foote & Morrison, 1987). ACh-containing axons innervate the hippocampus and developing cortex early in ontogeny and appear to modulate synaptic plasticity early in neocortical development, reaching functional maturity by early childhood (Yan, 2003). The anatomical organization of the cholinergic system supports its role in cortical activation and arousal, and compelling evidence implicates the cholinergic system in learning, memory, and the control of attention and vigilance (Richardson & DeLong, 1988; Perry et al., 1999). Large neurons within the NbM contain choline-acetyltransferase (ChAT), the biosynthetic enzyme for ACh production. Following release by the presynaptic neuron, ACh is degraded in the synaptic cleft by the enzyme acetylcholinesterase (AChE). Acetylcholinesterase inhibitors (AChEI) reduce the degradation of ACh, thus increasing synaptic availability at postsynaptic receptor sites to augment cholinergic signaling. The integrity of cholinergic function present early in life has not been determined with certainty in individuals with DS (Casanova et al., 1985; Kish et al., 1989; Bar-Peled et al., 1991). By middle age, however, cholinergic neurons in the NbM and other midbrain and brainstem nuclei show evidence of atrophy (Mann et al., 1987), and in elderly adults, declining ACh levels correlate with cortical changes of Alzheimer-type dementia (Yates et al., 1983).

Cholinergic medications

Four AChEIs (tacrine, donepezil, rivastigmine, and galantamine) have been approved by the FDA for the symptomatic treatment of cognitive and functional deficits in Alzheimer's disease (AD). Donepezil is a selective AChEI whereas rivastigmine exhibits dual cholinesterase inhibitory function owing to its action on butyrylcholinesterase. Based on these pharmacological properties, the expected cholinergic deterioration in older adults, and incomplete knowledge regarding the integrity of cholinergic function in children and young adults with DS, exploratory clinical trials have been pursued enthusiastically. Although AChEIs are commonly used in medical practice to manage symptoms of age-related cognitive decline in elderly persons with DS, clinical benefit is difficult to determine in any individual.

Donepezil in adults

There are two small studies regarding use of donepezil in aged persons with DS and Alzheimer's dementia. Lott et al. (2002) reported on the open-label use in nine DS subjects (mean 52.3 yr) treated with 5–10 mg donepezil for 3–5 months. Compared to untreated historical DS controls, the treated group showed a significant 6.1 point improvement (P = 0.03) on the Down Syndrome Dementia Scale (DSDS). No data on tolerability were reported. Prasher et al. (2002) recorded results from a double-blind, placebo-controlled study of 14 DS subjects (mean 54.6 yr) who received 5–10 mg donepezil for 24 weeks. Fifty percent of treated subjects showed less deterioration from baseline on the Dementia Scale for Mentally Retarded (DSMR), compared to 31% of the 13 placebo-treated subjects. Up to 50% of treated subjects experienced cholinergic side effects that were mild and transient, compared to 20% receiving placebo. Studies such as these are a challenge to interpret owing to the small sample size.

In non-demented adult DS subjects, Heller et al. (2006b) reported an open-label case series of six subjects (20–41 yr) receiving 5–10 mg donepezil over 24 weeks. Despite mild but transient side-effects (nausea, vomiting, diarrhea, anorexia, hypotension), all subjects tolerated the 10 mg dosage. Some improvement in expressive language function using the Test of Problem Solving (TOPS) at 12 (P = 0.01) and 24 weeks (P = 0.05) was seen. A minimal trend toward improvement on four subtests from the Clinical Evaluation of Language Function – Revised (CELF-R) was noted at 24 weeks. From an efficacy standpoint, studies such as this are essentially uninterpretable owing to an extremely small sample size, the frequency of repeated comparisons, and lack of an appropriate control group.

In a study designed to measure the safety and efficacy of donepezil in adults (18–35 yr) recruited across 24 centers in a 12-week double-blind, placebo-controlled study, 123 subjects received placebo or donepezil at 5 mg for 6 weeks, and 10 mg for the remaining 6 weeks (Kishnani et al., 2009). Using the Severe Impairment Battery Scales (SIB) as the primary outcome, significant improvement on SIB score was noted in both groups after 12 weeks of the double-blind phase. The Vineland Adaptive Behavior Scales (VABS) captured significant improvement only in donepezil-treated subjects during the same period. Secondary measures included the Rivermead Behavioral Memory Test for Children (RBMT-C) and the Clinical Evaluation of Language Fundamentals (CELF-P). On both measures, a positive trend was reported for the donepezil-treated group after 12 weeks, which was not significantly different between groups. Of the 123 subjects, 87 continued their participation for another 12 weeks in an open-label extension study. Those subjects previously on placebo who then received donepezil showed an improvement in SIB scores, whereas subjects previously on donepezil who continued on donepezil retained stable SIB scores. Adverse events (AE) were more likely in donepezil-treated subjects in both the double-blind and open-label phases. No deaths or serious life-threatening events were reported in either group. Donepezil-treated subjects reported abdominal pain, nausea, vomiting, and insomnia at twice the rate of the placebo group. Most adverse effects were transient and only mildly or moderately impairing. Two subjects receiving donepezil experienced hypertension or emotional lability rated as severe by the investigators; these subjects were withdrawn from the double-blind phase.

Donepezil in children

A safety and efficacy study using donepezil in children (10–17 yr) recruited across multiple centers, in a 10-week double-blind, placebo-controlled study, has recently been published (Kishnani et al., 2010). In the largest, best designed randomized controlled trial (RCT) of its kind involving subjects with DS, 129 subjects received either placebo or donepezil at 2.5 mg starting dose, which was increased in 2.5 mg increments every 14 days to 10 mg. Using the Vineland-II Adaptive Behavior Scales (VABS-II) Parent–Caregiver Rating Form (PCRF) as the primary outcome, improvement in both treatment and placebo groups was observed. Given the brevity of the trial, and the need for retest, a practice effect may have contributed to the improvements observed. Secondary measures, including the Test of Verbal Expression and Reasoning (TOVER), also showed improvement with no between group differences. Average daily dosing was 5.0 mg in the donepezil group and 5.6 mg in the placebo group, with greater than 90% compliance in both groups. The most common AEs in the treatment group resulting from expected cholinergic overstimulation included diarrhea (12.5%), and vomiting (6.3%). The majority of AEs were mild or transient with no serious AEs reported. Only one subject receiving donepezil discontinued the study because of moderately disturbing urinary retention. This study also reported on the pharmacokinetics of AChE inhibition, and found that treated subjects were receiving an appropriate dose based on AChE inhibition assays in plasma. None of the placebo responders in the untreated group demonstrated the presence of the active drug, so medication error was ruled out.

Rivastigmine in adults

There is one study regarding the use of a dual cholinesterase inhibitor rivastigmine in aged persons with DS and Alzheimer's dementia. Prasher et al. (2005) provided data on the open-label use in 17 DS subjects (mean 53.2 yr) treated with 12 mg rivastigmine for 24 weeks. The untreated group showed 10.7% change in scores on the DSMR while the treated group showed 7.8%. Compared to 53% of the 13 untreated DS control subjects (mean = 54.9 yr), only 35% of treated subjects showed a >5 point decline from baseline on the DSMR.

Rivastigmine in children

Rivastigmine has also been examined in older children with DS. In a recent open-label study, Heller et al. (2006b) reported on the short-term safety and efficacy using a liquid formulation of rivastigmine in 11 subjects with DS, aged 10–17 years. There were 16 AEs related or possibly related to the study medication, with two subjects accounting for more than one half of the 16 recorded AEs. Twelve AEs occurred in the first eight weeks of the treatment (seven at the 1.5 mg and five at the 3 mg dosage), and four occurred in the second eight weeks of treatment at the 4.5 mg dosage. None of the AEs was unexpected and was related to cholinergic enhancement. Four subjects reported no AEs and five subjects reported one to three mild, transient AEs, including vomiting, diarrhea, stomach ache, fatigue, insomnia, and an instance of "defiant, sassy language" at school. None of the subjects experienced bladder or bowel incontinence.

Significant improvements in adaptive function while on medication were found on the VABS Adaptive Behavior Composite and on the Communication and Daily Living Skills domains. On average, there was a 5.4 point (6%) increase (P = 0.03) on the Daily Living Skills domain, and a 5.6 point (6%) increase (P = 0.01) on the Communication domain, corresponding to a seven-month gain in communication skill. At the end of the 16-week trial, significant language effects were noted on both the TOVER and the CELF-P. Performance on the TOVER showed a 5.2 point (30%) increase (P = 0.02) from baseline. On the CELF-P, overall language performance showed a 7.1 point (9%) increase (P = 0.01) from baseline. Subjects also showed improved attention on the Leiter-R Attention Sustained tests A and B. Performance on the test A increased 12% from a mean of 50.7 at baseline to 56.6 at week 16 (P = 0.01), as on test B, which showed an increase of 19% from a mean of 42.5 at baseline to 50.5 at week 16 (P = 0.02). Statistically significant gains were found on the two memory measures emphasizing language: (NEPSY) Narrative Memory and Immediate Memory for Names. A 63% increase (P = 0.02) in performance from 7.5 at baseline to 12.2 at week 16 was noted in Narrative Memory, and a 72% increase in performance from 8.1 at baseline to 13.9 at week 16 was noted in Immediate Memory for Names (P = 0.01). There have been no published RCTs using rivastigmine in children with DS.

Macrocircuits and pyramidal neurons: why all the excitement?

The amino acid glutamate is the primary excitatory neurotransmitter in the brain, localizing to pyramidal neurons in layers III–V of the neocortex. Pyramidal neurons contribute axons to the commissural and association fibers and the large cortical neurons that innervate the striatum and thalamus (Fagg & Foster, 1983; Cotman et al., 1987). Glutamate is utilized by over 50% of brain synapses (McDonald & Johnston, 1990). The hippocampus also receives an abundant glutamatergic input from the entorhinal cortex, which receives its inputs from functionally distinct regions of the neocortex (Cotman et al., 1987). Ionotrophic or ion channel-linked glutamate receptors are classified according to their preferred agonists as: N-methyl-D-asparte (NMDA), amino-3-hydroxy-5-methyl-4-izoxazole-proprionic acid (AMPA), and kainate (KA) (Greenmayre & Porter, 1994). The NMDA receptor complex, which regulates calcium influx, is essential for memory encoding in collaboration with AMPA receptors. Together they encode information to create memory, strengthen individual synapses, regulate synaptic development, and plasticity (Johnston et al. 2009). Our knowledge of metabotropic, or second messenger-linked glutamate receptors, and their role in the synaptic mechanisms of learning is also achieving critical threshold (Niswender & Conn, 2010).

Glutamate-based strategies

Therapies that target glutamate neurotransmission have been in the pipeline for almost two decades (Robbins & Murphy, 2006; Buchanan et al., 2007). Drugs which amplify physiological glutamate signaling in a precise, time-limited manner without overstimulating voltage-sensitive NMDA channels may be beneficial. Strategies to enhance glutamate neurotransmission have focused on decreasing the desensitization of AMPA receptors (Francotte et al., 2006) and modulation of the NMDA receptor complex using partial agonists (Francis, 2008). Potentiating the effects of endogenous glutamate signaling, during periods of heightened sensitivity, could improve dendrite outgrowth and postsynaptic spine function (Kleinschmidt et al., 1987; Mattson, 1988), resulting in stronger connections, and network stability. However, concerns about overstimulation of NMDA channels and excitotoxicity secondary to excessive calcium influx, may limit this approach (Choi, 1988; Hattori & Wasterlain, 1990; McDonald et al., 1991).

Nootropic medications

Nootropic drugs take their name from the Greek words *tropein* (toward) and *noos* (mind), because of their supposed unique psychotrophic properties (Poschel, 1988). Despite a substantial body of animal and human studies, nootropics have not gained acceptance in North America for the treatment of cognitive impairment because of their apparent lack of efficacy and poorly understood mechanism of action. Several nootropics, including piracetam, appear to have partial ampakine activity because of their action at AMPA glutamate receptors (Francotte et al., 2006). While their clinical utility for treating cognitive impairment appears minimal at best, these compounds serve as a prototype for research and development of more potent and efficacious memory-enhancing compounds (Malykh & Sadaie, 2010).

Piracetam in children

Piracetam, the prototype for nootropic drugs, is perhaps the best studied. During the 1970–1980s, clinical trials performed in children with language-based learning disabilities suggested some benefit at doses ranging from 80 to 120 mg/kg per day, without significant side effects (Capone, 1998). This literature on piracetam was rediscovered during the mid-1990s, and gained enormous visibility within the DS parent community. Because it was being used among preschool and school-aged children with DS, it became necessary to study its effects in this population. A double-blind, placebo-controlled, crossover study assessing the cognitive and behavioral effects of piracetam given at 80–100 mg/kg per day in 18 DS subjects (7–13 yr) failed to demonstrate any benefit on a range of over 30 tests measuring attention, memory, and learning, in addition to several parent and teacher behavioral scales (Lobaugh et al., 2001). Treatment-emergent side effects including irritability, agitation, aggressiveness, sexual arousal, or poor sleep were reported in 7/18 (39%) subjects during the treatment arm, but did not result in withdrawal from the study.

In a double-blind, placebo-controlled feasibility trial conducted between 1997 and 1998, our research group studied 10 DS subjects (6–10 yr) who received placebo or piracetam (100 mg/kg per day), divided into two doses, for 48 weeks (Capone, unpublished). At the end of the trial, both groups showed an apparent improvement on the Total and Receptive portions of the Pre-School Language Scales-3 (PLS-3) without any significant between-group differences. No difference was observed in general intelligence (composite score) from the Stanford Binet Intelligence Scales-IV (SB-IV), and neither the verbal (digit recall) or nonverbal (hand movement task) memory portions of the Kaufman Assessment Battery for Children (KABC) showed any difference. Only spatial working memory (multiple boxes task) demonstrated some trend toward improvement in treated subjects after 48 weeks. Side effects were seen in one of the piracetam-treated subjects. Irritability, emotional lability, and sleep problems were observed at 100 mg/kg per day, which dissipated when the dose was lowered to 65 mg/kg per day and returned when the dosage was again increased. These symptoms indicate the central nervous system effects of piracetam, which may result from overstimulation of glutamate receptors.

Microcircuits and interneurons: inhibitory tendencies

Gamma-aminobutyric acid (GABA) functions as the primary inhibitory neurotransmitter in the hippocampus and cerebral cortex, and may be utilized by up to 30%–40% of cortical synapses (Krieger, 1983). GABA localizes to the small interneurons, which are widely distributed throughout all cortical layers, especially layers II and IV. GABAergic neurons provide inhibitory input to pyramidal neurons, the main source of excitatory output from the cortex and hippocampus (Ben-Ari et al., 2004; Markram et al., 2004). Microcircuits composed of a pyramidal neuron and one or more interneurons modulate cortical excitability and higher-order processing. GABAergic neuron dysfunction has been implicated in a number of neurodevelopmental disorders associated with cognitive disorganization or impairment (Stafstrom, 1993; Levitt et al., 2004; Kato, 2006; Woo & Lu, 2006; Gonzalez-Burgos et al., 2010). In the dorsolateral prefrontal cortex, GABAergic neurons modulate the excitatory activity of pyramidal neurons involved with pro-cognitive functions, such as response inhibition and working memory (Goldman-Rakic, 1995).

In Down syndrome brain congenital depletion of neurons and dysgenesis is evident in all cortical layers with an often striking paucity of small interneurons from layers II/III and IV, and pyramidal neurons from layers III and V (Ross et al., 1984; Wisniewski et al., 1986). The ratio of interneurons to pyramidal neurons differs among individuals with trisomy 21 but always results in some degree of inhibitory dysfunction. Furthermore, reduction in the number or efficiency of microcircuits below a critical threshold undermines the establishment of synchronicity, which drives cortical circuit development and maturation during prenatal and early postnatal periods (Grillner et al., 2005; Hensch, 2005). Vertically organized modules or physiological units, which in the aggregate process real-time data-streams, are reduced in the DS neocortex (Buxhoeveden et al., 2002) and altered in persons with autism (Casanova et al., 2003). Inconsistent or too little inhibitory modulation of pyramidal cell function may underlie the complex evolution of cognitive dysfunction and/or disorganization observed in children with DS across the first decade. In the absence of sufficient GABA-synthesizing neurons, modulation of $GABA_A$ receptors on postsynaptic pyramidal neurons becomes a worthy strategy for cognitive enhancement. Currently in the pharmaceutical pipeline are a number of drugs designed to modulate $GABA_A$ receptors, which offers some promise for the treatment of cognitive disorders, schizophrenia (Vinkers et al., 2010), and other neurodevelopmental conditions characterized by interneuron pathology.

Targeting the prefrontal cortex in Down syndrome

At least five parallel circuits connecting the thalamus and basal ganglia with functionally distinct subdivisions of the frontal cortex represent the anatomical substrate for the central executive, ideomotor, and volitional control of motor action and behavior (Cummings, 1993). Higher cortical function emerges as a result of functional integration between subcortical circuits in coordination with prefrontal activity, essential for planning, attending, shifting, organizing, and working memory (Barbas, 2000; Fuster, 2000). Dopamine (DA)-synthesizing neurons located in the ventral tegmental area (VTA) of the midbrain, innervate limbic and frontal cortices, respectively, to constitute the mesolimbic and mesocortical DA systems (Foote & Morrison, 1987). The prefrontal cortex, primary motor, and sensory association areas receive a particularly dense contribution of DA-containing fibers, which synapse on both pyramidal neurons (layer III) and interneurons (layers II/IV) (Goldman-Rakic et al., 2000). Dopamine, acting at D1 receptors, enhances working memory in a dose-dependent fashion and follows a classic, inverted U-shape curve. Moderate levels of DA enhance glutamate input to pyramidal neurons, leading to increased delay activity and improved working memory. At higher DA levels, glutamate input is enhanced to both pyramidal neurons and interneurons, leading to a reduction in working memory function. Dopamine synapses undergo a complex evolution and reorganization in the brain, not reaching complete functional maturity in the prefrontal cortex until adulthood (Spear, 2000), which presents the intriguing possibility that these circuits can be pharmacologically modified up until the time of puberty (Benes et al., 2000). Catecholamine-specific projection neurons and/or their postsynaptic receptors are already targets of numerous pharmacological agents intended to alleviate disabling psychiatric and cognitive symptoms (Nieoullon, 2002; Del Arco & Mora, 2009; Robbins & Arnsten, 2009). Dopamine and noradrenaline (norepinephrine) enhancing agents that are capable of improving inattention, impulsivity, and working memory if administered at the right time in neurodevelopment could produce a lasting imprint on prefrontal circuits, thereby directing subsequent prefrontal maturation and executive control function (Andersen, 2003, Andersen & Navalta, 2004). The consequence of such treatment in young children with DS has not yet been explored.

Psychotropic medication in persons with Down syndrome

There are several small case series reporting clinical success using psychotropic medications (lithium, anticonvulsant mood stabilizers, benzodiazepines, tricyclic antidepressants, selective serotonin reuptake inhibitors, first and second generation antipsychotics) for the treatment of mood-anxiety disorders, obsessive-compulsive disorder, agitation, functional decline, and psychosis in adults with DS (Duggirala et al., 1995; Myers & Pueschel, 1995; Geldmacher et al., 1997; Pary et al., 1999; Sutor et al., 2006). Virtually no literature exists on the pharmacological treatment of neurobehavioral disorders of childhood onset. It has been our observation that many children with DS and symptoms of attention deficit hyperactive disorder (ADHD) do not tolerate stimulant medications at commonly prescribed doses when anxiety, perseveration, or repetitive behaviors are also present. There exists a need for efficacy data, including both behavioral and cognitive outcomes; tolerability data, including dose-related adverse events; as well as studies using rational polypharmacy to guide physicians on the best use of psychostimulants and α_{2A}-adrenergic agonists for inattention, impulse dyscontrol, hyperactivity, and associated problems with behavioral regulation in children with DS.

Physiologically impairing symptoms

Targeting the physiological regulation of mood, emotion, and behavioral self-control is the mainstay of child psychiatry. While not typically considered under the domain of cognitive function, problems with hyperactivity, impulsivity and attention control, irritable mood, perseveration, and stereotypy may be prominent in a subset of children with DS (Capone et al., 2006). Such behaviors interfere with experience-dependent learning and the acquisition of adaptive skills (Hagerman, 1999). High levels of internalizing maladaptive behavior are inversely associated with cognitive function in children with DS (Capone, 2009). Estimates vary, but an estimated 5%–15% of prepubertal children with DS appear to meet criteria for an autism spectrum disorder using current diagnostic algorithms (DiGuiseppi et al., 2010).

Children with DS and autism phenotype are more likely to manifest severe ID and highly maladaptive behaviors (Capone et al., 2005). Could reduction in neurophysiological symptoms associated with irritability, stereotypy, and perseveration have a positive effect on both behavior and long-term developmental outcomes in affected children? For the point of discussion, assume the answer to be a qualified "yes." What, then, are the prospects for such intervention?

Strategies to reduce physiologically impairing symptoms

In some children, early-onset internalizing behaviors appear to diminish with neuromaturation, especially when comorbid medical conditions, environmental variables, and child–parent interactions are fully addressed. At other times, internalizing behaviors appear to be so physiologically driven as to intensify and interfere with the acquisition of other developmental skills. Considering the class of medications known as second-generation antipsychotics currently approved to alleviate autism-associated behaviors in older children (i.e. risperidone or aripiprazole), should a preemptive strike be considered in younger children who demonstrate a high burden of symptoms early in life? The short- and long-term effects of treating young children with DS in such circumstances remain largely unexplored. In children, unanticipated pharmacological effects should be expected when any medication gains access to the developing brain (Thompson & Stanwood, 2009); and not always for the worse, this sword cuts in both directions. In considering the risk for undesirable treatment emergent effects, it is important to know if measureable, long-term benefits might outweigh such risks. There is reason to believe that under certain circumstances this may be so.

Recently, we reported data from an open-label, naturalistic study, using risperidone to treat disruptive behaviors and self-injury in children with DS, severe ID, and autism phenotype (Capone et al., 2008). Subjects were children (mean age 7.8 ± 2.6 yr), consisting of 20 males and 3 females identified through our Down Syndrome Clinic. Using the Aberrant Behavior Checklist (ABC) as the primary outcome measure, all five subscales showed significant improvement following treatment. The mean duration of treatment was 95.8 ± 16.8 days, and the average total daily dosage was 0.66 ± 0.28 mg/day. The Hyperactivity, Stereotypy and Lethargy subscale scores showed the most significant reduction ($P < 0.001$), followed by Irritability ($P < 0.02$), and Inappropriate Speech ($P < 0.04$). Children with disruptive behavior and self-injury showed the greatest improvement. Sleep quality also improved for 88% of subjects with preexisting sleep disturbance. Subjects for whom a follow-up weight was available showed an average weight increase of 2.8 ± 1.5 kg during the treatment period. Low-dose risperidone was well tolerated, although concerns about weight gain and metabolic alterations may limit its long-term usefulness in some children. The ABC findings supported our clinical impressions of improvement on important target behaviors such as aggression, self-injury, stereotypy, and social withdrawal. It is unknown if treatment responsive subjects with DS and autism phenotype have a different functional outcome compared to non-responders or untreated subjects over a longer period of follow-up.

The urgency of reducing physiologically impairing symptoms

It could be argued that internalizing behavior as a physiological symptom is associated with heightened background noise that interferes with a clean stream of information signal processing. In this scenario, the usual pattern of synaptic overproduction, selection, and strengthening are undermined to the detriment of neocortical organization. Stated otherwise, "psychopathology itself can be neurotoxic, and should not be left untreated" (Vitiello, 1998). Failure to acquire requisite joint attention, social reciprocity, or communication skills and the likelihood of serious maladaptive behavior appears to argue in favor of using extraordinary intervention methods. Any willingness on the part of physicians to recognize and treat impairing symptoms in preschool-aged children in the absence of a formal ICD, DSM, or DM-ID psychiatric disorder might appear novel or too forward. Perhaps it is inconsistent with present clinical constructs about to whom, when, and under what circumstances we offer pharmacological interventions. Among conservative practitioners a more familiar and recognizable pattern of symptoms, informed by a positive family history, is required. However, to wait for that level of clinical symptomatology to emerge may be to forfeit the opportunity to sculpt the developing brain *in situ* (Johnston et al., 2001) in children at highest risk.

Concerns about moving forward

Given concerns about safety and residual long-term effects, it would require substantial clinical research support and a ground shift in opinion to advance such a practice, especially at most pediatric medical centers. Yet this is what appears to be occurring in some pediatric psychiatry programs (DeBar et al., 2003; Zito et al., 2003; Luby, 2007), which are modeled on an adult psychiatry approach of early symptom management (Slaby & Tancredi, 2001). Off-label prescribing supported by open-label studies partially address the clinical imperative to do something in children with unusual physiology or *forme fruste* autism phenotype in evolution. The value-added concept of medication as a pharmacological probe also invites further exploration of complex neurobehavioral syndromes, hopefully leading to more rigorous investigation. If the details of brain chemistry and organization remain unknowable for any particular child, then clinical experience, good judgment, and lucid decision making must prevail. Cognitive, emotive, and behavioral indicators become proxy markers for presumptive circuit dysfunction; if only we are wise enough to see and understand it. Such is the current dilemma of clinical practice. Fortunately, practice guidelines have been developed for the use of psychotrophic medications in young children (Gleason et al., 2007).

An analogy to current trends in adult psychiatry is enlightening. Early psychiatric intervention using cognitive–behavioral strategies and psychotropic medications to delay or prevent the onset of schizophrenia in ultra high-risk patients is underway (Larson et al., 2010; Mittal et al., 2010). Newer antipsychotic medications, which have proven so versatile in the treatment of depression and schizophrenia, are beginning to make achieving prevention of symptomatic expression a realistic target. We now appreciate that in addition to their complex receptor-binding profile (Meltzer, 1991), atypical antipsychotic medications and several antidepressants have a sustained influence on cell signaling and gene expression to function as potent pro-proliferative, pro-plasticity agents in the adult brain (Dranovsky & Hen, 2006; Newton & Duman, 2007; Calabrese et al., 2009; Molteni et al., 2009). Such observations may be the harbinger of novel therapeutic strategies just over the horizon.

Futuristic notions of biological therapy

Facilitation of functionally mature synapses, while an important strategy toward cognitive enhancement in trisomy 21, represents but one of several possible therapeutic approaches. Synaptic alteration and diminished synaptic density within the context of cortical dysgenesis may also be an indirect consequence of reductions in cell number throughout the fetal cortex. When stem cell or neuroblast proliferation is restricted owing to prolongation of the cell cycle early in embryonic development, the laminar organization of hippocampal and cortical structures become compromised (Contestabile et al., 2010). With fewer neurons and attendant glial support elements, cortical network capacity is diminished, resulting in oscillatory asynchrony and subsequent disorganization (Ben-Ari et al., 2004; Uhlhaas et al., 2009). Over time, these imperfect, tenuous connections, which depend on trophic support for their maintenance, can lose their resiliency and entire circuits become vulnerable to dissolution (Geschwind & Levitt, 2007). If such events are indeed operative in DS, it suggests that a different, more ambitious strategy founded on building a better brain early in development would be rational. This will likely require some combination of neurogenerative, neurotrophic, and neuroprotective strategies to potentiate neurogenesis in the embryonic brain, and buffer canalized developmental pathways from the multitude of deleterious consequences of trisomy 21. Biologically assisted neuromaturation could represent the Holy Grail of brain-based intervention for children with trisomy 21. If only we knew how to do this, we could debate if in fact we should, under what circumstances, and the reasons why or why not. Cell-based therapies engender the possibility of directing neurodevelopment along a more sustained pro-maturational trajectory, intent on generating network complexity, enhanced performance, and long-term stability. We are not even close to testing such ideas in humans.

Merging biological and educational strategies

A comprehensive cognitive research agenda would include enhancement and preservation of neurobiological function during critical or sensitive periods of development, without disrupting the precisely orchestrated sequence of events that unfolds during ontogeny (Levitt, 2003; Capone & Kaufmann, 2007). Safety is an obvious concern. For any pro-maturational biological intervention to be successful, benefits would need to include improvement in experience-dependent learning and adaptive behavior in real time. Furthermore, such therapies must be compatible with existing developmentally based education and behavior programs. Indeed, novel behavioral and educational programming, including computer simulation designed to utilize the very same brain circuits targeted for pharmacological enhancement, would be an important component of any comprehensive approach to early intervention specific to trisomy 21 (Fidler & Nadel, 2007; and other chapters in this book).

The Ts65Dn mouse model of Down syndrome

Animal models of trisomy using Ts65Dn mice are available to study the neurobiological and behavioral consequences of trisomy 21-related gene dosage imbalance (Davisson et al., 1993; Reeves et al., 1995). Ts65Dn mice are particularly useful for studying fetal and early postnatal brain development and for preclinical screening of pharmacological compounds that modulate hippocampal-dependent learning and memory (Wang et al., 2006; Gardiner, 2009; Contestabile et al., 2010). However, trisomy 21 in humans is orders-of-magnitude more complex than the Ts65Dn mouse model would suggest, especially as it pertains to cognitive functions requiring an exquisite degree of emotional and behavioral control for their execution. Despite the high degree of molecular conservation in signaling pathways utilized in mammalian brain development, learning and memory, the human attributes regarded as higher cortical function, and their dissolution in children with trisomy 21 are unlikely to be recapitulated using *Mus musculus*. Thus, clinical research and human drug trials remain a necessary part of the discovery process itself, which together with preclinical testing can inform and guide the drug discovery enterprise. Ts65Dn models have been used with notable success during the last decade, and there is cause for guarded optimism that new therapies will soon emerge. A summary of this exciting work has appeared in recent reviews (Reeves & Garner, 2007; Gardiner, 2009; Contestabile et al., 2010).

Summary

The field of cognitive pharmacology for children with intellectual disability (ID) does not yet exist, but recent research developments toward this goal appear promising. Neuroscience-informed investigation into the neurobiological basis of ID in Down syndrome (DS) and other neurogenetic conditions is beginning to accumulate the critical mass of research focus needed in order to move forward. Pharmacological agents that target GABA and glutamate receptors and dopamine transporters hold promise for advancement toward clinical testing. Cell-based therapies and related biological interventions are still in the preclinical discovery and testing stage; and the infrastructure and resources required to support such research efforts in children have been less than forthcoming, which hampers advancement in this field. The ability to translate breakthroughs from neuropharmacology and cognitive neuroscience into targeted therapies that improve the lives of children with trisomy 21 will thus remain a significant challenge.

References

Andersen, S. L. (2003). Trajectories of brain development: point of vulnerability or window of opportunity? *Neuroscience and Biobehavioral Reviews*, **27**, 3–18.

Andersen, S. L. & Navalta, C. P. (2004). Altering the course of neurodevelopment: a framework for understanding the enduring effects of psychotropic drugs. *International Journal of Developmental Neuroscience*, **22**, 423–440.

Baddeley, A. & Jarrold, C. (2007). Working memory and Down syndrome. *Journal of Intellectual Disability Research*, **51**, 925–931.

Bar-Peled, O., Israeli, M., Ben-Hur, H., et al. (1991). Developmental pattern of muscarinic receptors in normal and Down's syndrome fetal brain – an autoradiographic study. *Neuroscience Letters*, **133**, 154–158.

Barbas, H. (2000). Connections underlying the synthesis of cognition, memory, and emotion in primate prefrontal cortices. *Brain Research Bulletin*, **53**, 319–330.

Barsalou, L., Breazeal, C., Smith, L. (2007). Cognition as coordinated non-cognition. *Cognitive Process*, **8**, 79–91.

Beauchaine, T. P., Neuhaus, E., Brenner, S. L., Gatzke-Kopp, L. (2008). Ten good reasons to consider biological processes in prevention and intervention research. *Developmental Psychopathology*, **20**, 745–774.

Bell, M. A. & Deater-Deckard, K. (2007). Biological systems and the development of self-regulation: integrating behavior, genetics, and psychophysiology. *Journal of Developmental & Behavioral Pediatrics*, **28**, 409–420.

Ben-Ari, Y., Khalilov, I., Repressa, A., Gozlan, H. (2004). Interneurons set the tune of developing networks. *Trends in Neurosciences*, **27**, 422–427.

Benes, F. M., Taylor, J. B., Cunningham, M. C. (2000). Convergence and plasticity of monoaminergic systems in the medial prefrontal cortex during the postnatal period: implications for the development of psychopathology. *Cerebral Cortex*, **10**, 1014–1027.

Bito, H. (2010). The chemical biology of synapses and neuronal circuits. *Nature Chemical Biology*, **6**, 560–563.

Buchanan, R. W., Freedman, R., Javitt, D. C., Abi-Dargham, A., Lieberman, J. A. (2007). Recent advances in the development of novel pharmacological agents for the treatment of cognitive impairments in schizophrenia. *Schizophrenia Bulletin*, **33**, 1120–1130.

Buxhoeveden, D., Fobbs, A., Roy, E., Casanova, M. (2002). Quantitative comparison of radial cell columns in children with Down syndrome and controls. *Journal of Intellectual Disability Research*, **46**, 76–81.

Calabrese, F., Molteni, R., Racagni, G., Riva, M. A. (2009). Neuronal plasticity: a link between stress and mood disorders. *Psychoneuroendocrinology*, **34**(Suppl 1), S208–S216.

Capone, G. (1998). Drugs that increase intelligence? Application for childhood cognitive impairment. *Mental Retardation and Developmental Disabilities Research Reviews*, **4**, 36–49.

Capone, G. T. (2009). Behavioral phenotypes in Down syndrome: a probabilistic model. In B. K. Shapiro & P. J. Accardo (eds.), *Neurobehavioral Disorders: Science and Practice*, pp. 53–69. Baltimore: Brookes.

Capone, G., Goyal, P., Ares, W., Lannigan, E. (2006). Neurobehavioral disorders in children, adolescents, and young adults with Down syndrome. *American Journal of Medical Genetics. Part C, Seminars in Medical Genetics*, **142C**, 158–172.

Capone, G., Grados, M., Goyal, P., Smith, B., Kammann, H. (2008). Risperidone use in children with Down syndrome, severe intellectual disability and co-morbid autistic spectrum disorder. *Journal of Developmental and Behavioral Pediatrics*, **29**, 106–116.

Capone, G. T., Grados, M. A., Kaufmann, W. E., Bernad-Ripoll, S., Jewell, A. (2005). Down syndrome and comorbid autism-spectrum disorder: characterization using the aberrant behavior checklist. *American Journal of Medical Genetics. Part A*, **134**, 373–80.

Capone, G. & Kaufmann, W. E. (2007). Human Brain Development. In P. J. Accardo (ed.), *Neurodevelopmental Disabilities in Infancy and Childhood*, pp. 27–57. Baltimore: Brookes.

Carr, J. (1988). Six weeks to twenty-one years old: A longitudinal study of children with Down's syndrome and their families. *Journal of Child Psychology and Psychiatry*, **29**, 407–431.

Carroll, J. B. (1993). *Human Cognitive Abilities*. Cambridge: Cambridge University Press.

Casanova, M. F., Buxhoeveden, D., Gomez, J. (2003). Disruption in the inhibitory architecture of the cell minicolumn: implications for autism. *Neuroscientist*, **9**, 496–507.

Casanova, M., Walker, L., Whitehouse, P., Price, D. (1985). Abnormalities of the nucleus basalis in Down's syndrome. *Annals of Neurology*, **18**, 310–313.

Castillo, H., Patterson, B., Hickey, F., et al. (2008). Difference in age of regression in children with autism with and without Down Syndrome. *Journal of Developmental and Behavioral Pediatrics*, **29**, 89–93.

Choi, D. W. (1988). Glutamate neurotoxicity and diseases of the nervous system. *Neuron*, **1**, 623–634.

Contestabile, A., Benfenati, F., Gasparini, L. (2010). Communication breaks-Down: from neurodevelopment defects to cognitive disabilities in Down syndrome. *Progress in Neurobiology*, **91**, 1–22.

Cotman, C. W., Monaghan, D. T., Ottersen, O. P., Storm-Mathisen, J. (1987). Anatomical organization of excitatory amino-acid receptors and their pathways. *Trends in Neuroscience*, **10**, 273–279.

Cummings, J. (1993). Frontal-subcortical circuits and human behavior. *Archives of Neurology*, **50**, 873–880.

Davisson, M., Schmidt, C., Reeves, R., et al. (1993). Segmental trisomy as a mouse model for Down syndrome. In C. Epstein (ed.), *The Phenotypic Mapping of Down Syndrome and Other Aneuploid Conditions*, pp. 117–133. New York: Wiley-Liss.

DeBar, L., Lynch, F., Powell, J., Gale, J. (2003). Use of psychotropic agents in preschool children. *Archives of Pediatric and Adolescent Medicine*, **157**, 150–157.

Del Arco, A. & Mora, F. (2009). Neurotransmitters and prefrontal cortex-limbic system interactions: implications for plasticity and psychiatric disorders. *Journal of Neural Transmission*, **116**, 941–952.

Deng, W., Aimone, J. B., Gage, F. H. (2010). New neurons and new memories: how does adult hippocampal neurogenesis affect learning and memory? *Nature Reviews in Neuroscience*, **11**, 339–350.

DiGuiseppi, C., Hepburn, S., Davis, J. M., et al. (2010). Screening for autism spectrum disorders in children with Down syndrome: population prevalence and screening test characteristics. *Journal of Developmental and Behavioral Pediatrics*, **31**, 181–191.

Dranovsky, A. & Hen, R. (2006). Hippocampal neurogenesis: regulation by stress and antidepressants. *Biological Psychiatry*, **59**, 1136–1143.

Duggirala, C., Cooper, S., Collacott, R. A. (1995). Schizophrenia and Down's syndrome. *Irish Journal of Psychological Medicine*, **12**(1), 30–33.

Dykens, E. & Hodapp, R. (2007). Three steps toward improving the measurement of behavior and behavioral phenotype research. *Child and Adolescent Psychiatric Clinics of North America*, **16**, 617–630.

Edgin, J. O., Pennington, B. F., Mervis, C. B. (2010). Neuropsychological components of intellectual disability: the contributions of immediate, working, and associative memory. *Journal of Intellectual Disability Research*, **54**, 406–417.

Fagg, G. E. & Foster, A. C. (1983). Amino acid neurotransmitters and their pathways in the mammalian central nervous system. *Neuroscience*, **9**, 701–719.

Fidler, D. J. (2005). The emerging Down Syndrome behavioral phenotype in early childhood. *Infants & Young Children*, **18**, 86–103.

Fidler, D. J. & Nadel, L. (2007). Education and children with Down syndrome: neuroscience, development, and intervention. *Mental Retardation and Developmental Disability Research Reviews*, **13**, 262–271.

Foote, S. L. & Morrison, J. H. (1987). Extrathalamic modulation of cortical function. *Annual Reviews of Neuroscience*, **10**, 67–95.

Francis, P. T. (2008). Glutamatergic approaches to the treatment of cognitive and behavioural symptoms of Alzheimer's disease. *Neurodegenerative Disease*, **5**, 241–243.

Francotte, P., de Tullio, P., Fraikin, P., et al. (2006). In search of novel AMPA potentiators. *Recent Patents in CNS Drug Discovery*, **1**, 239–246.

Fuster, J. M. (2000). Memory networks in the prefrontal cortex. *Progress in Brain Research*, **122**, 309–316.

Gardiner, K. J. (2009). Molecular basis of pharmacotherapies for cognition in Down syndrome. *Trends in Pharmacological Sciences*, **31**, 66–73.

Geldmacher, D., Lerner, A., Voci, M., et al. (1997). Treatment of functional decline in adults with Down syndrome using selective serotonin-reuptake inhibitor drugs. *Journal of Geriatric Psychiatry and Neurology*, **10**, 99–104.

Geschwind, D. H. & Levitt, P. (2007). Autism spectrum disorders: developmental disconnection syndromes. *Current Opinion in Neurobiology*, **17**, 103–111.

Gleason, M. M., Egger, H. L., Emslie, G. J., et al. (2007). Psychopharmacological treatment for very young children: contexts and guidelines. *Journal of the American Academy of Child & Adolescent Psychiatry*, **46**, 1532–1572.

Goldman-Rakic, P. (1995). Cellular basis of working memory. *Neuron*, **14**, 111–117.

Goldman-Rakic, P. S., Muly III, E. C., Williams, G. V. (2000). D1 receptors in prefrontal cells and circuits. *Brain Research Reviews*, **31**, 295–301.

Gonzalez-Burgos, G., Hashimoto, T., Lewis, D. A. (2010). Alterations of cortical GABA neurons and network oscillations in schizophrenia. *Current Psychiatry Reports*, **12**, 335–344.

Greenmayre, J. & Porter, R. (1994). Anatomy and physiology of glutamate in the CNS. *Neurology*, **44**, S7–S13.

Grillner, S., Markram, H., De Schutter, E., Silberberg, G., LeBeau, F. E. (2005). Microcircuits in action–from CPGs to neocortex. *Trends in Neurosciences*, **28**, 525–533.

Hagerman, R. (1999). Psychopharmacological interventions in Fragile X syndrome, Fetal alcohol syndrome, Prader-Willi syndrome, Angelman syndrome, Smith-Magenis syndrome and Velocardiofacial syndrome. *Mental Retardation and Developmental Disabilities Research Reviews*, **5**, 305–313.

Hagerman, R. J., Berry-Kravis, E., Kaufmann, W. E., et al. (2009). Advances in the treatment of fragile X syndrome. *Pediatrics*, **123**, 378–390.

Hattori, H. & Wasterlain, C. G. (1990). Excitatory amino acids in the developing brain: ontogeny, plasticity, and excitotoxicity. *Pediatric Neurology*, **6**, 219–228.

Heller, J. H., Spiridigliozzi, G. A., Crissman, B. G., et al. (2006a). Clinical trials in children with Down syndrome: issues from a cognitive research perspective. *American Journal of Medical Genetics. Part C, Seminars in Medical Genetics*, **142C**, 187–195.

Heller, J. H., Spiridigliozzi, G. A., Crissman, B. G., et al. (2006b). Safety and efficacy of rivastigmine in adolescents with Down syndrome: a preliminary 20-week, open-label study. *Journal of Child and Adolescent Psychopharmacology*, **16**, 755–765.

Hensch, T. K. (2005). Critical period plasticity in local cortical circuits. *Nature Reviews in Neuroscience*, **6**, 877–888.

Heuss, C. & Gerber, U. (2000). G-protein-independent signaling by G-protein-coupled receptors. *Trends in Neurosciences*, **23**, 469–475.

Johnston, M. V. (2006). Fresh ideas for treating developmental cognitive disorders. *Current Opinion in Neurology*, **19**, 115–118.

Johnston, M. V. (2009). Plasticity in the developing brain: implications for rehabilitation. *Developmental Disabilities Research Reviews*, **15**, 94–101.

Johnston, M. V., Ishida, A., Ishida, W. N., et al. (2009). Plasticity and injury in the developing brain. *Brain Development*, **31**, 1–10.

Johnston, M., Nishimura, A., Harum, K., Pekar, J., Blue, M. (2001). Sculpting the developing brain. *Advances in Pediatrics*, **48**, 1–38.

Jung, R. & Haier, R. (2007). The parieto-frontal integration theory (P-FIT) of intelligence: converging neuroimaging evidence. *Behavioral and Brain Sciences*, **30**, 135–154.

Karmiloff-Smith, A. (2006). The tortuous route from genes to behavior: a neuroconstructivist approach. *Cognitive, Affective & Behavioral Neuroscience*, **6**, 9–17.

Kato, M. (2006). A new paradigm for West syndrome based on molecular and cell biology. *Epilepsy Research*, **70**(Suppl 1), S87–S95.

Kish, S., Karlinsky, H., Becker, L., et al. (1989). Down's syndrome individuals begin life with normal levels of brain cholinergic markers. *Journal of Neurochemistry*, **52**, 1183–1187.

Kishnani, P. S., Heller, J. H., Spiridigliozzi, G. A., et al. (2010). Donepezil for treatment of cognitive dysfunction in children with Down syndrome aged 10–17. *American Journal of Medical Genetics. Part A, Seminars in Medical Genetics*, **152**(12), 3028–3035.

Kishnani, P. S., Sommer, B. R., Handen, B. L., et al. (2009). The efficacy, safety, and tolerability of donepezil for the treatment of young adults with Down syndrome. *American Journal of Medical Genetics, Part A*, **149**, 1641–1654.

Kleinschmidt, A., Bear, M., Singer, W. (1987). Blockade of NMDA receptors disrupts experience-dependent plasticity of kitten striate cortex. *Science*, **238**, 355–358.

Krieger, D. T. (1983). Brain peptides: what, where and why? *Science*, **222**, 975–985.

Larson, M. K., Walker, E. F., Compton, M. T. (2010). Early signs, diagnosis and therapeutics of the prodromal phase of schizophrenia and related psychotic disorders. *Expert Reviews in Neurotherapy*, **10**, 1347–1359.

Lauder, J. (1993). Neurotransmitters as growth regulatory signals: role of receptors and second messengers. *Trends in Neurosciences*, **16**, 233–240.

Levitt, P. (2003). Structural and functional maturation of the developing primate brain. *Journal of Pediatrics*, **143**, S35–S45.

Levitt, P., Eagleson, K. L., Powell, E. M. (2004). Regulation of neocortical interneuron development and the implications for neurodevelopmental disorders. *Trends in Neurosciences*, **27**, 400–406.

Lobaugh, N., Karaskov, V., Rombough, V., et al. (2001). Piracetam does not enhance cognitive functioning in children with Down syndrome. *Archives of Pediatric and Adolescent Medicine*, **155**, 442–448.

Lott, I. T., Osann, K., Doran, E., Nelson, L. (2002). Down syndrome and Alzheimer disease: response to donepezil. *Archives of Neurology*, **59**, 1133–1136.

Luby, J. (2007). Psychopharmacology of psychiatric disorders in the preschool period. *Journal of Child and Adolescent Psychopharmacology*, **17**, 149–272.

Ma'ayan, A., Gardiner, K., Iyengar, R. (2006). The cognitive phenotype of Down syndrome: insights from intracellular network analysis. *Journal of the American Society for Experimental Neurotherapeutics*, **3**, 396–406.

Malykh, A. G. & Sadaie, M. R. (2010). Piracetam and piracetam-like drugs: from basic science to novel clinical applications to CNS disorders. *Drugs*, **70**, 287–312.

Mann, D. M. A., Yates, P. O., Marcynicuk, B., Ravindra, C. R. (1987). Loss of neurones from cortical and subcortical areas in Down's syndrome patients at middle age. *Journal of the Neurological Sciences*, **80**, 79–89.

Markram, H., Toledo-Rodriguez, M., Wang, Y., et al. (2004). Interneurons of the neocortical inhibitory system. *Nature Reviews Neuroscience*, **5**(10), 793–807.

Mattson, M. P. (1988). Neurotransmitters in the regulation of neuronal cytoarchitecture. *Brain Research Reviews*, **13**, 179–212.

McDonald, J. W., Garofalo, E. A., Hood, T., et al. (1991). Altered excitatory and inhibitory amino acid receptor binding in hippocampus of patients with temporal lobe epilepsy. *Annals of Neurology*, **29**, 529–541.

McDonald, J. W. & Johnston, M. V. (1990). Physiological and pathophysiological roles of excitory amino acids during central nervous system development. *Brain Research Reviews*, **15**, 41–70.

Meltzer, H. (1991). The mechanism of action of novel antipsychotic drugs. *Schizophrenia Bulletin*, **17**, 263–287.

Merovingian. (2003). *Matrix Reloaded*. Warner Brothers.

Mishkin, M. & Appenzeller, T. (1987). The anatomy of memory. *Scientific American*, **256**(6), 80–89.

Mittal, V. A., Walker, E. F., Bearden, C. E., et al. (2010). Markers of basal ganglia dysfunction and conversion to psychosis: neurocognitive deficits and dyskinesias in the prodromal period. *Biological Psychiatry*, **68**, 93–99.

Molteni, R., Calabrese, F., Racagni, G., Fumagalli, F., Riva, M. A. (2009). Antipsychotic drug actions on gene modulation and signaling mechanisms. *Pharmacology and Therapeutics*, **124**, 74–85.

Myers, B. A. & Pueschel, S. M. (1995). Major depression in a small group of adults with Down syndrome. *Research in Developmental Disabilities*, **16**, 285–299.

Newton, S. S. & Duman, R. S. (2007). Neurogenic actions of atypical antipsychotic drugs and therapeutic implications. *CNS Drugs*, **21**, 715–725.

Nieoullon, A. (2002). Dopamine and the regulation of cognition and attention. *Progress in Neurobiology*, **67**, 53–83.

Niswender, C. M. & Conn, P. J. (2010). Metabotropic glutamate receptors: physiology, pharmacology, and disease. *Annual Reviews in Pharmacology and Toxicology*, **50**, 295–322.

Pary, R. J., Friedlander, R., Capone, G. (1999). Bipolar disorder and Down syndrome: six cases. *Mental Health Aspects of Developmental Disabilities*, **2**, 1–5.

Perry, E. K., Walker, M., Grace, J., Perry, R. (1999). Acetylcholine in mind: a neurotransmitter correlate of consciousness? *Trends in Neurosciences*, **22**, 273–280.

Poschel, B. (1988). New pharmacologic perspectives on nootropic drugs. In L. Iversen, S. Iversen, S. Snyder (eds.), *Handbook of Psychopharmacology*, pp. 437–469. New York: Plenum Press.

Prasher, V. P. (2004). Review of donepezil, rivastigmine, galantamine and memantine for the treatment of dementia in Alzheimer's disease in adults with Down syndrome: implications for the intellectual disability population. *International Journal of Geriatric Psychiatry*, **19**, 509–515.

Prasher, V. P., Fung, N., Adams, C. (2005). Rivastigmine in the treatment of dementia in Alzheimer's disease in adults with Down syndrome. *International Journal of Geriatric Psychiatry*, **20**, 496–497.

Prasher, V. P., Huxley, A., Haque, M. S. (2002). A 24-week, double-blind, placebo-controlled trial of donepezil in patients with Down syndrome and Alzheimer's disease - pilot study. *International Journal of Geriatric Psychiatry*, **17**, 270–278.

Reeves, R. & Garner, C. (2007). A year of unprecedented progress in Down syndrome basic research. *Mental Retardation and Developmental Disabilities Research Reviews*, **13**, 215–220.

Reeves, R., Irving, N., Moran, T., et al. (1995). A mouse model for Down syndrome exhibits learning and behavioral deficits. *Nature Genetics*, **11**, 177–183.

Richardson, R. T. & DeLong, M. R. (1988). A reappraisal of the functions of the nucleus basalis of Meynert. *Trends in Neurosciences*, **11**, 264–267.

Robbins, T. W. & Arnsten, A. F. (2009). The neuropsychopharmacology of fronto-executive function: monoaminergic modulation. *Annual Reviews in Neuroscience*, **32**, 267–287.

Robbins, T. W. & Murphy, E. R. (2006). Behavioural pharmacology: 40+ years of progress, with a focus on glutamate receptors and cognition. *Trends in Pharmacological Sciences*, **27**, 141–148.

Roizen, N. J. (2005). Complementary and alternative therapies for Down syndrome. *Mental Retardation and Developmental Disabilities Research Reviews*, **11**, 149–155.

Ross, M., Galaburda, A., Kemper, T. (1984). Down's syndrome: is there a decreased population of neurons? *Neurology*, **34**, 909–916.

Rynders, J. (1987). History of Down Syndrome. In S. Pueschel (ed.), *New Perspectives on Down Syndrome*, pp. 1–17. Baltimore: Brookes.

Sabbagh, M. N. (2009). Drug development for Alzheimer's disease: where are we now and where are we headed? *American Journal of Geriatric Pharmacotherapy*, **7**, 167–185.

Salman, M. (2002). Systematic review of the effect of therapeutic dietary supplements and drugs on cognitive function in subjects with Down syndrome. *European Journal of Pediatric Neurology*, **6**, 213–219.

Scerif, G. & Karmiloff-Smith, A. (2005). The dawn of cognitive genetics? Crucial developmental caveats. *Trends in Cognitive Sciences*, **9**, 126–135.

Sigman, M. & Ruskin, E. (1999). Continuity and change in the social competence of children with autism, Down syndrome and developmental delays. *Monographs of the Society for Research in Child Development*, **64**, 1–113.

Slaby, A. E. & Tancredi, L. R. (2001). Micropharmacology: treating disturbances of mood, thought, and behavior as specific neurotransmitter dysregulations rather than as clinical syndromes. *Primary Psychiatry*, **8**, 28–32.

Spear, L. P. (2000). The adolescent brain and age-related behavioral manifestations. *Neuroscience and Biobehavioral Reviews*, **24**, 417–463.

Stafstrom, C. E. (1993). Epilepsy in Down syndrome: clinical aspects and possible mechanisms. *American Journal on Mental Retardation*, **98**, 12–26.

Sutor, B., Hansen, M. R., Black, J. L. (2006). Obsessive compulsive disorder treatment in patients with Down syndrome: a case series. *Down Syndrome Research and Practice*, **10**, 1–3.

Thompson, B. L. & Stanwood, G. D. (2009). Pleiotropic effects of neurotransmission during development: modulators of modularity. *Journal of Autism and Developmental Disorders*, **39**, 260–268.

Uhlhaas, P. J., Roux, F., Singer, W., et al. (2009). The development of neural synchrony reflects late maturation and restructuring of functional networks in humans. *Proceedings of the National Academy of Sciences of the United States of America*, **106**, 9866–9871.

Vicari, S. (2004). Memory development and intellectual disabilities. *Acta Paediatrica Supplement*, **93**, 60–63; discussion 63–64.

Vicari, S., Caselli, M. C., Tonucci, F. (2000). Asynchrony of lexical and morphosyntactic development in children with Down syndrome. *Neuropsychologia*, **38**, 634–644.

Vicari, S., Marotta, L., Carlesimo, G. A. (2004). Verbal short-term memory in Down's syndrome: an articulatory loop deficit? *Journal of Intellectual Disability Research*, **48**, 80–92.

Vinkers, C. H., Mirza, N. R., Olivier, B., Kahn, R. S. (2010). The inhibitory GABA system as a therapeutic target for cognitive symptoms in schizophrenia: investigational agents in the pipeline. *Expert Opinion in Investigational Drugs*, **19**(10), 1217–1233.

Vitiello, B. (1998). Pediatric psychopharmacology and the interaction between drugs and the developing brain. *Canadian Journal of Psychiatry*, **43**, 582–584.

Wang, H., Hu, Y., Tsien, J. Z. (2006). Molecular and systems mechanisms of memory consolidation and storage. *Progress in Neurobiology*, **79**, 123–135.

Wetmore, D. Z. & Garner, C. C. (2010). Emerging pharmacotherapies for neurodevelopmental disorders. *Journal of Developmental and Behavioral Pediatrics*, **31**, 564–581.

Wisniewski, K. (1990). Down syndrome children often have brain with maturation delay, retardation of growth, and cortical dysgenesis. *American Journal of Medical Genetics*, **7**, 274–281.

Wisniewski, K. E., Laure-Kamionowska, M., Connell, F., Wen, G. Y. (1986). Neuronal density and synaptogenesis in the postnatal stage of brain maturation in Down syndrome.

In C. J. Epstein (ed.), *The Neurobiology of Down Syndrome*, pp. 29–45. New York: Raven Press.

Woo, N. H. & Lu, B. (2006). Regulation of cortical interneurons by neurotrophins: from development to cognitive disorders. *Neuroscientist*, **1**, 43–56.

Worley, P. F., Baraban, J. M., Snyder, S. H. (1987). Beyond receptors: multiple second-messenger systems in brain. *Annals of Neurology*, **21**, 217–229.

Yan, J. (2003). Canadian Association of Neuroscience Review: development and plasticity of the auditory cortex. *Canadian Journal of Neurological Science*, **30**, 189–200.

Yates, M., Simpson, J., Maloney, A. F. J., et al. (1983). Catecholamines and cholinergic enzymes in pre-senile and senile Alzheimer-type dementia and Down's syndrome. *Brain Research*, **280**, 119–126.

Zito, J., Safer, D., Dosreis, S., et al. (2003). Psychotropic practice patterns for youth. *Archives of Pediatric and Adolescent Medicine*, **157**, 17–25.

Section 3 Pharmacological and medical management and treatment

Chapter

8

Early medical caretaking and follow-up

Alberto Rasore Quartino

Introduction

Down syndrome (DS) is caused by trisomy of chromosome 21 and is the most common autosomal disorder in man, occurring in approximately 1/1000 newborns. Main phenotypic traits are cognitive and language impairment, neuromotor dysfunction, growth reduction, congenital heart disease, immune dysfunction and autoimmune disorders, early ageing and pathological ageing. These traits can be associated with various diseases that are partly responsible for shorter life in people with DS and for the appearance of secondary disability, which greatly affects their well-being.

The main concern of clinicians who care for children with DS is to prevent or to treat these diseases, as early as possible, in order to hamper the appearance of severe clinical consequences.

The concept of early caretaking in its common meaning is early in life – even in prenatal life, as it has been recently suggested – but another meaning can be important as well: that of early medical intervention in relation to the course of the diseases.

In the last 30 to 40 years, DS experienced outstanding changes in quality and duration of life, the causes of which are numerous and can be exemplified in early rehabilitation, in more diffuse social integration, including life in one's own family, participation in mainstream schooling and employment, and last but not least, in more sensible and accurate medical care from birth and throughout life.

A brief survey of some of the most common diseases and their treatment, pointing out early medical intervention and its meaning, follows.

Congenital malformations

Congenital malformations are an important item in DS healthcare. Luckily at present, they are easily diagnosed through echocardiography, even before birth.

Congenital heart disease is the most frequent among the known malformations in DS, appearing in 40%–50% of DS newborns (less than 1% in non-trisomic infants). In mosaic cases, congenital heart disease is less frequent (30%) and less severe (Marino & DeZorzi, 1993). Atrioventricular canal defect is the prevailing form (36%–47%). Early diagnosis is essential, as almost all forms are successfully treated by surgical correction.

Neurocognitive Rehabilitation of Down Syndrome, eds. Jean-Adolphe Rondal, Juan Perera, and Donna Spiker. Published by Cambridge University Press. © Cambridge University Press 2011.

Increased pulmonary flux is the main characteristic of the cardiac anomalies in DS. Symptoms develop early and pulmonary hypertension is a rapidly ensuing consequence; cardiomegaly, hepatic cirrhosis, and heart failure follow. Obstructive pulmonary vascular disease is the most severe complication, occurring earlier than in non-DS children and preventing surgical correction of the underlying heart defect. Surgery should therefore be performed as early as possible after birth, as soon as the clinical conditions allow it. Today surgical mortality is greatly reduced to approximately the same level as that obtained in children without DS, and the long-term prognosis is good.

Congenital heart disease in DS is less severe and more predictable than in other infants and often results of surgery are even more favorable than those obtained in patients with the same malformation, but without DS (Marino et al., 2004).

Gastrointestinal malformations have an increased incidence in DS as well. Duodenal stenosis (4%–7%) represents nearly half of all the congenital duodenal stenoses. Hirschprung's disease occurs in 3%–4% of DS newborn infants versus 0.02% in other neonates. Relatively frequent are pancreas annulare and anal imperforation. Diagnosis at birth is easy, through accurate clinical examination and ecography. Timely surgical correction must follow.

Malformations of the urinary tract (congenital hydronephrosis, obstructive uropathy) are less frequent but must be kept in mind.

Sensory defects

Ocular abnormalities are more frequent in DS than in other children, averaging 38% from birth to one year of age. The percentage increases up to 80% before puberty. Some of these abnormalities do not have any pathological connotation, like Brushfield nodules and epicanthal folds. Of clinical importance, however, are refractory defects (either hypermetropia or myopia), strabismus, and cataract, because they all decrease normal visual acuity, adding an organic defect to the preexisting cognitive impairment. Early diagnosis is crucial, in order to correct the anomaly in time, preventing the subsequent deterioration and the secondary consequences on intellectual development. Correction is done mainly through spectacles that can be well tolerated, even by infants, who receive a real benefit. Surgical correction should be taken into account, when and if necessary, as for strabismus and cataract.

DS children who are affected by hearing abnormalities are not able to use the necessary strategies to make up for their deficiency, so that their global cognitive development will be impaired. Data on the frequency of hearing defects in DS are controversial, but it is thought that nearly 80% of people at any age have a partial or total hearing defect, mostly a conductive one. There exists an excess of middle ear pathology, which is commonly the consequence of a typically serous otitis beginning in early age. Owing to its scarce and usually non-specific symptoms, it can persist for a very long time. Because therapy is often neglected, hearing defects are long-term unwanted consequences.

A preventive approach to hearing problems in DS children must be considered and periodic checks should be done regularly in order to help them to maintain good communication ability and satisfying socialization. Hearing should be checked at birth through otoacustic emissions that do not require active participation of the infant. More sophisticated and accurate techniques, such as auditory evoked potentials, should be used later for a specific diagnosis.

Immune disorders and autoimmune diseases

Noncontroversial immunological defects in DS are the following: a small thymus with structural anomalies and lymphocyte depletion, increased antibody levels, altered maturation of T-lymphocytes, and a high number of functionally deficient NK-cells.

Several tentative therapies for enhancing organic defenses have been proposed over the years. Zinc supplementation showed a positive variation of some immune parameters and a reduction of recurrent infections (Franceschi et al., 1988; Licastro et al., 1994). Selenium supplementation would reduce the rate of infections in DS children, with a possible immunoregulatory mechanism (Annerén et al., 1990). Further investigations are needed before using these and other substances as routine therapy in DS children.

Frequent autoimmune diseases in DS are: thyroiditis (15%), celiac disease (CD) (6%), diabetes mellitus type I (1%), juvenile idiopathic arthritis (1%), and thrombocytopenia. Hypothyroidism is frequent in DS, even if most people with DS have a normally functioning thyroid. Primary persistent congenital hypothyroidism affects 0.7%–1.0% of DS newborns (0.015%–0.20% of normal neonates). Acquired hypothyroidism varies between 13% and 54% in DS versus 0.8%–1.1% in the general population. Increased values of thyroid autoantibodies are found as well in about 30% (13%–34%) of people with DS.

The pathogenesis of hypothyroidism is a result of either autoimmunity or progressive gland hypofunction and hypoplasia. Autoimmune thyroiditis is uncommon before eight years of age, becoming more frequent thereafter (Karlsson et al., 1998). Generally, the disease is asymptomatic in the beginning, showing increased values of thyroid stimulating hormone (TSH) while the levels of thyroid hormones (T3 and T4) remain within normal limits. Clinical symptoms appear progressively when hormone values decrease to subnormal. The symptoms (reduced growth velocity, weight increase, constipation, dry skin, hair loss, developmental problems, learning difficulties, easy fatigue, mood changes, and depression) in DS are often difficult to diagnose because they can be confused with some neurological and behavioral aspects of the syndrome itself.

Because hypothyroidism interferes with normal neuronal metabolism causing permanent damage and making early clinical diagnosis not particularly easy, periodic laboratory tests are strongly recommended; there is still no consensus on the age at which they should start or on their periodicity. It is suggested that these tests begin after the first year of life and continue with yearly checks at least until adolescence. Substitutive therapy with thyroxine should be started as soon as the diagnosis of hypothyroidism is made and carried on throughout life.

Compensated hypothyroidism or hyperthyrotropinemia (elevated TSH and normal free T3/T4) is considered a benign condition that mostly precedes frank hypothyroidism. Moreover, in DS increased TSH is often transient and reversible. Some authors have found significantly reduced intelligence quotients (IQs) in people with isolated hyperthyrotropinemia. One third of these patients, with positive thyroid antibodies, will in time develop true hypothyroidism. Therefore, pharmacological treatment of these cases is advisable – it can have a protective effect on the thyroid and also prevent, or at least slow down, the appearance of the disease.

Celiac disease, or gluten intolerance, is an autoimmune disorder, causing serious damage to intestinal mucosa. Gluten is a component of wheat, rye, barley, spelt, kamut, and triticum; it is absent in maize, rice, buckwheat, manioc, millet, sorghum, and quinoia. CD develops in early childhood, some time after the introduction of gluten into the diet. Its severe form, which today is rather uncommon, manifests with diarrhea, bulky stools, prominent abdomen, and poor growth. At present, possibly associated with the late introduction of gluten in alimentation, more frequent, moderate, or atypical forms are described, appearing late in childhood or in adolescence and even in adulthood. The patients show hypovitaminosis, sideropenic anemia, stunted growth, and scarce or absent intestinal symptoms. Asymptomatic or silent cases are observed as well. Prevalence of CD in the general population is 1/133 (Fasano et al., 2003). In DS the prevalence is definitely higher, varying from 5% to 15%, as shown in different population studies (Bonamico et al., 2001).

The clinical diagnosis of CD in DS is not easy, therefore laboratory screening tests are usually required. They consist of dosage of antiendomysial and/or transglutaminase antibodies and screening of total IgA levels. The diagnosis is confirmed by intestinal biopsy that shows different degrees of flattening of the jejunal mucosa and lymphocyte infiltration.

The elimination of gluten from the diet, which results in complete recovery, is the only treatment. The gluten-free diet must be kept up for an indefinite period. Therefore, high levels of commitment and continuous surveillance are required from patients and their relatives, as compliance is usually difficult to obtain.

Cancer

Although cancer is of uncommon occurrence in DS, basic research has revealed interesting biological specificities and strong correlations between chromosome 21 and leukemia. The tumor profile of DS is unique and not shared with other genetic conditions. It displays a significant incidence of some cancers, while others are rare.

There is a reduced risk of solid tumors in DS, except for testicular tumors that have been estimated to be 50-fold more frequent (Satgé et al., 1997). Retinoblastoma seems to be more frequent as well (10-fold more). Ovarian cancer could be slightly over-represented (Satgé et al., 2006). Neuroblastoma and medulloblastoma, which are frequently reported in children, are rare in DS (Satgé & Bénard, 2008). On the other hand, in children with DS there is a 20-fold increased risk of developing leukemia (Goldacre et al., 2004). DS children account for about 3% of children with acute lymphoblastic leukemia (ALL) and for 5%–8% of children with acute myeloblastic leukemia (AML); 20% of leukemias of DS are acute megakaryoblastic leukemia (AMKL), an otherwise very unusual form of leukemia, which among DS is 500-times more frequent.

An increased sensitivity to chemotherapy is observed in DS (Ravindranath, 2003). However, the outcome of ALL in DS children is equivalent or slightly inferior to that in non-DS children. This observed poorer outcome is possibly a result of a greater infection rate or to less intensive salvage offered to DS children in relapse. In these patients, great attention should be paid to methotrexate dosage because of its significant treatment-related toxicity. This could occur owing to its reduced clearance and also to increased intracellular transport.

On the contrary, AML (particularly AMKL) in DS children has an extremely high event-free survival (80%–100%) and lower relapse rate (<15%), compared to that in non-DS children, who show a very poor outcome with a lower than 25% cure (Taub & Ge, 2005). This better outcome of AMKL is of multifactorial origin.

One of the most singular expressions of DS is the so-called transient leukemia (TL), which is characterized by the accumulation of immature megakaryocytes in peripheral blood, bone marrow, and liver (Zipursky, 2003). TL is detected in approximately 10% of DS newborn infants, and might not be recognized in mild cases without the careful observation of peripheral blood smears, being largely clinically silent. Only about 10% of cases are routinely diagnosed (Bradbury, 2005). TL has a high incidence of spontaneous remissions, but in some instances it is life threatening; the infant may be born with *hydrops fetalis* and may show evidence of pulmonary hypertension, respiratory failure, hepatic failure, and multiorgan failure. Prenatal and neonatal mortality may range from 11% to 55%. Up to 30% of those who achieve spontaneous remission will subsequently develop a severe form of AMKL within the first four years of life (Massey, 2005).

No therapy is generally required as most cases of TL recover spontaneously, but it is not clear yet whether patients with particularly severe forms of TL should be treated and how. Repeated courses of low-dose cytosine arabinoside have been used successfully in a small number of children (Cominetti et al., 1985; Zipursky, 1996). This raises the intriguing possibility that such treatment may prevent the subsequent occurrence of AMKL (Ravindranath, 2005).

Musculoskeletal disorders

Musculoskeletal problems are often present in DS. Muscular hypotonia is almost constant and is commonly considered of central origin. General hypotonia is significantly related to a number of medical conditions, like recurrent dislocation of the hip, subluxation and dislocation of the patella, genu valgum, and pes planus. These conditions are important causes of walking problems and sometimes of severe static problems, such as scoliosis and kyphosis. Prevention is essential and is performed through yearly clinical follow-up, early and correct mobilization, active life, and sport activities. Surgical correction of the underlying conditions may be required as well.

In recent years, atlanto-axial instability (AAI) has received great attention, although this condition is not specific to DS, where AAI is present in 10% to 20% of cases (Pueschel & Schola, 1987; Menzes & Ryken, 1992). Instability of the atlanto-axial joint occurs when the distance between the first two cervical vertebrae that form the joint is greater than 4.5 mm on lateral cervical spine radiographs taken in flexion, neutral, and extension. The instability is generally asymptomatic, but an increased risk of subluxation and dislocation exists after cervical or head traumas, sudden and rough movements of the head, or neck manipulation during surgical procedures (Mitchell et al., 1995). Neurological complications because of cervical cord compression can follow. Symptoms can be variable and often are difficult to diagnose. Staggering gait, head tilt, torticollis, neck pain, hyperreflexia, urinary incontinence, paraplegia, or quadriplegia, alone or in combination, can be found. Accurate clinical observation is of paramount importance for the early diagnosis of subluxation.

Screening procedures to detect individuals at risk were recommended. It is suggested that a set of lateral cervical spine radiographs are performed when the child is between three and five years of age. The prognostic value of the radiographic diagnosis has been challenged, because AAI only rarely (2%) will progress to subluxation, but for the moment it seems prudent to continue the current recommendation (Cohen, 2006). Children at risk should not be allowed to practice sports where cervical injuries are possible, like somersaulting, trampolining, diving, boxing, etc. In symptomatic cases, vertebral fusion is recommended (Aicardi, 1992).

Short stature

Short stature is characteristic of children and adults with DS. Commonly, stature stabilizes at minus 2–3 standard deviations on normal growth charts. The mechanisms responsible for short stature are not completely explained yet. Most authors have confirmed normal or subnormal growth hormone (GH) secretion. Nevertheless, therapy with human recombinant GH (hrGH) has been proposed for DS children with impaired growth, irrespective of their GH and insulin-like growth factor-I (IGF-I) levels. Acceleration of growth velocity and increase of stature were obtained, but after cessation of treatment, growth velocity slowed down. The risk of complications related to prolonged administration (hypertension, diabetes mellitus, intracranial neoplasia) (Monson, 2003) has not been sufficiently evaluated (Lanes, 2004). Recent studies seem to exclude significant side effects after long-term treatment (Pallotti et al., 2002), but further observations are needed. At present hrGH therapy has no indication in DS children without GH deficiency (Annerén et al., 2000).

Sleep problems

Disruption of the sleep cycle in DS has been reported in numerous studies. Its commonest form is obstructive sleep apnea (OSA), occurring in 20%–50% of people with DS. It develops for a combination of causes, including small upper airway, midfacial hypoplasia, micrognatia, adenotonsillar hypertrophy, and muscular hypotonia causing glossoptosis. In DS, central sleep apneas are increased as well, possibly related to a dysfunction of the central respiratory control at the brainstem level (Ferri et al., 1997). Repeated bouts of apnea during sleep result in persistent oxygen desaturation, which may have dramatic consequences in brain functions leading to cognitive impairment, reduced memory, depression, and early ageing. There is an obvious relationship between the number of apneas and cognitive impairment: the more apneas a subject has, the more difficulties he/she has in visuoperceptual skills, including orientation (Andreou et al., 2002). Overnight polysomnography is the technique of choice to diagnose the number and extent of sleep apneas. Surgery is the preferred treatment for the correction of the underlying defect that favors the occurrence of the airways obstruction and, hence, the apneas. Adenotonsillectomy generally improves the respiratory condition. Recently introduced for patients with neuromuscular diseases, continuous positive pressure ventilation is a noninvasive therapy that has been tentatively applied in DS, with apparently good results (Anzai et al., 2006).

Seizure disorders

Historically, epilepsy has not been considered a major component of DS. Its prevalence ranges from 8% to 10%. Pueschel et al. (1991) studied a large cohort of people with DS (405 subjects) and found that 8.1% had seizure disorders with two peaks at onset: 40% of the patients began the epileptic activity before one year of age while a further 40% had seizures between 20 and 30 years old. In the first group, infantile spasms and tonic–clonic seizures with myoclonus were observed; in the young adult group, generalized tonic–clonic seizures and partial seizures were most frequent.

Late-onset epilepsy shows an age-related increase in DS, being present in 11.4% of aged people. Seizures are often an early sign of Alzheimer's disease (AD) and represent a severe complication of the condition. Up to 84% of DS people with AD have seizure disorders (McCarron et al., 2005).

Drug treatment is the major form of therapy for people with seizure disorders, but the management of epilepsy is not limited to the prescription of drugs. Education and support of parents and relatives, counseling and help with educational problems in children, and management of behavioral difficulties in all patients may be important as well.

Normal and pathological ageing

A very important and up-to-date issue concerning DS is ageing, as survival of people with the syndrome has greatly increased through the years: now people with DS can reach 60 years old and over. Early ageing is a constant in DS adults, who may show physical signs of senescence as much as 20 years earlier than non-DS people (Service & Hahn, 2003). A constant but variable intellectual decline is observed, consisting mainly in a reduction in the ability to elaborate abstract thought. Memory, mental status, and psychomotor function show a slight progressive decrease.

Chronic oxidative stress may be the main cause of early ageing in DS. Its progressive increase with advancing age may be related to the lesions of AD that appear in approximately 30% of DS people after the age of 50 years. This form of dementia combines disorders of cognitive functions and behavior, modifying the personality. Affected people show a deterioration of mental and emotional responses, abnormal excitation or apathy, and loss of the acquired vocabulary. The course of the disease is more rapid than in non-DS people.

Prevention and treatment of premature normal and pathological senescence in DS is definitely a difficult task. The ageing in DS people is very sensitive to their environment, and cognition, autonomy, and behavior, therefore assigning great value to the role played by families and caregivers in helping them to maintain or even enhance their abilities in adult life.

The use of antioxidants like nicotinamide, L-carnitine, lipoic acid and dehydroascorbic acid, and some nutrients has been proposed, but with meager practical results. The efficacy on ageing of antioxidant substances extracted from green tea (epigallocatechin-3-gallate) and from gingko biloba is currently being investigated (Mazza et al., 2006; Nagle et al., 2006; Zaveri, 2006). Very exciting results have been obtained recently in animal studies: it has been demonstrated that epigallocatechin-3-gallate administration is effective in rescuing the main neurological features in transgenic mice (Guedj et al., 2009).

A specific pharmacological approach for AD has been attempted with drugs acting on the cholinergic system. This approach is aimed at containing cognitive impairment through these molecules, based on the hypothesis that a functional deficit in that system is responsible for the cognitive impairment observed (Coyle et al., 1983). Acetylcholinesterase inhibitors (donezepil, rivastigmine, and galantamine) as well as memantine are the most promising drugs at present and could improve the cognitive function and behavioral disorders of AD. Their action is limited in time and side effects are observed in some patients. Even if the results obtained in AD seem promising, the samples studied are still limited and therefore more extended investigations are required. It should be noted that the use of donepezil has been extended to aged DS people without dementia, with positive results (Heller et al., 2003, Johnson et al., 2003). Interestingly, preliminary clinical trials have shown improvement of language, memory, and attention in small numbers of children and adolescents with DS given rivastigmine (Heller et al., 2006) or donepezil (Spiridigliozzi et al., 2007).

Nutritional problems

Great attention has been given to nutritional problems in DS for multiple reasons: the presence of considerable obesity among people with DS, of the possible existence of food intolerance or allergy, and of vitamin deficiencies.

Although obesity was considered a common problem in children and adults with DS, presently its frequency is markedly reduced. Prevention begins early and consists of a balanced diet, accompanied by correct physical activity. Treatment should not restrict food and energy intake excessively, but should work out a balanced diet and increase motor and sport activities.

No specific food allergies or intolerances exist in people with DS. As regards definite vitamin and mineral deficiencies, many studies exist in the scientific literature but results are mostly contradictory (Pueschel & Pueschel, 1992). On the premise of real or supposed vitamin deficiencies, high-dose vitamin and mineral supplementations have been proposed for many years. The main goal was not only to correct the deficiency, but also to improve the cognitive and behavioral situations of affected people. We must recall that vitamin action is effective at very low doses. At high doses, they no longer act as vitamins, but as true drugs. In this way, they can be toxic and also interfere with the action of other vitamins or drugs. A summary of the toxic effects of vitamins can be seen in Rasore Quartino (2007).

Unconventional therapies have been proposed for a long time, often without a scientific basis, in order to enhance cognitive functions of children with DS and even to modify their phenotypic aspects.

Sicca cell therapy consisted in injections of fetal tissue of sheep, goats, and rabbits.

The U-series proposed by Turkel in 1975 consisted of numerous different compounds, including vitamins, minerals, thyroid hormone, enzymes, and medications, to be administered several times a day. Vitamin and mineral mixtures in very high doses (up to 333 times the recommended doses) were proposed by Harrel et al. in 1981.

Pituitary extracts, 5-hydroxytryptophan (a precursor of serotonin, the blood levels of which are reduced in DS), glutamic acid, dimethyl-sulfoxide (a solvent extracted from the wood pulp), piracetam (a derivative of gamma-amino butyric acid), Prozac (an antidepressive drug), and Focalin (generally used in the treatment of attention deficit and hyperactivity disorders) are only some of the many substances that have been administered to children with DS in the last 30 years (Rasore Quartino, 2007). Although exceptional results have been claimed by the proposers, repeated scientific controls did not show any effect on intellectual development or behavioral activities (Salman, 2002).

Basic research is proceeding actively and is currently working on approaches that are of great interest. Therapeutic strategies are envisaged in the field of genetic disorders such as those encountered in trisomy 21, but without significant practical results to date. Pathological changes can be the consequence of the global effect of a supplementary chromosome fragment; the hypothesized treatment should be effected by removing the chromosome. In case there is a direct relationship between the increased expression of one gene or of a few genes and a given phenotype, it should be necessary to regulate the altered gene or the protein dosage, or to regulate the altered pathway. Primary targets of therapeutic interventions should be genes on chromosome 21, and secondary target genes on other chromosomes or downstream pathways. Current investigations on polymorphisms in the genes involved in folate metabolism agree that abnormal folate metabolism is an increased risk factor for having a child with DS. Until now, periconceptional folic acid supplementation did not show any reduction in the births of affected children.

In conclusion, experience has shown that most diseases in children and adults with DS can definitely be prevented and currently take advantage of medical intervention, especially if proposed early in age. The results obtained are still unsatisfactory, but we must persevere in these studies to further improve the lives of people with DS.

Healthcare guidelines should be greatly expanded, as should practical prevention measures like correct alimentation, hygienic procedures, and vaccinations. Multicenter and multidisciplinary clinical and biological investigations are required to accomplish the task. Scientific studies are underway to increase the knowledge of the biological basis of trisomy 21.

Basic research also currently envisages promising lines of investigation. Various methods of correcting the effects of the supernumerary chromosome during prenatal life are under study in many laboratories and practical results are expected in the near future.

Summary

Down syndrome (DS) is associated with congenital malformations, immune deficiencies, leukemia, and cognitive impairment. In recent years, therapies have been sought in order to improve the clinical conditions and reduce the cognitive impairment of the affected people. Long years of experience have confirmed that early medical intervention is more effective in both the cure and the prevention of secondary disabilities. Moreover, it is essential for the success of rehabilitation and social integration, resulting in a better quality of life of affected persons.

The surgical approach to congenital heart disease and gastrointestinal malformations is discussed, as well as pharmacological treatments for thyroid disorders, leukemia, short stature, and other conditions of medical interest. Early intervention for correction of sensory defects is examined. Early diagnosis of celiac disease and subsequent dietary changes can avoid serious consequences. Suggestions for appropriate diet and vitamin and mineral supplementations are given. Moreover, the importance of following healthcare guidelines is emphasized.

Unconventional therapies are briefly discussed. These therapies have been advocated with the object of remedying the intellectual impairment or phenotypic features: to date, unfortunately, they have not shown any positive results, but only negative effects on patients and always severe disappointments for the parents. Lastly, the principles of new research on molecular biology of chromosome 21 are noted.

References

Aicardi, J. (1992). *Diseases of the Nervous System in Childhood*. London: McKeith Press.

Andreou, G., Galanopoulou, C., Gourgoulianis, K., Karapetsas, A., Molyvdas, P. (2002). Cognitive status in Down syndrome individuals with sleep disorders breathing deficits (SDB). *Brain and Cognition*, **50**, 145–149.

Annerén, G., Magnusson, C. G. M., Nordvall, S. L. (1990). Increase in serum concentrations of IgG2 and IgG4 by selenium supplementation in children with Down's syndrome. *Archives of Disease in Childhood*, **65**, 1353–1355.

Annerén, G., Tuvemo, T., Gustafsson, J. (2000). Growth hormone therapy in young children with Down and Prader-Willi syndromes. *Growth Hormone & IGF Research*, **10**(Suppl B), S87–S91.

Anzai, Y., Ohya, T., Yanagi, K. (2006). Treatment of sleep apnea syndrome in a Down syndrome patient with behavioural problems by non-invasive positive pressure ventilation: a successful case report. *No To Hattatsu/Brain and Development*, **38**, 32–36.

Bonamico, M., Mariani, P., Danesi, H. M., et al. (2001). Prevalence and clinical picture of celiac disease in Italian Down syndrome patients: a multicenter study. *Journal of Pediatric Gastroenterology and Nutrition*, **33**, 139–143.

Bradbury, J. (2005). High leukaemia cure rate in Down's syndrome explained. *Lancet*, **6**, 134.

Cohen, W. I. (2006). Current dilemmas in Down syndrome clinical care: celiac disease, thyroid disorders and atlanto-axial instability. *American Journal of Medical Genetics. Part C, Seminars in Medical Genetics*, **142C**, 141–148.

Cominetti, M., Rasore Quartino, A., Acutis, M. S., Vignola, G. (1985). Neonato con sindrome di Down e leucemia mieloide acuta. Difficoltà diagnostiche fra forma maligna e sindrome mieloproliferativa. *Pathologica*, **77**, 625–630.

Coyle, J. T., Price, D. L., DeLong, M. R. (1983). Alzheimer's disease: a disorder of cholinergic innervation. *Science*, **219**, 1184–1190.

Fasano, A., Berti, I., Gerarduzzi, T., et al. (2003). Prevalence of celiac disease in at-risk and not-at-risk groups in the United States: a large multicenter study. *Archives of Internal Medicine*, **163**, 286–292.

Ferri, R., Curzi-Dascalova, L., Del Gracco, S., Elia, M., et al. (1997). Respiratory patterns during sleep in Down's syndrome: importance of central apnoeas. *Journal of Sleep Research*, **6**, 134–141.

Franceschi, C., Chiricolo, M., Licastro, F., et al. (1988). Oral zinc supplementation in Down's syndrome: restoration of thymic endocrine activity and of some immune defects. *Journal of Mental Deficiency Research*, **32**, 169–181.

Goldacre, M. J., Wotton, C. J., Seagrott, V., Yeates, D. (2004). Cancer and immune related diseases associated with Down's syndrome: a record linkage study. *Archives of Disease in Childhood*, **89**, 1014–1017.

Guedj, F., Sébrié, C., Rivals, I., et al. (2009). Green tea polyphenols rescue of brain defects induced by overexpression of DYRK1A. *PLoS ONE*, **4**, e4606.

Harrel, R. J., Capp, R. H., Davis, D. R. (1981). Can nutritional supplements help mentally retarded children? *Proceedings of the National Academy of Sciences United States of America*, **78**: 574–578.

Heller, J. H., Spiridigliozzi, G. A., Crissman, B. G., et al. (2006). Safety and efficacy of rivastigmine in adolescents with Down syndrome: a preliminary 20-week, open-label study. *Journal of Child and Adolescent Psychopharmacology*, **16**, 755–765.

Heller, J.H., Spiridigliozzi, G. A., Sullivan, J. A., et al. (2003). Donepezil for the treatment of language deficits in adults with Down syndrome. A preliminary 24-week open trial. *American Journal of Medical Genetics. Part A, Seminars in Medical Genetics*, **116A**, 111–116.

Johnson, N., Fahey, C., Chicoine, B., Chong, G., Gitelman, D. (2003). Effects of donepezil on cognitive functioning in Down syndrome. *American Journal on Mental Retardation*, **108**, 367–372.

Karlsson, B., Gustafsson, J., Hedow, G., Ivarsson, S. A., Annerén, G. (1998). Thyroid function in children and adolescents with Down syndrome in relation to age, sex, growth velocity and thyroid antibodies. *Archives of Disease in Childhood*, **79**, 242–245.

Lanes, R. (2004). Long-term outcome of growth hormone therapy in children and adolescents. *Treatments in Endocrinology*, **3**, 53–66.

Licastro, F., Chiricolo, M., Moccheggiani, E., et al. (1994). Oral zinc supplementation in Down's syndrome subjects decreased infections and normalized some humoral and cellular immune parameters. *Journal of Intellectual Disability Research*, **38**, 149–162.

Marino, B., Assenza, G., Mileto, F., Digilio, M. (2004). Down syndrome and congenital heart disease. In J. A. Rondal, A. Rasore-Quartino, S. Soresi (eds.), *The Adult with Down Syndrome. A New Challenge for Society*, pp. 39–50. London: Whurr .

Marino, B. & DeZorzi, A. (1993). Congenital heart disease in trisomy 21 mosaicism. *Journal of Pediatrics*, **122**, 500–501.

Massey, G.V. (2005). Transient leukaemia in children with Down syndrome. *Blood Cancer*, **44**, 29–32.

Mazza, M., Capuano, A., Bria, P., Mazza, S. (2006). Gingko biloba and donepezil: a comparison in the treatment of Alzheimer's dementia in a randomized placebo-controlled double-blind study. *European Journal of Neurology*, **13**, 981–985.

McCarron, M., Gill, M., McCallion, P., Begley, C. (2005). Health co-morbidities in ageing persons with Down syndrome and Alzheimer's dementia. *Journal of Intellectual Disability Research*, **49**, 560–566.

Menzes, A. H. & Ryken, T. C. (1992). Craniovertebral anomalies in Down's syndrome. *Pediatric Neurosurgery*, **18**, 24–33.

Mitchell, V., Howard, R., Facer, E. (1995). Down's syndrome and anaesthesia. *Pediatric Anesthesia*, **5**, 379–384.

Monson, J.P. (2003). Long-term experience with GH replacement therapy: efficacy and safety. *European Journal of Endocrinology*, **148**(Suppl 2), S9–S14.

Nagle, D. G., Ferreira, D., Zhou, Y. D. (2006). Epigallocatechin-3-gallate (EGCG): chemical and biomedical perspectives. *Phytochemistry*, **67**, 1849–1855.

Pallotti, S., Giuliano, S., Giambi, C. (2002). Growth disorders in Down's syndrome: growth hormone treatment. *Minerva Endocrinologica*, **27**, 59–64.

Pueschel, S. M., Louis, S., McKnight, P. (1991). Seizure disorders in Down syndrome. *Archives of Neurology*, **48**, 318–320.

Pueschel, S. M. & Pueschel, J. K. (1992). *Biochemical Concerns in Persons with Down's Syndrome*. Baltimore: Brookes.

Pueschel, S. M. & Schola, F. H. (1987). Atlantoaxial instability in individuals with Down syndrome: epidemiologic, radiographic and clinical studies. *Pediatrics*, **80**, 555–560.

Rasore Quartino, A. (2007). Medical therapies in the lifespan. In J. A. Rondal & A. Rasore Quartino (eds.), *Therapies and Rehabilitation in Down Syndrome*, pp. 43–62. Chichester: Wiley.

Ravindranath, Y. (2003). Down syndrome and acute myeloid leukaemia: the paradox of increased risk for leukaemia and heightened sensitivity to chemotherapy (Editorial). *Journal of Clinical Oncology*, **21**, 3385–3387.

Ravindranath, Y. (2005). Down syndrome and leukaemia: new insights into the epidemiology, pathogenesis and treatment. *Pediatric Blood Cancer*, **44**, 1–7.

Salman, M. S. (2002). Systematic review of the effect of therapeutic dietary supplements and drugs on cognitive function in subjects with Down syndrome. *European Journal of Pediatric Neurology*, **6**, 213–219.

Satgé, D. & Bénard, J. (2008). Carcinogenesis in Down syndrome: what can be learned from trisomy 21? *Seminars in Cancer Biology*, **18**, 365–371.

Satgé, D., Honoré, L., Sasco, A. J., et al. (2006). An ovarian dysgerminoma in Down syndrome. Hypothesis about the association. *International Journal of Gynecologic Cancer*, **16**(Suppl 1), 375–379.

Satgé, D., Sasco, A. J., Cure, H., Sommelet, D., Vekemans, M. J. (1997). An excess of testicular germ cell tumors in Down syndrome. Three cases and literature review. *Cancer*, **80**, 929–935.

Service, K. P. & Hahn, J. A. (2003). Issues in aging. The role of the nurse in the care of older people with intellectual and developmental disabilities. *Nursing Clinics of North America*, **38**, 291–312.

Spiridigliozzi, G. A., Heller, J. H., Crissman, B. G., et al. (2007). Preliminary study of the safety and efficacy of donepezil hydrochloride in children with Down syndrome. *American Journal of Medical Genetics. Part A, Seminars in Medical Genetics*, **143A**, 1408–1413.

Taub, J. V. & Ge, Y. (2005). Down syndrome, drug metabolism and chromosome 21. *Pediatric Blood Cancer*, **44**, 33–39.

Turkel, H. (1975). Medical amelioration of Down's syndrome incorporating the orthomolecular approach. *Journal of Orthomolecular Psychiatry*, **4**, 102–115.

Zaveri, N. T. (2006). Green tea and its polyphenolic catechins: medicinal uses in cancer and noncancer applications. *Life Science*, **78**, 2073–2080.

Zipursky, A. (1996). The treatment of children with acute megakaryoblastic leukaemia who have Down syndrome. *Journal of Pediatric Haematology and Oncology*, **18**, 59–62.

Zipursky, A. (2003). Transient leukaemia – a benign form of leukaemia in newborn infants with trisomy 21. *British Journal of Haematology*, **120**, 930–938.

Chapter

9

Evaluation and management of cardiovascular diseases in Down syndrome

Guy Dembour and Stephane Moniotte

Introduction

Down syndrome (DS) is the most common chromosomal anomaly. Its overall worldwide prevalence is approximately 10 per 10,000 live births, a number which tended to increase over the recent years. The increasing average maternal age at childbirth mostly explains the elevated prevalence of the syndrome. In the Netherlands, the prevalence of DS was estimated to be 16 per 10,000 live births in 2003 (Weijerman et al., 2008). Similarly, DS accounts for up to 8% of all registered cases of congenital anomalies in Europe (De Walle & Cornel, 1995).

Historically, the association between DS and congenital heart disease (CHD) was described very early on. Down, in his original description of 1866, mentioned the possibility of cardiac disease and reported that "the circulation is feeble."

In 1894, Garrod reported the association between DS and CHD. In the early twentieth century, the presence of CHD was used as a feature to distinguish DS from cretinism. The specific association between DS and atrioventricular septal defect (AVSD) was reported by Ablert in 1924 and more accurately by Helen Taussig in 1947. The incidence of CHD in DS was first described with very wide variations, from 16% to 62% (Berg et al., 1960). The current observations demonstrate that infants with DS have a 40%–50% risk of CHD (Wells et al., 1994; Marino, 1996; Stoll et al., 1998; Freeman et al., 2008; Weijerman et al., 2008). The prevalence of CHD is much lower in infants with a mosaic DS. Marino and DeZorzi (1993) described such a subgroup of 27 patients with a mosaic syndrome, only eight patients (29.6%) presenting a CHD, which in general seemed less severe than in patients with complete trisomy 21. This difference in phenotypic expression could possibly be explained by a partial aneuploidy.

The most frequently reported CHDs in DS do not have the same distribution as in the general population. Atrioventricular septal defects are clearly the most commonly observed lesions in Europe and North America, accounting for approximately 50% of all cardiac anomalies in patients with DS. The other cardiac malformations encountered in DS are ventricular septal defects (VSDs), in about 30% of affected patients, secundum atrial septal defects (ASDs), isolated tetralogy of Fallot (TOF), and patent ductus arteriosus (PDAs). The incidence of these CHDs varies in the other regions of the world: in Asia and in Central and South America, AVSDs are far less frequent, VSD being identified in about 40% of the cases, and AVSD being the second most common lesion (Lo et al., 1989; Hoe et al., 1990; Jacobs

Neurocognitive Rehabilitation of Down Syndrome, eds. Jean-Adolphe Rondal, Juan Perera, and Donna Spiker. Published by Cambridge University Press. © Cambridge University Press 2011.

et al., 2000). In Mexico, secundum ASD is the most frequent defect (about 40%), while complete AVSD is reported in only 8% of DS children (Figueroa et al., 2003).

Other types of CHD are less frequent in DS infants: pulmonary and aortic stenosis or atresia, double outlet right ventricle, and isolated coarctation of the aorta. Interestingly, some other defects are almost never observed in DS: viscero-atrial situs anomalies, atrioventricular valve atresia, and truncus arteriosus or transposition of the great arteries. Ongoing efforts to delineate the role of specific genes in the distribution of each defect in these various populations should, in the near future, allow us to better understand the molecular mechanisms underlying DS.

The sex ratio in DS is approximately three males for two females (De Grouchy & Turleau, 1982; Stoll et al., 1998; Frid et al., 1999), but females seem to be more often affected by CHD (Pinto et al., 1990; Freeman et al., 2008). The genetic substrate for this sexual dimorphism is not really understood.

The presence of CHD in DS is sometimes associated with congenital anomalies of the gastrointestinal system. In 1999, Torfs and Christianson described a cohort of 687 DS infants: 385 of them (56%) had CHD, and 52 presented various gastrointestinal malformations. Among them, 24 infants out of 28 (85.7%) with duodenal atresia and 7 infants out of 10 (70%) with Hirschprung disease had a CHD.

A number of authors have studied the association between maternal risk factors and DS. If maternal age is a well-known factor, consanguinity also seems to increase the incidence of DS, while the role of maternal diabetes remains controversial. The possible interactions between trisomy 21 and environmental factors as an additional risk factor for associated defects were also studied. It appears that maternal smoking could be associated with an increased frequency of some CHDs (AVSD and TOF). In contrast, alcohol consumption during gestation, the mother's ethnic origin, age, and parity were not found to be significant risk factors for CHD (Torfs & Christianson, 1999).

From a surgical perspective and until the early 1990s, postoperative morbidity and mortality following AVSD repair was high, to the point that some centers questioned the advisability of repairing these defects, even in the general population. However, important advances in the preoperative assessment, surgical management, and postoperative intensive care have occurred over the last 15 years and DS is no longer considered as a risk factor for surgical repair. The mid- and long-term advantages obtained with surgery versus a limited medical therapy of DS patients with AVSD are no longer discussed. The current practice favoring early (4–6 months of age) cardiac repair allowed a tremendous and objective improvement of their prognosis and quality of life. Furthermore, a similar improvement in the management of associated malformations, a broader use of antibiotics, and specific preventive healthcare programs for DS children worked as supplementary positive factors to explain their improved overall outcome. It is therefore not surprising to see a substantial increase of life expectancy in DS patients, with a median age of death of 25 years in an American series from 1983 and 47 years in a cohort from 1997 (Yang et al., 2002). A similar study from Israel reported a death rate of 57% at 14 years in 1979, a number reduced to only 10.5% in 1996 (Merrick, 2000).

Pathophysiology of cardiovascular disease in Down syndrome

Complete AVSDs and large VSDs, independently of their genetic substrate, are responsible for massive left-to-right shunts leading to pulmonary arterial hypertension. In this situation, the most significant risk is the mid- to long-term development of pulmonary vascular obstructive disease. Pulmonary vascular obstructive disease is a major determining factor of the surgical outcome of DS children with CHD. The pulmonary vascular disease begins at birth when the vasculature fails to adapt normally to extrauterine life. Because of the high pulmonary blood flow, the tunica media of large arteries progressively increases in thickness as smooth muscle cells hypertrophy and excessive connective tissue is deposited in the tunica media and tunica adventitia of the vessels. The normal postnatal increase in contractile myofilaments is accelerated, and there is evidence of early endothelial dysfunction. In the small muscular arteries, intimal proliferation narrows the lumen. This progressive fibrous vascular occlusion coincides with increased pulmonary arterial resistance. After a few months, with a precise delay that can vary from patient to patient, the phenomenon becomes fixed and irreversible, with an elevated pulmonary vascular resistance prohibiting surgical management of the disease. Interestly, this complication tends to occur earlier in unrepaired infants with DS than in the general population with similar defects.

In the general population, infants with AVSD develop severe medial hypertrophy and intimal proliferation earlier and more severely than those with isolated large VSDs, usually by six to nine months of age. In DS, pulmonary vascular obstructive disease could occur even earlier. For that reason, complete AVSD repair should be scheduled in early infancy, before six months of age, or even before four months as performed in experienced surgical centers.

Large VSDs should also be addressed surgically before the age of six months, although with medium-sized VSDs a minimal follow-up period is mandatory to follow the natural evolution of pulmonary arterial pressures and confirm or refute the indication for surgery. The natural course of unrepaired AVSDs is a progression toward pulmonary vascular obstructive disease with progressively increasing pulmonary vascular resistance. Pulmonary arterial and right ventricular pressures ultimately become higher than systemic pressures measured in the left ventricle; the left-to-right interventricular shunt becomes bidirectional and then reversed (right-to-left). This situation is defined as the Eisenmenger's syndrome: the pulmonary hypertension rises to reach systemic levels; because of a reversed shunt, central cyanosis is constant and progressive clubbing, polycythemia, exercise intolerance, and finally dyspnea with minimal effort will develop.

The pulmonary arterial pressure can be indirectly determined by Doppler echocardiography, based on the tricuspid regurgitation jet or the interventricular septum geometry. To accurately measure the pulmonary arterial pressure and estimate pulmonary arterial resistance, cardiac catheterization is mandatory. This investigation is particularly indicated in cases of late assessment in DS children with AVSD or large VSD to confirm that the patient's physiology remained compatible with a complete surgical correction of the cardiac malformation. Cardiac catheterization estimates the pulmonary arterial resistance (normal <1.5 Wood units) in room air and in the presence of 100% oxygen and/or 20–80 ppm inhaled nitric oxide (iNO). These two agents are potent vasodilators, producing a fall in arterial resistance in patients with elevated but not fixed pulmonary vascular resistance.

A patient with a left-to-right shunt is considered suitable for surgery if his/her pulmonary vascular resistance is low or moderately high but reversible with oxygen and NO (<4 Wood units).

It is important to note that pulmonary vascular obstructive disease can develop in DS children who have minor or no cardiac defects. Chronic upper airway obstruction, including upper airway obstruction secondary to obstructive sleep apnea (OSA) can explain such development of pulmonary hypertension. Macroglossia, glossoptosis, muscular hypotonia, tonsillar and adenoidal hypertrophy, and laryngomalacia contribute to the relatively high incidence of OSA in DS children. In a recent prospective study (Shott et al., 2006), it was estimated to affect 50% to 80% of DS children, independently of a history of snoring. In a selected cohort of 33 snoring DS children (mean age: 4.9 years), 97% presented OSA and oxygen desaturations (average fall of 4% in O_2 saturation) (Fitzgerald et al., 2007). In another study including 19 DS children (between 3 and 18 years), a 79% prevalence of OSA was found despite a previous adenotonsillectomy in 40% of the cohort (Dyken et al., 2003).

In DS children, adenotonsillar hypertrophy alone is not a major determinant of OSA and severe airway obstruction may be caused by other physiological and anatomical factors. Donnelly et al. (2004) demonstrated a higher prevalence of OSA during the first years of life, indicating that other craniofacial or functional anomalies in conjunction with adenotonsillar hypertrophy might be responsible for OSA. If the upper airway obstruction is not relieved by adenotonsillectomy, continuous positive airways pressure (CPAP) may be indicated to prevent OSA and their deleterious consequences: pulmonary hypertension, higher prevalence of behavioral problems, and neurocognitive impairment (attention deficit disorders, somnolence, depression). As a whole, this explains why most authors recommend polysomnography for all DS children, especially when snoring is reported.

Congenital heart diseases in Down syndrome

Atrioventricular septal defect

Atrioventricular septal defect is characterized by the abnormal development of the atrioventricular valves with persistence of the atrial ostium primum and a VSD.

Atrioventricular septal defect accounts for about 3%–5% of congenital cardiac defects at birth in the general population but up to 70% of patients with complete AVSD are affected by DS (Al-Hay et al., 2003; Formigari et al., 2004). Although there is a strong genetic correlation between AVSD and DS, this defect is also described in a variety of other syndromes. In addition, there is a significant sex ratio shift and ethnic characteristics in patients with AVSDs, with twice as many affected females, twice as many Blacks and half as many Hispanics (Freeman et al., 2008). AVSD is found in approximately 40%–50% of DS children in Europe and North America. In Asia, AVSD is the second most common CHD, after the various VSDs. In Mexico, AVSDs are reported in only 8% of DS children (Figueroa et al., 2003), and Vida et al. (2005) described 54.1% of 349 DS children in Guatemala with associated CHDs (28.6% with isolated PDA, 27.5% with VSD, 12.7% with ASD, and 9.5% with ASVD). Freeman et al. (2008) reported an AVSD rate of 19.2% among the North American white DS population, compared to 29.5% among the North American black population, 11.6% among Hispanics, and 11.1% among Asians. Of note, black women born outside of the United States are more likely to have a DS child with AVSD than black mothers born in the country. Finally, the maternal age per se does not seem to play a role in the prevalence of AVSD by comparison with other CHDs.

Within the AVSDs, there is a large spectrum of anatomical variations, from very large atrial and ventricular defects with a common undivided atrioventricular valve to a mild abnormality of the mitral valve (e.g. cleft in the anterior leaflet). Therefore, we can grossly distinguish two groups of AVSDs: complete and partial AVSD.

In complete AVSD (CAVSD), there is a common atrioventricular valve with large communications between the atria and ventricles (Figure 9.1). The common atrioventricular valve has five leaflets: two confined to the right ventricle, one exclusively in the left, and two crossing the ventricular septum with attachments to both ventricles. The last two leaflets are called

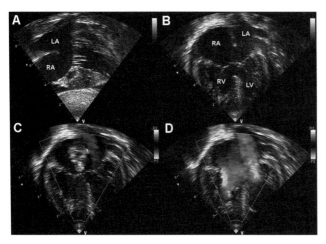

Figure 9.1 Echocardiographic assessment of complete atrioventricular septal defects. Two-dimensional echocardiographic sub-xiphoid (A) and four-chamber (B) views in a complete atrioventricular septal defect, showing the primum atrial septal defect, common atrioventricular valve, and large ventricular septal defect. The Doppler echocardiography in the apical four-chamber view allows evaluation of the degree of common atrioventricular valve regurgitation (C), and clearly shows the major blood mixing across the primum ASD and large VSD (D). LA: left atrium; RA: right atrium; RV: right ventricle; LV: left ventricle.

superior and inferior bridging leaflets. The classification proposed in 1966 by Rastelli et al. is based largely on the anatomy of the superior bridging leaflet (SBL; Figure 9.2). Complete AVSDs are more frequently associated with DS (60%–80%)

In partial AVSDs, the atrioventricular valves are more completely formed with valve tissue attached to the crest of the interventricular septum. This atrioventricular valve tissue can produce different degrees of occlusion of the ventricular defect. When the ventricular defect is completely occluded, there is a residual ostium primum atrial communication; when the ventricular occlusion is partial with a persistent ventricular restrictive shunt, the defect is described as an intermediate AVSD. Partial and intermediate AVSDs are more prevalent in the absence of chromosomal abnormalities.

Other anatomical characteristics of AVSDs have been described. The left ventricular outflow tract (LVOT) is longer, more anterior, and narrower than normal (explaining the "gooseneck" image on angiography) with an added risk of associated LVOT obstruction, in both partial and complete forms of AVSD. The atrioventricular conduction system is also abnormal, located posteriorly to the ventricular defect, in a course particularly at risk for postoperative atrioventricular blocks.

Associated cardiac anomalies observed in children with CAVSD include: (1) a right ventricular outflow obstruction (RVOT) and pathophysiology similar to the TOF, owing to anterior malalignment of the infundibular septum; (2) coarctation of the aorta; (3) unbalanced ventricles (of asymmetrical sizes), most frequently with a right ventricular dominance, and sometimes with a very hypoplastic left ventricle unsuitable for a biventricular repair; (4) other malformations of the left atrioventricular valve (double orifice, single papillary muscle, valvular dysplasia); (5) a patent ductus arteriosus; and (6) less frequently, a pulmonary valve stenosis. In DS children, the most frequent associated malformation is RVOT obstruction (from 6% to 18% of patients), while in the absence of trisomy 21, LVOT obstruction, unbalanced ventricles, and mitral valve abnormalities are more common.

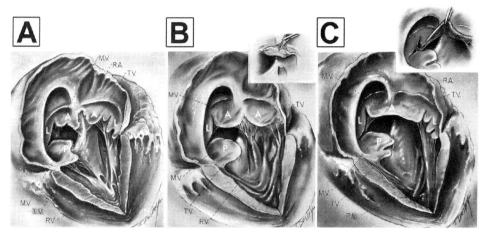

Figure 9.2 Rastelli classification of complete atrioventricular septal defects (AVSDs). The Rastelli classification only refers to the anatomy of the superior bridging leaflet (SBL) of the common atrioventricular valve. (A): Rastelli type A has an SBL divided into two parts, with chordal attachments to the crest of the muscular interventricular septum. (B): Rastelli type B has an SBL partly divided into two parts, but not attached to the interventricular septum. Instead, it is attached to an anomalous right ventricular papillary muscle that arises from the right ventricular septal surface. (C): Rastelli type C has an SBL that is undivided and unattached to the crest of the ventricular septum. The interventricular communication is usually larger than in type A and extends to the vicinity of the aortic cusps. In the absence of trisomy 21, type A is the most common and type C is the second most common variant of AVSD; type B is rare. In DS children, type C is the more frequent (36% vs. 23% in the normal population) and type B is more common (4% vs. 1%) (Lange et al., 2007). (Reproduced from Rastelli, G. C., et al. (1967), with permission.)

Ventricular septal defect

Ventricular septal defect is the second most common defect in DS children in Europe and North America (about 30%); and it is even more frequent than AVSD in Asia and Central America. Different types of VSD are described according to the localization of the defect in the ventricular septum (Figure 9.3).

The membranous portion of the ventricular septum deficient in perimembranous VSDs is located in the superior portion of the septum. In perimembranous inlet VSD, the defect occurs in the posterior area next to the atrioventricular valve; in perimembranous outlet VSD, the defect is located in the anterosuperior area next to the aortic valve.

Muscular VSDs, in the muscular portion of the ventricular septum, lie in the inferior part of the septum and are more prone to spontaneous closure over time.

Doubly-committed subarterial VSDs are defects in which the aortic-to-pulmonary valve continuity constitutes the rims of the defect; the defect is both subpulmonary and subaortic.

In DS infants, a membranous VSD is frequently seen in the inlet segment of the ventricular septum (30%, in a study by Marino et al. [1990], vs. 4% in the general population), sometimes in combination with secundum ASDs and PDAs, with a major left-to-right shunt and early signs of heart failure.

In clinical practice, the majority of VSDs diagnosed in DS infants are large and encompass both the inlet and outlet segments of the membranous septum. Large muscular or doubly-committed subarterial VSDs are less common in DS infants and muscular VSDs are often associated with more complex lesions. A cleft in the mitral valve is a frequent additional malformation, often in association with membranous inlet VSD. By contrast, LVOT

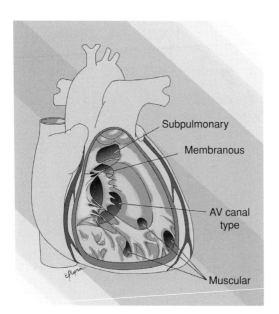

Figure 9.3 Ventricular septal defect subtypes as viewed from the right ventricle. (Reproduced from Keane et al. (2006), with permission.)

obstruction, mitral stenosis, and aortic coarctation are rarely associated with VSD in DS patients.

Tetralogy of Fallot

This malformation is the only conotruncal anomaly occurring in DS infants, encountered in 2.7%–7% of children with CHD (Wells et al., 1994; Källen et al., 1996; Freeman et al., 2008). The four classic hallmarks of TOF are: (1) a right-sided aorta overriding (2) a malalignment VSD; (3) a variable degree of infundibular/valvular pulmonary stenosis resulting from the anterior deviation of the conal septum; and (4) right ventricular hypertrophy. The severity of this condition depends mostly on the degree of infundibular pulmonary stenosis. If mild, the hemodynamic situation is similar to an isolated VSD with preferential left-to-right shunt. When moderate, the shunt is bidirectional with mild cyanosis (SpO_2 around 85%), but in severe RVOT obstruction, the shunt becomes preferentially right-to-left, with marked cyanosis and episodes of hypoxic spells. When the patient appears very hypoxic in the neonatal period, a Blalock shunt (between the subclavian artery and ipsilateral pulmonary artery) is mandatory to achieve a sufficient pulmonary blood flow and systemic oxygenation.

The more common isolated TOFs with mild or moderate infundibular pulmonary stenosis are rarely symptomatic early in life, and a complete repair can be electively scheduled between four and six months of age. In the association of TOF and complete AVSD, a Blalock shunt is frequently proposed as an initial palliative surgery in the first weeks of life, and the complete repair of the CHD is performed later, as the pulmonary vasculature is protected by the RVOT obstruction.

Hopefully, some of the more complex cardiac anomalies commonly observed in association with TOF in the general population (pulmonary atresia, absent pulmonary valve, discontinuity of the pulmonary arteries, and multiple aortopulmonary collaterals) are rarely found in DS children.

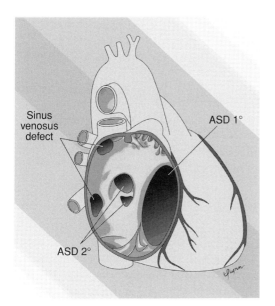

Figure 9.4 Atrial septal defect subtypes. An ostium primum defect (ASD 1°) is located immediately adjacent to the mitral and tricuspid valves. Ostium secundum defects (ASD 2°) are located near the fossa ovalis in the center of the atrial septum. Sinus venosus defects are located in the area derived from the embryological sinus venosus. (Reproduced from Keane et al. (2006), with permission.)

Atrial septal defect

Ostium secundum ASD is the most frequent CHD in the general population, while such isolated lesions are less frequently encountered in DS children. The majority of these can be closed percutaneously in the catheterization laboratory by a variety of specifically designed prostheses. Surgery remains indicated in the absence of margins around the defect(s) to anchor the devices. In sinus venosus ASD, a defect rare in association with trisomy 21, percutaneous closure is impossible because of its superoposterior location, and surgery is indicated at about three to four years of age. Ostium primum ASD is considered as a partial form of AVSD and is very often associated with a mitral valve cleft. These various types of ASDs are described in Figure 9.4.

Patent ductus arteriosus and aortic arch malformations

The ductus arteriosus is a remnant of the portion of the sixth aortic arch connecting the future main pulmonary artery to the aorta in the embryo. During fetal life, lungs are not aerated and the pulmonary arteries are poorly perfused, the ductus allowing the blood to shunt from the right ventricle to the descending aorta, thereby bypassing the pulmonary circulation. After birth, closure of the ductus must occur in the first days/weeks of life, although it is often delayed in premature babies. When hemodynamically significant, a ductus can be closed pharmacologically (e.g. with ibuprofen) or by surgical clipping or section (by lateral thoracotomy or minimally invasive thoracoscopy).

In DS infants, the isolated persistence of the ductus arteriosus is observed in 2%–5% of patients in Europe (Stoll et al., 1998), but significantly more frequently in Central America (28%) (Vida et al., 2005). Should the PDA be responsible for enlargement of left-sided cavities, percutaneous closure is indicated, at around 12 months of age or sometimes earlier.

An aberrant right subclavian artery (also called *arteria lusoria*) is an anomaly in which the right subclavian artery arises from the aortic arch distal to the left subclavian

Table 9.1 Congenital heart diseases reported in 106 Down syndrome children who underwent cardiac surgery

	Number of patients	%
Complete AVSD	50	47.1
VSD	31	29.2
Partial AVSD (primum ASD)	10	9.4
Isolated tetralogy of Fallot	6	5.6
Secundum ASD	4	3.7
Sinus venosus ASD	1	0.9
Persistent ductus arteriosus	2	1.9

AVSD: atrioventricular septal defect; VSD: ventricular septal defect; ASD: atrial septal defect.

artery and crosses the midline behind the esophagus. Prevalence of this anomaly seems to be higher in DS children than in the general population. It has been suggested that the prenatal occurrence of this *arteria lusoria* is up to 19%–36% in DS fetuses (Chaoui et al., 2005). In most cases, this anomaly is asymptomatic; but in 10%–20% of the cases (Bakker et al., 1999), it induces feeding problems, with impaired swallowing and frequent vomiting caused by posterior compression of the esophagus, particularly after the introduction of solid food. A barium-contrast esophagogram will help to identify the posterior compression of the esophagus and chest computerized tomography (CT) imaging can confirm the diagnosis and describe the anatomy of the arch and great vessels. Surgery performed through a thoracotomy is necessary to relieve the esophageal compression.

Surgical experience at the Cliniques universitaires Saint-Luc, Brussels

A retrospective study evaluated the risks and benefits of cardiac surgery in DS children in our institution between January 1992 and May 2008 (1992 corresponding to the arrival of a new surgical team).

During the study period, 106 DS children, with 58 females (55%) and 48 males (45%), underwent cardiac surgery. Thirty-five more patients were not included in the study, because they were from North African countries and were lost for follow-up. The different types of CHDs observed in the remaining 106 DS patients included in the study are described in Table 9.1.

Six other DS children had an interventional catheterization (two for ASD closure and four for PDA closure) during the same period and were not included in the study. A total of 99 children (93.3%) had a primary repair; seven children (6.7%) had palliative surgery in the neonatal period [including three with a complete AVSD and coarctation of the aorta, who underwent a coarctation repair and a pulmonary banding (to prevent chronic pulmonary arterial hypertension and pulmonary vascular obstructive disease); three children with an unbalanced AVSD and relative hypoplasia of the left ventricle incompatible with a complete repair; and one child with a complete AVSD and TOF, who underwent a Blalock shunt]. From the seven children who had palliative surgery, six ultimately had a complete repair after an

Table 9.2 Median age at the time of surgical correction

Defect	Age at surgery (months)	Range (months)
Complete AVSD (primary repair)	5.7	1–78
Complete AVSD (s/p shunt palliation)	18.1	6–53
VSD	10.1	2–78
Partial AVSD (primum ASD)	60.5	3–188
Isolated tetralogy of Fallot	7.2	5–9.5
Secundum ASD	21	6.5–34

AVSD: atrioventricular septal defect; s/p: status post; VSD: ventricular septal defect; ASD: atrial septal defect.

average of 12.4 months following palliation. The two-patch technique was routinely used by our surgeons for a complete AVSD repair, at an average age of 5.7 months (Table 9.2). The median follow-up time for the entire cohort was 8.35 years (range: 8 months–16 years).

Results

The early postoperative mortality (30-day mortality) was 5.6% (six patients); two late deaths occurred secondary to extracardiac causes (one following a bronchopulmonary infection; one owing to an associated cystic fibrosis). Interestingly, five patients died early after a CAVSD repair in the initial study period from 1992 to 2000, but none in the next period from 2001 to 2008. One patient died (from intractable pulmonary hypertension) following a VSD repair in 2002. Early postoperative morbidity was transient in most of the cases. Pericardial effusion was frequent (10.6%); severe but reversible pulmonary hypertension was reported in 4.5% of cases; chylothorax or sepsis were both described in 3% of the cases; and transient hemiparesia was observed in one patient. Long-term complications were experienced in only three patients: two with a complete atrioventricular block requiring a permanent pace-maker and one with hemiplegia. Four patients needed reoperation after AVSD repair; three of them for moderate to severe residual mitral valve insufficiency, and one for subaortic stenosis (requiring two reoperations). One patient needed four operations: a Blalock shunt for an associated right ventricular obstruction; a complete repair at 15 months of age; a reoperation for residual mitral valve regurgitation and a residual VSD; and finally a percutaneous closure of a large residual VSD. The global incidence of reoperation was 4% for all CHDs; and 8.8% for CAVSD patients only.

Long-term follow-up showed moderate mitral valve regurgitation in 12 patients following AVSD repair. Severe mitral valve incompetence was diagnosed in five patients, currently requiring chronic medical management, but possibly to be addressed surgically in the future.

In conclusion, this study showed that 83% of all DS patients undergoing cardiac surgery had a primary repair without major complications; the early postoperative mortality was 5.6% for all patients, and 10% for CAVSD only.

Discussion

The 10% mortality rate observed after CAVSD repair seems to be high in comparison with other recent studies, but we noticed that all our patients who died after CAVSD repair were operated on between 1992 and 2000. Since then, only one child, who had a VSD repair, died.

Similarly, Al-Hay et al. (2003) observed a 30-day mortality of 16% in a group of 106 DS children operated on in London between 1986 and 1998. In a cohort including 341 DS children operated on in Münich between 1974 and 2005, the early mortality rate was 5.3% (Lange et al., 2007), and as low as 4.6% in a study by Formigari et al. (2004), with 131 DS patients operated on in Rome between 1992 and 2002.

These three studies did not find any statistically significant difference between DS children and non-DS children in terms of early mortality after surgery. In the German study, the actuarial survival of 20 years after CAVSD repair was 84% in the DS group and 75% in the non-DS group with a lower need for reoperation (11.1% vs. 22.7%). Formigari et al. (2004) reported, after 12 years of following up a similar 94% actuarial survival in DS patients (compared with 86% in the general population) and a need for reoperation in 5.4% of DS patients (compared with a higher rate of 18.6% in the non-DS group). Interestingly, Al-Hay et al. (2003) also observed a lower rate of reoperations in the DS group (17% vs. 32%). Together, these studies suggest that DS children have a lower probability of reintervention for residual mitral valve regurgitation. This could be explained by a different amount and quality of valvular tissue available from the atrioventricular valve to reconstruct a competent mitral valve and, possibly, less friable valves in trisomy 21. As a whole, this tends to demonstrate that the presence of DS in children with CAVSD is no longer a risk factor for surgical repair. Strikingly, DS seems to be associated with a better long-term survival and a lower morbidity after cardiac surgery in comparison with non-DS children presenting with the same cardiac defects. These favorable results are probably linked to the specific anatomy observed in DS, with a lower prevalence of left-sided obstructions, right ventricular dominance, and complex anomalies of the mitral valve (such as the presence of a double orifice) (Formigari et al., 2004; Alexi-Meskishvili et al., 1996). As an example, Alexi-Meskishvili et al. found complex mitral anomalies in 10.6% of DS children compared with 17.6% in those without DS. Al-Hay et al. (2003) also confirmed the lower rate of mitral valve dysplasia among DS children (3%) than among non-DS children (24%). As expected, the increased rate of reoperation could be related to the severity of the preoperative mitral valve regurgitation (Michelon et al., 1997). In our study, the three children who presented with CAVSD and unbalanced ventricles underwent a pulmonary banding operation before a complete biventricular repair, on average 12 months later. Another patient with the same malformation had a pulmonary banding in 2002; although his anatomy was initially considered as unsuitable for complete biventricular repair, he was reevaluated by cardiac catheterization at the age of five years, to measure the pulmonary arterial pressures and describe both ventricular components. Considered as a good candidate for biventricular repair, he was successfully corrected as such. In our series, no patient needed a univentricular palliation with the Fontan operation.

The median age at CAVSD repair was 5.7 months; timing in line with other studies. It is known that DS children with CAVSD are at greatest risk of pulmonary vascular obstructive disease, and that fixed pulmonary vascular disease could develop as early as six months of age. In a study from 2007, Kobayashi et al. described two in-hospital deaths in children at 5.2 and 5.9 months of age, who both already had significant pulmonary arterial obstructive disease and postoperatively presented major pulmonary hypertensive crises.

Finally, Michelon et al. (1997) and Suzuki et al. (1998) presented another argument for early repair. They showed that early primary repair might prevent mitral valve regurgitation from annular dilatation and degenerative changes in the valve. The same trend (although not reaching statistical significance) for repair (before three months of age) as a protective factor against the need for mitral valve reoperation was also described by Al-Hay et al. (2003). In a Dutch study (Kortenhorst et al., 2005), DS children with CAVSD were reported as being progressively younger at the time of surgical correction (median age 43 weeks in the 1980s; 24 weeks in the 1990s; and 13 weeks in the 2000–2003 period), with a similarly decreasing mortality rate.

In conclusion, over the last 15 years, we have accomplished many significant improvements in the management of CDHs in patients with DS. Not only prenatal and neonatal diagnosis, but also surgical techniques and postoperative intensive care were drastically improved in most referral institutions. Early and late postoperative mortality and morbidity decreased significantly and are still improving. The diagnosis of DS is no longer considered as a risk factor for CAVSD repair. According to recent publications, early surgical correction before four months of age combines the best results and low risk, at least in experienced hands. In addition, improvements in interventional catheterization and hybrid surgery techniques enable percutaneous or preoperative device closure of moderate-sized VSDs and could reduce the need for pump surgery and circulatory arrest in some patients. We believe that these advances will contribute to a better quality of life for DS children and their families.

Summary

Down syndrome (DS) is frequently (40%–50% of DS patients) associated with congenital heart defects.

Until the early 1990s, cardiac surgery in these patients was considered as a high-risk procedure. At that time, some cardiology centers questioned the advisability of repairing complete atrioventricular septal defects (CAVSD), the most frequent cardiac lesion in DS, because of the high postoperative mortality rate.

Over the last 15 years, we have achieved many significant improvements in the management of congenital heart diseases (CHDs) in patients with DS. Not only prenatal and neonatal diagnosis but also surgical techniques and postoperative intensive care were drastically improved in most referral institutions. Early and late postoperative mortality and morbidity decreased very significantly and are still improving. The diagnosis of DS is no longer considered as a risk factor for CAVSD repair. We believe that these advances will contribute to a better quality of life for DS children and their families.

References

Alexi-Meskishvili, V., Ishino, K., Dänert, I., et al. (1996). Correction of complete atrioventricular septal defects with the double patch technique and cleft closure. *Annals of Thoracic Surgery*, **62**, 519–525.

Al-Hay, A. A., MacNeill, S. J., Yacoub, M., Shore, D. F., Shinebourne, E. A. (2003). Complete atrioventricular septal defect, Down syndrome, and surgical outcome: risk factors. *Annals of Thoracic Surgery*, **75**, 412–421.

Bakker, D., Berger, R., Witsenburg, M., Bogers, A. (1999). Vascular rings: a rare cause of common respiratory symptoms. *Acta Paediatrica*, **88**, 947–952.

Berg, J. M., Crome, L., France, N. E. (1960). Congenital cardiac malformations in mongolism. *British Heart Journal*, **22**, 331–346.

Chaoui, R., Hering, K., Sarioglu, N., et al. (2005). Aberrant right subclavian artery as a new cardiac sign in second and third trimester fetuses with Down syndrome. *American Journal of Obstetrics and Gynaecology*, **192**, 257–263.

De Grouchy, J. & Turleau, C. (1982). *Atlas des maladies chromosomiques.* (2nd edn.), pp. 340–351. Paris: Expansion scientifique.

De Walle, H. E. & Cornel, M. C. (1995). Survival rates of children with Down syndrome in the northern Netherlands, 1981–1991. *Tijdschrift of Kindergeneeskunde*, **63**, 40–44.

Donnelly, L. F., Shott, S. R., LaRose, C. R., et al. (2004). Causes of persistent obstructive sleep apnea despite previous tonsillectomy and adenoidectomy in children with Down syndrome as depicted on static and dynamic cine MRI. *American Journal of Roentgenology*, **183**, 175–181.

Down, J. L. (1866). Observations on an ethnic classification of idiots. *London Hospital Clinical Lecture*, **3**, 259–262.

Dyken, M. E., Lin-Dyken, D. C., Poulton, S., Zimmerman, M. B., Sedars, E. (2003). Prospective polysomnographic analysis of obstructive sleep apnea in Down syndrome. *Archives of Pediatric and Adolescence Medicine*, **157**, 655–660.

Figueroa, J., Magana, B., Hach, J., Jimenez, C., Urbina, R. (2003). Heart malformations in children with Down syndrome. *Revista Española de Cardiología*, **56**, 894–895.

Fitzgerald, D. A., Paul, A., Richmond, C. (2007). Severity of obstructive apnea in children with Down syndrome who snore. *Archives of Disease in Childhood*, **92**, 423–425.

Formigari, R., Di Donato, R. M., Gargiulo, G., et al. (2004). Better surgical prognosis for patients with complete atrioventricular septal defect and Down syndrome. *Annals of Thoracic Surgery*, **78**, 66–72.

Freeman, S. B., Bean, L. H., Allen, E. G., et al. (2008). Ethnicity, sex, and the incidence of congenital heart defects: a report from the National Down Syndrome Project. *Genetic Medicine*, **10**(3), 173–180.

Frid, C., Drott, P., Lundell, B., Rasmussen, F., Anneren, G. (1999). Mortality in Down syndrome in relation to congenital malformations. *Journal of Intellectual Disabilities Research*, **43**(3), 234–241.

Garrod, A. E. (1894). On the association of cardiac malformations with other congenital defects. *St Bartholomew's Hospital Report*, **30**, 53.

Hoe, T. S., Chan, K. C., Boo, N. Y. (1990). Cardiovascular malformations in Malaysian

neonates with Down syndrome. *Singapore Medical Journal*, **31**, 474–476.

Jacobs, E. G., Leung, M. P., Karlberg, J. (2000). Distribution of symptomatic congenital heart disease in Hong Kong. *Pediatric Cardiology*, **21**, 148–157.

Källen, B., Mastroiacovo, P., Robert, E. (1996). Major congenital malformations in Down syndrome. *American Journal of Medical Genetics*, **65**, 160–166.

Keane, J., Fyler, D., Lock, J. (2006). *Nada's Pediatric Cardiology* (2nd edn.), Oxford: Elsevier.

Kobayashi, M., Takahashi, Y., Ando, M. (2007). Ideal timing of surgical repair of isolated complete atrioventricular septal defect. *Interactive Cardiovascular Thoracic Surgery*, **6**(1), 24–26.

Kortenhorst, M. S., Hazekamp, M. G., Rameloo, M. A., Schoof, P. H., Ottenkamp, J. (2005). Complete atrioventricular septal defect in children with Down syndrome: good results of surgical correction at younger and younger ages. *NederlandseTijdschrift of Geneeskunde*, **149**, 589–593.

Lange, R., Guenther, T., Busch, R., Hess, J., Schreiber, C. (2007). The presence of Down syndrome is not a risk factor in complete atrioventricular septal defect repair. *Journal of Thoracic and Cardiovascular Surgery*, **134**, 304–310.

Lo, N. S., Leung, P. M., Lau, K. C., Yeung, C. Y. (1989). Congenital cardiovascular malformations in Chinese children with Down syndrome. *Chinese Medical Journal*, **102**, 382–386.

Marino, B. (1996). Patterns of congenital heart disease and associated cardiac anomalies in children with Down syndrome. In B. Marino & S. M. Pueschel (eds.), *Heart Disease in Persons with Down Syndrome*, pp. 133–140. Baltimore: Brookes.

Marino, B. & DeZorzi, A. (1993). Congenital heart disease in trisomy 21 mosaicism. *Journal of Pediatrics*, **122**, 500–501.

Marino, B., Papa, M., Guccione, P., et al. (1990). Ventricular septal defect in Down syndrome. Anatomic types and associated malformations. *American Journal of Diseases in Childhood*, **144**, 544–545.

Merrick, J. (2000). Incidence and mortality in Down syndrome. *Israel Medical Association Journal*, **2**(1), 25–26.

Michielon, G., Stellin, G., Rizzoli, G., Casaroto, D. C. (1997). Repair of complete common atrioventricular canal defects in patients younger than 4 months of age. *Circulation*, **96**(II), 316–322.

Pinto, F. F., Nunes, L., Ferraz, F., Sampayo, F. (1990). Down syndrome: different distribution of congenital heart diseases between the sexes. *International Journal of Cardiology*, **27**, 175–178.

Rastelli, G. C., Kirklin, J. W., Titus, J. L. (1966). Anatomic observations on complete form of persistent common atrioventricular canal with special reference to atrioventricular valves. *Mayo Clinic Proceedings*, **41**, 296–308.

Rastelli, G. C., Wallace, R. B., Ongley, P. A., McGoon, D. C. (1967). Replacement of mitral valve in children with persistent common atrioventricular canal associated with severe mitral incompetence. *Mayo Clinic Proceedings*, **42**, 417–422.

Shott, S. R., Amin, R., Chini, B. (2006). Obstructive sleep apnea: should all children with Down syndrome be tested? *Archives of Otolaryngology Head and Neck Surgery*, **114**, 1640–1648.

Stoll, C., Alembik, Y., Dott, B., Roth, M. P. (1998). Study of Down syndrome in 238, 942 consecutive births. *Annals of Genetics*, **41**, 44–51.

Suzuki, K., Tatsuno, K., Kikuchi, T., Mimori, S. (1998). Predisposing factors of valve regurgitation in complete atrioventricular septal defect. *Journal of American College of Cardiology*, **32**, 1449–1453.

Torfs, C. P. & Christianson, R. E. (1999). Maternal risk factors and major associated defects in infants with Down syndrome. *Epidemiology*, **10**, 267–270.

Vida, V. L., Barnoya, J., Larrazabal, L. A., et al. (2005). Congenital cardiac disease in children with Down syndrome in Guatemala. *Cardiology in the Young*, **15**, 286–290.

Weijerman, M., Marceline van Furth, A., Vonk Noordegraaf, A., et al. (2008). Prevalence, neonatal characteristics, and first-year mortality of Down syndrome: a national study. *Journal of Pediatrics*, **152**, 15–19.

Wells, G. L., Barker, S. E., Finley, S. C., Colvin, E. V., Finley, W. H. (1994). Congenital heart disease in infants with Down syndrome. *Southern Medical Journal*, **87**, 724–727.

Yang, Q., Rasmussen, S. A., Friedman, J. M. (2002). Mortality associated with Down syndrome in the USA from 1983 to 1997: a population-based study. *Lancet*, **359**, 1019–1025.

Chapter

10

Developmental models as frameworks for early intervention with children with Down syndrome

Jacob A. Burack, Katie Cohene, Heidi Flores

Our contribution to this book is the outline of a developmental approach that can be used to guide early intervention for individuals with Down syndrome (DS). For this task, we come fortified with frameworks, models, and paradigms from general developmental theory and research to guide our perspective on intervention. With this background and these resources, we suggest a universal context that is premised on the overwhelming similarities in underlying developmental processes that are observed among children, regardless of disability, and ability levels or individual experiences, as a first step to understanding intervention for children with DS from as early as birth and how it can be impacted by various direct and indirect factors (Hodapp & Burack, 1990). The emphasis on the commonalities of development does not obscure the obvious and important differences across etiologies, families, and individuals, but rather provides a framework of the whole child within which these differences can be discussed and understood (Zigler, 1967, 1969; Hodapp et al., 1990). Contemporary developmentalists celebrate differences at all levels of the human experience as essential, but not sole contributors, to developmental outcomes and behavior. Thus, the extensive understanding of universal trajectories of development and the ways that they are maintained or affected by cultural, societal, communal, familial, and individual differences is an organizing framework for understanding the relevance of the family, the individual, and outside influences to positive outcomes for children with DS (Hodapp, 1990; Hodapp & Burack, 2006). The developmental models of Werner, Piaget, Zigler, Cicchetti, Bronfenbrenner, and other developmentalists help serve as conceptual frameworks to guide the understanding of factors that influence development for children with DS.

The notion of a single developmental framework is illusory as models and theories abound, and the terms development and developmental have become so much a part of the common nomenclature that they may be deemed meaningless. Yet, classic developmental theories are premised on certain fundamentals – development needs to be universal, directional, organized, systemic, and orderly, and the organism (i.e. child) needs to be an active participant in the process. In this sense, classic developmental theories are essentially frameworks of meaning or systems that are governed by rules that need to be maintained across persons and situations. Early developmental theorists focused on delineating frameworks for understanding typical children and largely were able to smooth over individual differences in order to formulate coherent and universal guidelines. The exceptions to the theories were

Neurocognitive Rehabilitation of Down Syndrome, eds. Jean-Adolphe Rondal, Juan Perera, and Donna Spiker. Published by Cambridge University Press. © Cambridge University Press 2011.

typically thought of as antithetical to the cause of a developmental framework and, therefore, typically ignored (Burack, 1997). In particular, persons with atypical developmental histories, such as intellectual disabilities in general or genetic syndromes more particularly, and other atypicalities were considered outside the sphere of traditional developmental thought. Although not necessarily the first to broaden the notion of developmental theory, Werner (Werner, 1948, 1957; Werner & Wapner, 1949) fueled the application of typical developmental frameworks to persons with intellectual disabilities, psychiatric disorders, and other examples of psychopathology. His mentee, Zigler (Zigler 1967, 1969; Zigler & Balla, 1982; Zigler & Hodapp, 1986), extended this approach by applying developmental theory to the study of persons with intellectual disabilities, as he and colleagues considered issues such as cognitive rates, sequences, structures, as well as social and personality development within the context of the whole person. Cicchetti and colleagues (Cicchetti & Sroufe, 1978; Cicchetti & Pogge-Hesse, 1982; Cicchetti & Beeghly, 1990) further fine-tuned this application in their arguments for an expansion of the developmental approach, based on their work with persons with DS in which apparently unique aspects of DS are informative about the extents and limits of developmental processes (also see Hodapp & Burack, 1990; Hodapp & Zigler, 1990).

Werner and the universality of development

Werner's perspective on development entails a global approach. His research on the commonalities of development led to the orthogenetic principle. The idea is that "wherever development occurs it proceeds from a state of relative globality and lack of differentiation to a state of increasing differentiation, articulation, and hierarchic integration ... " (Werner, 1957, p. 126). Werner's idea of the notion of percepts is a clear example of how development follows an orderly sequence of stages. In a first stage, perception is global such that the individual views whole qualities. The second stage is analytical, whereby the component perceives the component parts of an event. Finally in the synthetic stage, the individual sees how the parts of an event become integrated within the whole (Werner, 1957).

The development of children with DS can be viewed conceptually within this framework. As with typically developing individuals, cognitive structures and developmental processes unfold from simple to more complex systems. Individuals with DS will exhibit more complex behaviors and thought structures as they mature and interact with the surrounding world, both inanimate and animate (Cicchetti & Beeghly, 1990). Although their development may unfold at a slower pace than in typically developing individuals and with evidently different profiles of strengths and weaknesses, progression occurs from being stimulus bound to increased shaping or control over their environment. Responses to the environment, in turn, change as their understanding of the surrounding systems become more differentiated, abstract, and integrated (Cicchetti & Beeghly, 1990).

Werner introduced the notion of equifinality, in which development begins with varying characteristics and leads to the same outcome versus multiformity, in which similar paths may lead to very different outcomes. In this context, he differentiates between ability and outcome to the extent that greater ability in certain areas may actually lead to a lower developmental level on specific tasks. For example, Werner (1957) found that when asked to construct squares and rectangles out of irregular pieces from which the shapes were originally cut, eight-year-old children without intellectual disabilities performed at a lower level than eight-year-old children with intellectually disabilities, owing to their inclination to try and relate the figuratively unrelated pieces to the end form they pictured in their minds. In contrast, the children with intellectual difficulties performed significantly better as they worked at a more mechanical level and focused on matching same length pieces. He concluded that "a thinker oriented toward and capable of highly abstract thought may be at a disadvantage in certain concrete tasks of concept formation, compared with a concretely thinking person" (Werner, 1957, p. 133).

Werner also introduced the notion that development is both gradual and smooth (the notion of continuity) as well as having abrupt stops, changes, and regression (the notion of discontinuity). Here, discontinuity is expressed by two characteristics. The first is the emergence; for example, the irreducibility of a later stage to an earlier stage and later forms; the second is gappiness, which is best described as the lack of stages between earlier and later stages. However, for Werner, the latter might be attributed largely to an inability to see the smaller, more subtle changes that occur between those larger more measurable forms (Werner, 1957). Development may also follow more circumscribed and fixed levels (the notion of unlinearity), or more mobile and differentiated levels (the notion of multilinearity). Werner concluded that developmental processes are characterized by regular and invariant sequences leading to an endpoint (see Cicchetti & Beeghly 1990).

Developmental sequences

Although Piaget himself did not work with individuals with disabilities, his research of developmental sequences provides researchers with guidelines of development that can serve as a comparison for individuals with atypical development. Piaget's ideas of development were eventually extended to work with children with intellectual disabilities by his student, Barbel Inhelder (1968), who suggested that children with intellectual disabilities followed the same sequence of development, although they never obtain the highest or formal operational stage of development. These assertions were based on Piaget's 1970 notion of stages that outline development in invariant sequences leading to an endpoint. The changes that can be observed in the child's development reflect changes in mental structures. Behavior is therefore a reflection of these underlying changes. In the sensorimotor stage (birth to two years of age), infants use their senses and motor abilities to experience the world. In this stage, if an infant cannot touch, see, or smell an object, that infant will not attempt to search for it. In the preoperational stage (two to seven years of age), children will begin to express language or other symbols to represent objects. Children during this stage will begin to group objects and understand various types of conservation. During the concrete operations stage (seven to eleven years of age), children are beginning to be able to think and make rational judgments on more abstract concepts. In the final stage called the formal operational stage (adolescence and beyond), individuals are capable of higher-order thinking. There is no longer a dependence on concrete objects; the mind is able to manipulate information without the presence of physical objects. Clearly, to Piaget, development is orderly. Functioning evolves and transforms in a consistent way whereby earlier and simpler abilities are the foundations for later complex skills. These developmental sequences can be observed in an individual's behavior as the process of development is reflected in behavior (Hodapp et al., 1998).

Piaget also saw the child as an active participant in his/her learning. The perception was that the child is a little scientist exploring the world and that learning occurs through a process of accommodation and assimilation (Piaget, 1970). Like typically developing children, children with DS will experience the world through trial-and-error. The sequences predescribed by Piaget are a frame of reference for the cognitive processes that children will generally experience through development. The emergence of new skills can only occur when the child is ready. Consequently, children with DS will loosely follow these patterns at their own pace and this developmental pattern will be affected by the numerous other factors that will be discussed in the following sections.

Universality and uniqueness

Within his developmental approach to disabilities, Zigler (1967, 1969) focused on several factors that influence development of the whole child including personality, motivation, and the commonalities and differences between diverse etiologies. A developmental perspective is based on the idea that there are two distinct types of disability (Zigler, 1969). In Zigler's earlier research of this two-group approach (1969), he states:

If the etiology of the phenotypic intelligence (as measured by an IQ) of two groups differs, it is far from logical to assert that the course of development is the same, or that even similar contents in their behaviors are mediated by exactly the same cognitive processes. (p. 533)

Subsequently, Burack et al. (1998) differentiated among the many different etiologies that comprise this so-called organic group and argued that each different etiology was composed of separate etiology-related trajectories and behaviors. As DS is easily identifiable and the most common of the genetic syndromes, specific behavioral, cognitive, and developmental patterns have long been recognized. The uniqueness of the profiles is pronounced in some areas and more subtle in others. From a developmental perspective, they all point to a system that is intrinsically interrelated and organized (Cicchetti & Pogge-Hesse, 1982).

For example, research in early social communication skill development among individuals with DS suggests children with DS perform similarly to individuals of the same mental age, both with and without developmental delays in the areas of nonverbal joint attention and social interaction skills, but display deficits in nonverbal requesting that are associated with later difficulties in expressive language acquisition (Mundy & Sheinkopf, 1998).

An understanding of the overarching similarities within etiologies can provide valuable information about treatment and overall developmental milestones and trajectories. Within this developmental approach, there has been a focus on the ways that individuals with various disabilities develop in comparison to typical developmental trajectories. As patterns of strengths and weaknesses vary throughout the lifespan, the charting of developmental pathways can be informative about the focus and timing of intervention.

The notion of a whole child

Zigler (1971) promoted the need to consider the whole child and pay more attention to factors that influence behavior beyond just cognition. The emphasis was on taking into account and supporting the whole child. Zigler (1971) focused on many factors that can influence the personality and motivation of a child. He highlighted personality attributes including an overdependence on adults (positive reaction tendency), a wariness in initial reactions to adults (negative reaction tendency), a lowered expectancy of success, an overdependence on others to help solve problems (outerdirectness), a lack of pleasure gained from solving problems and a preference for more tangible rewards in contrast to verbal praise or other nontangible rewards (effectance motivation), and finally a less differentiated self-concept and lowered standards for their ideal self (Hodapp et al., 1998).

Zigler wondered why individuals matched according to mental age would not perform similarly on cognitive tasks (Weisz & Zigler, 1979). He concluded that a focus on the whole child, considering personality and motivational characteristics, is imperative in understanding the differences between two individuals that have a similar mental age but differ significantly in cognitive abilities. Zigler emphasized that life experiences such as repeated failure and social deprivation affects an individual's self-image and therefore impacts performance. For example, in a series of studies, Zigler and colleagues (Bybee & Zigler, 1992; for reviews, see Zigler & Hodapp, 1986; Merighi et al., 1990) found that individuals with disabilities often chose less difficult problems in later life, looked more to others for help, and also demonstrated less satisfaction in solving problem solving tasks. This is also evident in the relationship between school-aged children with DS and their parents who tend to be overly didactic and intrusive. This, in turn, translates into fewer opportunities for children with DS to problem-solve independently and gain pleasure from their successes. Thus, the development of intrinsic motivation can be impeded, setting the stage for reduced interest in solving problems and increased reliance on others (Hodapp & Fidler, 1999).

In response to this phenomenon, Bybee and Zigler (1992) presented the easy-to-hard principle and concluded that one way to increase intrinsic motivation is to provide problems of increasing difficulty at an earlier age. Understanding the cognitive level of the child helps guide the level of problem solving tasks. Just as the presentation of tasks that are too difficult leads to decreased motivation among children, the reverse is also true. The presentation of tasks that are too easy to accomplish decreases the pleasure derived from achieving the desired result. Confidence is built when children feel successful in completing tasks of increasing difficulty levels.

Unfortunately, the self-esteem of children with DS is often diminished as they are typically exposed to problems introduced by their mothers that are higher than their current cognitive level (Mahoney et al., 1990). This phenomenon results in repeated experiences in which the children are overtaxed and require additional support to complete tasks. Consequently, the children derive less pleasure owing to the exposure to repeated failed experiences. In addition, this reinforces children to take a more passive role in their activities and interactions. As their role in these interactions is more passive, they serve as an observer rather than an active explorer and problem-solver. Thus, when children are not given the opportunity to control their environment and become more active participants, this passive behavior will generalize to similar situations and contexts in later life (Hodapp & Fidler, 1999). Therefore, the type of early experiences that children with DS are exposed to may contribute to higher dependencies on adults and more reliance on external cues for solving problems as well as a lower expectancy of success (for a general discussion of these issues, see Merighi et al., 1990). For this reason, close attention to earlier experiences of success and failure are crucial in promoting a more positive self-image and work ethic.

Cicchetti and an expanded developmental approach

Cicchetti forwarded a more liberal developmental perspective that is based on an organizational approach in which development is viewed as "a series of qualitative reorganizations among and within behavioral and biological systems" (Cicchetti & Beeghly, 1990). According to this approach, development proceeds in accordance with the orthogenetic principle with three additional principles of change. Changes occur over time in the structure–function relationship, are both qualitative and quantitative in nature, and are best described as "a move towards increasing cortical control over the more diffuse, automatic behavioral centers" (Cicchetti & Beeghly, 1990, p. 32).

Cicchetti and his colleagues set out to clarify and elaborate on this notion of an organized developmental framework. In a series of studies by Cicchetti and Sroufe (1976, 1978) and Mans et al. (1978) on infants with DS, they highlighted consistency between this group and typically developing children with regard to the organization across domains and order of development, even if development proceeds at slower pace. Cicchetti and Sroufe (1976) found that infants with DS had a later onset of laughter than typically developing infants, which is problematic for long-term development as early laughter is a better predictor of later cognitive development. Similarly, Cicchetti and Sroufe (1978) found that infants with DS also displayed a delay in negative emotions such as crying and other signs of distress like an accelerated heart rate in experience with the visual cliff and approaching looming shadows in the collision course. Again, the onset of negative emotions was positively correlated with later cognitive functioning. The earlier the child shows negative emotions, the better the results found on later cognitive tests. Cicchetti and Pogge-Hesse (1982) also introduced a more liberal developmental approach in which the concept of developmental structure is provided more flexibility as it compensates for the uneven patterns of development found in individuals with exceptionalities. These patterns found in specific etiologies can help to understand the outer limits of which certain developmental links can be stretched but still maintained within organized developmental sequences (Wagner et al., 1990).

Cicchetti's (1984) dictum that "we can learn about the normal functioning of an organism by studying its pathology and, likewise, more about its pathology by studying its normal condition" (p. 1) is relevant to the study of family. The emphasis on studying the way in which functioning in typical families both influences the development of the child and can be influenced by the child is informative for studying families with children with DS (Cicchetti & Beeghly, 1990). Cicchetti and Beeghly concluded that research on the influence of family in development explains that the behaviors and attitudes of the parents affect the child's development and, conversely, the child's development influences parenting responses and the interaction between parent and child. These interactions between parenting styles and the child's development are clear examples of the necessity of considering multiple factors that influence development.

Ecological theory

Bronfenbrenner (1979, 1986, 1989) was able to conceptualize the impact of the outside systems surrounding the child and their development. He noted that research on child development was lacking as it did not take into account the larger system that influences the child and stated "It can be said that much of the developmental psychology is the science of the strange behavior of children in strange situations with strange adults for the briefest possible periods of time" (Bronfenbrenner, 1977, p. 513). An interest in the influences of outside systems surrounding the child such as the family, neighbors, the community, and the media became a major focus as he introduced the ecological theory.

Bronfenbrenner (1974) provided an argument for early intervention as he depicted, in the ecological theory, the impact of the family as an active agent for implementation of interventions. Burack et al. (1998) outlined the three major components of this approach. The first is the idea that the environment plays a significant role and has a substantial effect on development. Second, the interaction between the environmental effect and the developing individual varies from one individual to another. It may have a more or less substantial effect depending on the individual. Finally, the individual will also have an impact on the environment. In Bronfenbrenner's (1979, 1986, 1989) ecological theory, child development occurs within the context of environmental systems that contribute to or have an effect on the child. The environmental influence can be examined by looking at the interaction with all of the surrounding influential systems, the immediate setting including the child (microsystem), the interrelationships between settings whereby the child interacts (mesosystems), the larger structures in society that include the neighbors, the media, and governmental influences not necessarily including the child (macrosystems), and finally the larger cultural and societal value systems (exosystems) (Bronfenbrenner, 1979, 1986, 1989).

All of the systems have varying influences, both indirect and direct, on the individual's development. If we examine the direct influences on an infant, we can see many systems that could include the home, day care or nanny support, and the family. As the child gets older, the surrounding systems become more complex and comprehensive, as they would include not only the home environment but also the school peers, the teachers, neighbors, and closer friends. As the child develops into adolescence, the system broadens even more to include the family, school, and community, which can include family, peers, close friends, role models and teachers, and other influences such as spirituality. Stressors, changes, or other conflicts in the surrounding systems both indirectly and directly cause changes to a child's path of development. A change within one system will inevitably cause a change in the other surrounding systems.

Complex developmental trajectories

The consideration of the many factors in an individual's life is useful in understanding how developmental trajectories are maintained or affected by societal, familial, and individual differences, and influence positive outcomes for all children, including those with DS and intellectual disabilities (IDs). Developmental trajectories emerged with the transactions among various factors that can moderate and account for various outcomes in both indirect and direct ways.

As DS is associated with risk for negative outcomes in many areas, the most simple way to understand developmental trajectories for children with this condition is to assume that early predictors of problems in a domain may lead to later problems in that domain. For example, early challenges in achievement and motivation are thought to lead to later problems in school success. As a result of deficits in motivation that begin in infancy and early childhood owing to repeated failure and exposure to tasks above their cognitive level, children with DS often exhibit later difficulties in school achievement and problem solving capacity. The effects of low motivation and a lack of willingness to attempt new challenges limits the abilities of adults with DS to actualize their full potential. They learn that it is easier and safer to rely on the support of other individuals to accomplish tasks that they could and should be able to accomplish successfully independently. Thus, the children may stagnate developmentally as an effect of early challenges in a domain.

However, this is an oversimplified trajectory as early problems in one domain may also lead to later adaptations in that domain. Early problems in achievement and motivation may lead to early interventions, changes in parenting styles, increased supports, and adaptations of school programs that ultimately lead to relative school success. Conversely, early problems in a domain may underlie or contribute to further difficulties in achievement and motivation that can extend to more complex problems in another domain. As children with DS often have higher numbers of experiences of failure and therefore motivation deficits, this may lead to problems in self-esteem and peer relationships. Early predictors of adaptational deficits provide challenges in leading a more independent life and, consequently, participating in the work force may be compromised for individuals with DS. Repeated failures throughout infancy and early childhood can lead many individuals with DS to avoid situations where they may feel the potential to fail is elevated. This may impact significantly on their emotional and psychological development as they may become more isolated and, in turn, those around them may make fewer demands and have lower expectations. A downward spiral of negative outcomes that affect development may therefore stem from early problems in a domain and extend further into that and other domains (e.g. the school setting).

Alternatively, early problems in achievement and motivation may be associated with other forms of adaptation in later life. Here, problems in one domain can lead to later adaptations in one or more other domains. As children with DS may have difficulties in school achievement, programming that capitalizes on their individual strengths and characteristics can lead to alternate opportunities and increased success in less academically dependent areas. Individuals with DS are often described as having an outgoing and friendly disposition. These characteristics may be compensatory skills that have developed through reinforcement and refinement of skills that they demonstrated at a young age. When infants and young children with DS were consistently reinforced for being playful, outgoing, and sociable as infants and young children, they will have learnt how valuable these skills are and may make further use of this during adolescence and adulthood. These characteristics are often perceived by adults as making up for cognitive skills deficits and are more able to participate functionally in the community setting. However, the picture is more complex than both these examples as there are ongoing transactions among early predictors and developmental outcomes. Early predictors and later problems do not occur in isolation, and instead remain linked, continuously affecting each other and leading to multiple variations of outcomes.

This conceptual pattern of developmental outcomes can also be used as a model to understand early adaptations. In this case, early success in a domain leads to later adaptation in that domain. As children with DS may have the skills needed to succeed in some academic areas, this may predict better functioning in higher grade levels. They may be compliant and follow instructions from parents and teachers, and this may predict better functioning in school at a later age. However, early adaptation in a domain may also lead to later problems in another domain. In this case, dependency on adults for directions may be an indicator of early adaptation that can lead to later problems in independent living outside of the school domain, as persons with DS often lack self-determination skills such as choice making, taking the initiative, and autonomous problem solving in later life. Conversely, early adaptation in a domain may lead to later adaption in another domain. For example, following directions and cues from parents and teachers may promote the formation of the skills necessary to participate in the workforce. As with the previous example of early problems, the outcomes of early adaptation and later outcomes are complex, with an interaction between predictors and outcomes. Influencing factors happen simultaneously and are not independent of each other, with multiple moderating effects on outcomes.

The models and examples discussed here lack the complexity of the transaction among the levels of functioning of the individual, the environmental factors, and the relationships that together provide a more real-life pattern of developmental trajectories through the lifespan for individuals with DS. The different outcomes of individuals with similar early predictive and transactional factors suggest that certain characteristics can moderate outcomes at different developmental stages. In this way, a more comprehensive model for understanding developmental trajectories might have to:

account for competence in X, problem in Y, relationship with Z, in situation Q, at age A that are constantly changing, or interacting, individually and in relation to each other such that they need to be considered at A+1 minute, A+1 day, A+ the rest of the person's life with any number of different factors and combinations among them.

Clearly, no two individuals with DS share the exact same profile or are exposed to the same life events. Therefore, developmental trajectories are unique and continue to evolve over the lifespan for each individual despite similarities in etiological groups.

Implications of developmental models

In this chapter, we provide frameworks in which the role of many of the seemingly endless possible contributors to the developmental outcomes of children with DS can be considered, both individually and within the context of the meaningfully and continually evolving and transacting systems that are involved in virtually every aspect of the individual's life. Because the number of potentially relevant factors is infinite, as every aspect of the individual's being from the molecular to the societal and the specific etiology to the current moment's actions can be positively or negatively associated with different outcomes, the identification of the most essential ones are a necessary preliminary task. Therefore, an elaborate explanation of the universal trajectories of development and the ways that they are sustained or influenced by cultural, societal, communal, familial, and individual differences is presented as an organizing structure for considering and accounting for the relevance of the interactions with family, the individual differences between children with DS, and the various indirect and direct outside influences to positive developmental outcomes for children with DS. The developmental models of Werner, Piaget, Zigler, Cicchetti, and Bronfenbrenner together help guide our understanding of intervention. The understanding that intervention is not a construct that solely occurs in a school setting is imperative, as the developmental perspective explains that intervention includes all interactions affecting developmental outcomes, such as the complexity among the various factors in relation to issues of developmental level, individual characteristics, the various aspects of the environment, the individual's family, community, culture, and society.

Summary

We highlight the contributions of the developmental approach to understanding and intervening with children with Down syndrome (DS). Classic theories of development and their contemporary revisions are discussed with regard to their applicability to the study of persons with intellectual disabilities in general and to persons with DS more specifically. The emphasis is on the commonalities of development that are evident despite obvious and important differences across etiologies, families, and individuals. In this context, the focus is on the cognitive, social, emotional, behavioral whole child, who is continually transacting with the multi-layered universe in which he/she lives.

Acknowledgments

The work on this chapter was funded by an operating grant from the Social Sciences and Humanities Research Council of Canada to J. A. B. We thank Fabienne Bain, Alexandra

D'Arrisso, and Jacqueline Hodgson for their help in the preparation of the manuscript. We thank Drs. Juan Perera and Jean-Adolphe Rondal for the organization of the Down syndrome meeting in Palma de Mallorca and for their leadership in the field.

References

Bronfenbrenner, U. (1974). Developmental research, public policy, and the ecology of childhood. *Child Development*, **45**, 1–5.

Bronfenbrenner, U. (1977). Toward an experimental ecology of human development. *American Psychologist*, **32**, 515–531.

Bronfenbrenner, U. (1979). *The Ecology of Human Development: Experiments by Nature and Design*. Cambridge: Harvard University Press.

Bronfenbrenner, U. (1986). Ecology of the family as a context for human development: research perspectives. *Developmental Psychology*, **22**, 723–742.

Bronfenbrenner, U. (1989). Ecological systems theory. In R. Vasta (ed.), *Six Theories of Child Development: Revised Formulations and Current Issues*, Vol. 6. Greenwich: JAI Press.

Burack, J. A. (1997). The study of atypical and typical populations in developmental psychopathology: the quest for a common science. In S. S. Luthar, J. A. Burack, D. Cicchetti, J. R. Weisz (eds.), *Developmental Psychopathology Perspectives on Adjustment, Risk and Disorder*, pp. 139–165. New York: Cambridge University Press.

Burack, J. A., Hodapp, R. M., Zigler, E. (1988). Issues in the classification of mental retardation: differentiating among organic etiologies. *Journal of Child Psychology and Psychiatry*, **29**, 765–779.

Burack, J. A., Hodapp, R. M., Zigler, E. (eds.) (1998). *Handbook of Mental Retardation and Development*. New York: Cambridge University Press.

Bybee, J. & Zigler, E. (1992). Is outer directedness employed in a harmful or beneficial manner by students with and without mental retardation? *American Journal on Mental Retardation*, **96**, 512–521.

Cicchetti, D. (1984). The emergence of developmental psychopathology. *Child Development*, **55**, 1–7.

Cicchetti, D. & Beeghly, M. (eds.) (1990). *Children with Down Syndrome: A Developmental Approach*. New York: Cambridge University Press.

Cicchetti. D. & Pogge-Hesse, P. (1982). Possible contributions of organically retarded persons to developmental theory. In E. Zigler & D. Balla (eds.), *Mental Retardation: The Developmental-Difference Controversy*, pp. 277–318. Hillsdale: Erlbaum.

Cicchetti, D. & Sroufe, L. A. (1976). The relationship between affective and cognitive development in Down's syndrome infants. *Child Development*, **47**, 920–929.

Cicchetti, D. & Sroufe, L. A. (1978). An organizational view of affect: illustration from the study of Down's syndrome infants. In M. Lewis & L. A. Rosenblum (eds.), *The Development of Affect*. New York: Plenum.

Hodapp, R. M. (1990). One road or many? Issues in the similar sequence hypothesis. In R. M. Hodapp, J. A. Burack, E. Zigler (eds.), *Issues in the Developmental Approach to Mental Retardation*, pp. 49–70. Cambridge, England: Cambridge University Press.

Hodapp, R. M. & Burack, J. A. (1990). What mental retardation teaches us about typical development: the examples of sequences, rates, and cross–domain relations. *Development and Psychopathology*, **2**, 213–225.

Hodapp, R. M. & Burack, J. A. (2006). Developmental approaches to children with mental retardation: a second generation? In D. Cicchetti & D. J. Cohen (eds.), *Developmental Psychopathology (Volume 3): Risk, Disorder, and Adaptation*, pp. 235–267. New York: Wiley.

Hodapp, R. M., Burack, J. A., Zigler, E. (1990). The developmental perspective in the field of mental retardation. In R. M. Hodapp, J. A. Burack, E. Zigler (eds.), *Issues in the Developmental Approach to Mental Retardation*, pp. 3–26. New York: Cambridge University Press.

Hodapp, R. M., Burack, J. A., Zigler, E. (1998). Developmental approaches to mental retardation: a short introduction. In J. A. Burack, R. M. Hodapp, E. Zigler (eds.), *Handbook of Mental Retardation and Development*, pp. 3–19. New York: Cambridge University Press.

Hodapp, R. M. & Fidler, D. J. (1999). Special education and genetics: connections for the 21st century. *Journal of Special Education*, **33**, 130–137.

Hodapp, R. M. & Zigler, E. (1990). Applying the developmental perspective to individuals with Down syndrome. In D. M. Cicchetti & Beeghly (eds.), *Children with Down Syndrome*. New York: Cambridge University Press.

Inhelder, B. (1968). *The Diagnosis of Reasoning in the Mentally Retarded*. New York: Day. (Originally published, 1943.)

Mahoney, G., Fors, S., Wood, S. (1990). Maternal directive behavior revisited. *American Journal on Mental Retardation*, **94**, 398–406.

Mans, L., Cicchetti, D., Sroufe, L. A. (1978). Mirror reactions of Down's syndrome infants and toddlers: cognitive underpinnings of self-recognition. *Child Development*, **49**, 1247–1250.

Merighi, J., Edison, M., Zigler, E. (1990). Motivational factors in mentally retarded functioning. In R. M. Hodapp, J. A. Burack, E. Zigler (eds.), *Issues in the Developmental Approach to Mental Retardation*. Cambridge: Cambridge University Press.

Mundy, P. & Sheinkopf, S. (1998). Early communication skill acquisition and developmental disorders. In: J. A. Burack, R. M. Hodapp, E. Zigler. (eds), *Handbook of Mental Retardation and Development*. New York: Cambridge University Press.

Piaget, J. (1970). Piaget's theory. In P. H. Mussen & W. Kessen (eds.), *Handbook of Child Psychology: Vol. 1, History, Theory, and Methods*. New York: Wiley.

Wagner, S., Ganiban, J. M., Cicchetti, D. (1990). Attention, memory and perception in infants with Down syndrome: a review and commentary. In D. Cicchetti & M. Beeghly (eds.), *Children with Down Syndrome: A Developmental Perspective*, pp. 147–179. New York: Cambridge University Press.

Weisz, J. R. & Zigler, E. (1979). Cognitive development in retarded and nonretarded persons: Piagetian tests of the similar sequence hypothesis. *Psychological Bulletin*, **90**, 153–178.

Werner, H. (1948). *Comparative Psychology of Mental Development (Rev. edn.)*. New York: International Universities Press.

Werner, H. (1957). The concept of development from a comparative and organismic point of view. In D. Harris (ed.), *The Concept of Development*. Minneapolis: University of Minnesota Press.

Werner, H. & Wapner, S. (1949). Sensory-tonic field theory of perception. *Journal of Personality*, **18**, 88–107.

Zigler, E. (1967). Familial mental retardation: a continuing dilemma. *Science*, **155**, 292–298.

Zigler, E. (1969). Developmental versus difference theories of mental retardation and the problem of motivation. *American Journal of Mental Deficiency*, **73**, 536–556.

Zigler, E. (1971). The retarded child as a whole person. In H. E. Adams & W. K. Boardman (eds.), *Advances in Experimental Clinical Psychology*. New York: Pergamon.

Zigler, E. & Balla, D. (1982). Motivational and personality factors in the performance of the retarded. In E. Zigler & D. Balla (eds.), *Mental Retardation: The Developmental-Difference Controversy*, pp. 9–26. Hillsdale: Erlbaum.

Zigler, E. & Hodapp, R. (1986). *Understanding Mental Retardation*. New York: Cambridge University Press.

Aspects of motor development in Down syndrome

Naznin Virji-Babul, Anne Jobling, Digby Elliot, Daniel Weeks

Introduction

In the first year of life, typically developing infants make huge strides in motor development. They progress from a limited repertoire of spontaneous and reflex movements to more purposeful, goal-directed movements. Using their arms, they achieve greater balance in more upright positions and progress from sitting and crawling to standing and walking. The rate of motor development is influenced by a number of factors including the maturation of the nervous system, individual/genetic make-up, the ability to process sensory stimulation such as touch, sound, vestibular, muscle and joint sensations, and movement experience within different environmental contexts. While movement experience has always been recognized as important for motor learning, it is only recently that evidence of the central nature of action experience on cognitive development is being explored. As a consequence, there is increased appreciation that infants learn rapidly from active experience and are able to transfer this knowledge to viewing the actions of others (Sommerville et al., 2005).

The onset of locomotion is one of the major transitions in early development and results in changes not only in motor skill but also in perception, spatial cognition, and social and emotional development (Campos et al., 2000). As infants become more mobile and start to explore their environment, they learn not only about their own bodies but also about objects, places, and events that have consequences for mobile exploration. Walking has tremendous implications on all areas of development. The opportunities for exploration, play, and interaction with peers increase significantly. In addition, walking has an impact on the development of the perception of space and objects, and is a prerequisite for more advanced locomotor skills. Meltzoff and Brookes (2008) proposed that the information infants take from their own experience and from observing the actions of others is mapped onto a shared abstract framework. Meltzoff and Brookes reported that the infant's experience is informed by understanding similar experiences in others. Such an ability to form abstract representations of goal-directed actions would provide infants with a powerful learning mechanism by enabling them to rapidly transfer action information across modalities and from one agent to another, and thereby would provide the basis for the acquisition of a host of cognitive abilities that rely on recognizing goal structure in action.

For many infants and children with Down syndrome (DS), delays in motor development and postural control no doubt limit motor experiences and motor exploration. The question of whether and how these delays impact on perception and cognition has not been studied

Neurocognitive Rehabilitation of Down Syndrome, eds. Jean-Adolphe Rondal, Juan Perera, and Donna Spiker. Published by Cambridge University Press. © Cambridge University Press 2011.

directly. However, given the findings in the literature on typical development, it is reasonable to assume that motor delays will impact negatively on the overall movement experiences available to the infant with DS and this, in turn, will lead to some degree of change in perception, spatial cognition and motor learning, and development. The purpose of this chapter is to briefly review the literature on select motor development issues in DS and highlight some new research in relation to early intervention strategies. Finally, we discuss some recent trends in neuroscience that might inspire a new framework for understanding perception and action and, in turn, stimulate new directions for research on DS.

Fundamental perceptual–motor processes

There is now compelling evidence that children with DS exhibit both motor and perceptual difficulties that jointly impact on motor development. In this section, we briefly review two fundamental perceptual–motor skills that demonstrate such impact: the development of reach-to-grasp and locomotion.

Development of reach-to-grasp

The ability to successfully manipulate objects is highly dependent on the ability to reach and grasp. The characteristics of reach-to-grasp have been well documented and generally consist of two components: transport (brings the hand to the object) and manipulation (fingers are opened in readiness for the grasp and then closed to form an appropriate grasp) (Jeannerod, 1981, 1984). The reach-and-grasp must be coordinated in space and time so that the fingers remain open until the hand reaches the object. In typically developing children, functional reaching begins at about four months of age. Initially, reaches tend to be clumsy and circuitous and – within a few months – they become more coordinated and straight (Von Hofsten, 1991). Arbib (1981) has shown that the ability to adapt the grasp in relation to the object is one of the important features of mature reaching. Furthermore, he suggested that knowing the goal of the task together with the knowledge of the properties of the object to be grasped will determine hand posture and type of grasp.

There are a number of factors that can affect the development of reach-and-grasp in infants with DS. Hypotonia or low muscle tone can affect muscles throughout the body. Low muscle tone in the muscles of the trunk can impact on postural stability, thereby making it difficult to maintain balance while the infant is attempting to lean forward and reach for an object. In addition, hypotonia in the muscles around the shoulder joint, lower arm, and hand may result in increased co-contraction (Latash, 2000), making grasping and manipulating movements quite challenging.

One critical component in relation to grasping objects is hand size. Children with DS generally have smaller hands in comparison with children without DS (Chumlea et al., 1979). This may make it more difficult for infants to start to hold large objects and to perform manipulations, thus limiting the types of toys the infant chooses to handle. As the child matures, movements that need a larger finger span may also be more difficult. Savelsbergh and colleagues (2000) studied the grasping behavior of children with DS (aged 3–11 years). They reported that there was a significant difference between the finger spans of children with and without DS. Children with DS had an average finger span of 8.2 cm, while the children without DS had an average span of 9.9 cm. Children with DS used a one-handed grasping pattern less often than their age-matched peers. Interestingly, however, the differences in grasping patterns decreased when the size of the hand was taken into account. The authors stressed the importance of using objects that are scaled to the size of the hand to develop the skill of grasping. By providing appropriately scaled objects for the infant to grasp, the opportunities for increased manipulation increase. Infants may begin to use their hands more frequently to explore the world around them. Structuring the environment to increase the probability of manipulation will help to develop their perceptual–motor abilities.

Development of walking

Walking is an extremely complex skill and there are a multitude of factors that influence the development of walking in typically developing children. Successful locomotion requires the control and coordination of multiple joints, generation of appropriate forces, activation of specific patterns of muscles, modulation of changes in the center of gravity, and coordination of information from the visual, auditory, vestibular, and proprioceptive systems. These patterns must be coordinated with the appropriate timing and take into account the goal of the task and changes in the environment (Leonard, 1998). In addition, factors such as muscle strength, endurance, and fatigue all influence ambulation. Once achieved, walking has tremendous implications on all areas of development. The opportunities for exploration, play, and interaction with peers increase significantly, impacting on cognitive, language, and social development (Ulrich et al., 2001). In addition, walking has an impact on the development of the perception of space and objects, and promotes increased active participation.

Delays in the acquisition of this highly complex skill can therefore be a source of great anxiety for both parents and professionals. In children with DS, the wide range and combination of specific physical, cognitive, sensory, perceptual, and developmental changes can have a significant impact on the onset and development of walking. Independent walking can occur within a broad time-frame extending from 13 months to 48 months of age (Reid & Block, 1996). Decreased muscle strength and/or lack of postural control or balance skills are some of the factors that are thought to contribute to the delayed onset of walking (Dyer et al., 1990; Ulrich et al., 1992).

Ulrich and Ulrich (1995) compared the spontaneous leg movements of infants with and without DS. They did not observe significant differences between the frequencies of leg movements between the two groups. However, they did note that there were fewer occurrences of more complex patterns of leg movements such as kicking. Interestingly, they found that in both groups of infants, the frequency of kicking was significantly correlated with the age of onset of walking.

By looking at the postures assumed by infants in a variety of circumstances (i.e. postural reactions), Haley (1986, 1987) was able to establish a strong relationship between the system of postural control and the achievement of developmental motor milestones. Unlike typically developing children who develop a wide variety of postural reactions, these studies showed that infants with DS refined only those actions necessary for their immediate milestone phase.

The immature gait pattern observed in individuals with DS is thought to result from a poor heel–toe mechanism, which is in part a result of a dysfunction in the kinetics related to ankle movements (Parker & Bronks, 1980; Parker et al., 1986; Cioni et al., 2001). Compensatory movements observed in walking were correlated with an abnormal base of support and flat foot contact with the ground. Qualitatively, children with DS demonstrate poor heel-strike patterns and instability during the support phase of walking, where their weight is momentarily taken on one leg. Arm movements may also be poorly controlled and appear stiff.

In an analysis of the walking patterns of children with DS (five and seven years of age), Parker and Bronks (1980) reported that there were significant differences in gait pattern when compared with typically developing children. These differences were evident in the quality as well as in the form of the movements associated with walking (Parker et al., 1986). This finding was supported by MacNeill-Shea and Mezzomo (1985), who showed a lack of ankle joint strength and balance control in heel-down squatting. Recently, Galli and colleagues (2008) conducted a full 3D gait analysis in a large cohort of children with DS. Their analysis revealed increased joint stiffness at the hip joint with decreased stiffness at the ankle joint, suggesting that there may be a number of different compensatory responses occurring owing to muscle weakness and hypotonia that may have a significant influence on the development of fundamental motor skills.

Virji-Babul and Brown (2004) examined the movement strategies used by young children with DS as they crossed obstacles of two different heights – a subtle obstacle that was placed at a very minimum height off the floor and an obvious obstacle that was placed at a much greater height off the floor. Children with DS were able to successfully extract information about obstacle height and appropriately match this information to their movements. However, visual information about the obstacle was not consistently used to modulate movements early in the gait cycle. Greater step length variability was observed in response to the subtle obstacle suggesting that some form of anticipatory adjustments were being made. In contrast, there was very little variability observed in response to the higher obstacle. This finding, in combination with the observation that the children with DS stopped in front of the higher obstacle for long periods of time, indicated that children with DS may be unable to use early visual cues about negotiating an obstacle, and thus wait until they reach an obstacle to extract the visual information needed to appropriately modulate their actions. This conclusion corroborates the findings of Charlton et al. (2002) and others and provides further evidence of difficulties in perceptual–motor coupling in DS.

More recently, Virji-Babul et al. (2006) examined the influence of the environment in a playground setting on the movement strategies used by children with DS. They analyzed the level of motor engagement with playground equipment and within the playground environment. In this particular playground, the environment was classified according to the following categories: non-grass surface, uneven grass surface, and grass surface with an incline. Tasks were categorized into the following self-initiated motor tasks: walking, running, and walking and balancing on one foot (e.g. when climbing over an obstacle or toy).

Not surprisingly, the non-grass, even surface was more conducive to a larger range of motor skills such as walking, running, and climbing. As the surface became more challenging, the children had more difficulty. When walking and running on an uneven surface and going up or down an incline, many of the children walked with a wide-based gait or ran slowly. Balancing on one foot while climbing over an obstacle or getting into a stationary piece of playground equipment was particularly difficult, and all the children required external support (either from a parent or by holding on to the equipment) to balance on one foot while on an uneven surface.

The development of locomotion and of reach-to-grasp demonstrates the difficulties associated with the acquisition of skills that requires complex interactions, or couplings between perceptual processes. That such couplings may be uniquely compromised in persons with DS is a theme we shall return to later.

Early intervention

In an excellent review of the studies documenting the effects of early intervention for children with DS, Spiker and Hopmann (1997) stated that there is a general assumption that early intervention is of benefit to both infants with DS and their families. These benefits are believed, first, to relate directly to improving the rate of development of the infant and, second, to provide parents with emotional support, professional service, and education about DS. However, in reviewing studies from a broad range of interventions (i.e. language and communication, parent–child interaction, motor and physical development), the results remain unclear. In the area of motor development, Harris (1985) showed that while there were some benefits reported following specific motor therapies, the design of the studies was such that made the results questionable.

It is therefore important that careful planning of early intervention services be done so that the long-term needs of a child with DS are taken into account. Planning from the perspectives of the child, family, teacher, and service provider constitutes an essential part of early childhood intervention service provision.

Program planning

Presently, it is assumed that all program planning activities are highly individualized and respond to the unique needs and assets of children and their families (Lollar et al., 2000). A planning tool, such as the Individualized Family Service Plan (IFSP), is frequently used and goals, objectives, and the services or specific programs that children and families will receive as well as the specific curriculum are outlined. The use of specific instructional strategies may also be indicated. The IFSP should be flexible with an ongoing, decision-making process inherent. Programs should be implemented in a systematic manner that allows families to consider various service alternatives and the teacher to facilitate this process (Jobling & Gavidia-Payne, 2002).

A range of instructional approaches is generally used in early childhood intervention. These instructional strategies play a significant role in the teaching, maintenance, and generalization of skills in young children, and in meeting a full range of their needs. Wolery (1994) proposed four different instructional procedures:

1   Positive reinforcement is considered to be one of the most powerful strategies in changing human behavior and it is contingent on the presentation of a stimulus following a response that results in an increase in the future occurrence of the response. In early childhood settings, this procedure may be used to shape a particular behavior, such as a social skill, which could produce positive benefits for the child.
2   Naturalistic (milieu) strategies have mainly been used in the promotion of language and communication development. These strategies have the following characteristics: they are used during ongoing activities and interactions; they involve repeated use of brief interactions between children and adults; they are responsive to children's behavior; they involve giving children feedback and naturally occurring consequences; and they require purposeful planning on the part of adults (Jobling & Gavidia-Payne, 2002).
3   Peer-mediated strategies are used to promote social interaction in regular play settings. Peers are given consistent opportunities for using social, motor, and language skills with the teacher providing positive reinforcement when a goal is achieved. Motor skill activities provide many opportunities for the use of this strategy.

4   Prompting strategies involve the use of prompts to help a child perform a skill. They can be used to help children learn and then the prompts are systematically faded and positive reinforcement is used. Prompts may be given verbally, but with motor skill development may be given physically to assist the child to feel the movement.

No one strategy should be used exclusively by the teacher in an early childhood special education setting, as the use of a diverse set of strategies enables the teacher to cater for the specific characteristics of the child, the range of motor skill(s) that are to be taught, and the features of the child's environment.

Generalization of skills

One of the key issues in early intervention research is that of generalization to other situations. In her review, Henderson (1985) suggested that the motor skills learned in one situation should not be assumed to transfer to novel situations. This raises the question of how change is measured and what tools should be used to measure the success of early intervention programming.

For example, Ulrich and colleagues (Ulrich et al., 2001) recently conducted a study to determine if the practice of stepping on a motorized treadmill could help reduce the delay in walking onset in infants with DS. Infants were randomly assigned to two groups – a control group and an intervention group. All infants received traditional physical therapy at least every other week. Infants in the intervention group practiced stepping on specially engineered miniature treadmills five days per week, for eight minutes a day. The authors reported that the infants in the intervention group learned to walk earlier than the infants in the control group. These results are both interesting and encouraging but demand further study prior to broad adoption of the exercise as an intervention tool.

First, the long-term outcome of this intervention requires further evaluation. As mentioned in the earlier section, ambulation (the ability to walk) requires the integration of multiple inputs from the visual, proprioceptive, and vestibular systems. In addition, the pattern of ambulation is directly related to the task and the environment. Locomotion conducted on a treadmill involves an environment that is constant and requires no anticipatory postural adjustments. An obvious question is: what is the impact on the development of postural control? That is, how will the infants transfer the skills learned under very specific and controlled conditions to walking under very different environments – where the surface on which they are walking may change and where there are other people walking, or where there are obstacles to be negotiated?

The important point here is that research into early intervention needs to be directed at analysis of specific functional outcomes. The influence of the program on both the child and family must be addressed from this perspective. That is, do the skills that are emphasized in the intervention program generalize to situations at school, in the playground, and at home? As a consequence, it is critical to determine what elements of the programming have had the greatest impact on functional outcomes.

Guralnick (1997) suggested that early intervention programs should be flexible enough to consider both the individual child's need and the needs of the family. Although the overall framework of the program may remain consistent, the specific features within the program should be responsive to the changing needs of the family, as these features can influence developmental outcomes. For example, family stress and response to stressors (i.e. in relation to their child with a disability or other family circumstances) are key determinants of the early intervention approach used for a specific child. This is particularly relevant in light of recent work that suggests that the match between family and program characteristics is critical to the effectiveness of early intervention programming (Dunst, 2000).

One example of an early intervention program that is designed specifically for infants with DS and their caregivers is the Learn at Play Program (LAPP). LAPP prioritizes the goals of nurturing and shaping the development of interpersonal skills and social competence among children with DS (Iarocci et al., 2006). Within this framework the initial developmental tasks involved maximizing the quality of early dyadic interactions between infants with DS and their parents within a play context. As the children develop, the tasks are modified to reflect developmentally appropriate goals that emphasize the social and emotional skills that are essential for children during the preschool years and the transition into formal schooling. Interventions are designed to target the specific domains (e.g. motor, language, short-term memory) that are typically affected by DS within the broader context of social competence goals. The main components of LAPP include: relationship building, social communicative competence, triadic interactions (joint attention), imitative and social play, and social understanding and awareness of the child as a separate individual.

Recent research from neuroscience

As we noted in a previous section, one underlying factor that cuts across much of our own research (and our interpretation of much of the research literature) is the difficulty in perceptual–motor coupling that seems to accompany DS. Over the last decade, there have been some new developments in neuroscience that provide evidence for a possible neural mechanism for the functional relationship between perception and action. This neural substrate named the mirror neuron system was first discovered in the inferior prefrontal cortex (area F5) and inferior parietal lobule (area PF) in the monkey. Cell units in these areas were found to discharge both when the monkey produced an object-related action and when it observed another monkey or an experimenter performing the same or similar action (Gallese et al., 1996; Rizzolatti et al., 1996). This discovery has led to the hypothesis that action understanding may be achieved by mapping the visual representation of the observed action onto the observer's motor representation for the same actions (Buccino et al., 2001). In humans, evidence for mirror neurons that respond to both the observation and execution of an action has been associated with the ventral premotor cortex, the inferior parietal lobe (Rizzolatti & Craighero, 2004), and the superior temporal sulcus (STS) (Iacoboni et al., 2001). Given the difficulties in perceptual–motor processing evident in individuals with DS, we hypothesized that there may be a dysfunction in the mirror neuron system in DS. We investigated this hypothesis by asking adult participants with and without DS to make self-paced movements that involved reaching with the dominant hand to grasp and lift a cup and to observe an experimenter performing the same action. We imaged participants' brains under both conditions using magnetoencephalography (MEG) (Virji-Babul et al., 2008, 2010).

In the observation condition, cortical activity in the control group involved a network of areas including the right mid-temporal gyrus, premotor, and parietal regions. Of particular interest was that although there were strong activations observed in the right parietal, frontal, and bilateral temporal regions in the DS group, no significant peak activity was observed in the motor areas. Consistent with our hypothesis, the most significant finding of this study was the diminished correspondence between the networks involved in action execution and action observation in the group with DS.

These results suggest that at least some of the skill performance and acquisition challenges associated with DS may be related to impairments in those processes involved in extracting relevant visual cues from the environment and matching (or coupling) that information to their own movements. The impact of perceptual–/visual–motor coupling deficits is a relatively new idea and obviously has not been explicitly considered in traditional early intervention programs that often focus on facilitating movement within a typical developmental trajectory framework.

From our point of view, it may be that to facilitate early perceptual–/visual–motor competencies, individuals with DS may benefit from intervention experiences that emphasize the development of effective perceptual–/visual–motor coupling. This might include strategies to enhance the ability of infants to attend to salient features of objects, people, and the environment, and enhance active manipulation of toys. The goal is to increase active exploration of the environment and, in turn, facilitate generalization of skills through practice in different environmental contexts and under different conditions.

Conclusions

Parents and caregivers have a unique and integral role in any intervention and they require a good understanding of any specific aims, goals, and expected responses as well as the methods used to gain the desired outcome. Professionals such as therapists and teachers need to ensure that the focus is on the child within the family context, not on the program or any specific intervention. For example, as suggested by Lydic and Steele (1979) and Harris (1988), there are many daily activities such as feeding, changing, bathing, and playing that parents can be taught to use to facilitate normal postural responses and movement. In using this realistic and common-sense approach toward programming, interventions are not isolated from the child's environment or from the motor aspects of a functional task. Intervention is a process not a performance. As such, slow may be fast enough. It is important to recognize that the intervention/s for some children may be limited owing to the unique biological and behavioral properties of the syndrome, and there may be some basic anomalies in the central nervous and musculoskeletal systems that, at present, cannot be ameliorated.

The development of a movement language can assist in the association between the mover, the task, and the environment (Jobling et al., 2006). There is an inherent importance in the use of language – words, signs, and gestures – to enhance the visual images of movement and moving. Words can help children understand and frame their movement responses by drawing their attention to the actions that are required. Movement is dynamic and can be enlivened with words, sentences, rhymes, and conversations so that moving is not just the passage of a limb or body part from here to there, nor a succession of exercise activities or movement routines, but an expression of themselves to be participated in and enjoyed.

The study of motor development has a long history. However, intervention strategies for individuals with developmental challenges are still primarily based on our understanding of typical developmental trajectories. With new paradigms and techniques emerging from the movement sciences and neurosciences, it may soon be possible to tailor interventions that target the unique information processing profile and developmental trajectory associated with DS and other development disabilities.

Summary

For many infants and children with Down syndrome (DS), delays in motor skill acquisition and postural control limit the opportunities for movement experiences and exploration. As a consequence, this presents a significant challenge to optimizing their developmental trajectory. In this chapter we briefly review the literature on select motor development issues in DS and highlight some new research in relation to early intervention strategies. Finally, we discuss some recent trends in neuroscience that might inspire a new framework for understanding perception and action and, in turn, stimulate new directions for research on DS.

Author notes

Much of this chapter is adapted from the book *Down Syndrome: Play, Move and Grow* by Anne Jobling and Naznin Virji-Babul. Those interested in obtaining a copy of this book should visit the Down Syndrome Research Foundation website at www.dsrf.org.

References

Arbib, M. A. (1981). Perceptual structures and distributed motor control. In V. B. Brooks (ed.), *Handbook of Physiology – Section 1: The Nervous System, Vol. 2: Motor Control*, pp. 1449–1480. American Physiological Society.

Buccino, G., Binkofski, F., Fink, G. R., et al. (2001). Action observation activates premotor and parietal areas in a somatotopic manner: an fMRI study. *European Journal of Neuroscience*, 13, 400–404.

Campos, J. J., Anderson, D. I., Barbu-Roth, M. A., et al. (2000). Travel broadens the mind. *Infancy*, 1, 149–219.

Charlton, J., Ibsen, E., Lavelle, B. M. (2000). Control of manual skills in children with Down syndrome. In D. J. Weeks, R. Chua, D. Elliott (eds.), *Perceptual-Motor Behavior in Down Syndrome*, pp. 25–48. Champaign: Human Kinetics.

Chumlea, W. C., Malina, R. M., Rarick, G. L., Seefeldt, V. D. (1979). Growth of short-bones of the hand in children with Down's syndrome. *Journal of Mental Deficiency Research*, 23, 137–150.

Cioni, M., Cocilovo, A., Rossi, F., Paci, D., Valle, M. S. (2001). Analysis of ankle kinetics during walking in individuals with Down syndrome. *American Journal on Mental Retardation*, 106, 470–478.

Dunst, C. J. (2000). Revisiting "rethinking early intervention". *Topics in Early Childhood Special Education*, 20, 95–104.

Dyer, S., Gunn, P., Rauh, H., Berry, P. (1990). Motor development in Down's syndrome children: an analysis of the motor scale of the Bayley scale of infant development. In A. Vermeer (ed.), *Motor Development, Adapted Physical Activity and Mental Retardation*, pp. 7–20. Basel: Karger.

Gallese, V., Fadiga, L., Fogassi, L., Rizzolatti, G. (1996). Action recognition in the premotor cortex. *Brain*, 119(2), 593–609.

Galli, M., Rigoldi, C., Brunner, R., Virji-Babul, N., Albertini, G. (2008). Joint stiffness and gait pattern evaluation in children with Down syndrome. *Gait and Posture*, 28(3), 502–506.

Guralnick, M. J. (1997). Second generation research in the field of early intervention. In M. J. Guralnick (ed.), *The Effectiveness of Early Intervention*, pp. 271–305. Baltimore: Brookes.

Haley, S. M. (1986). Postural reactions in infants with Down syndrome: relationship to motor milestone development and age. *Physical Therapy*, 66, 17–22.

Haley, S. M. (1987). Sequence of development of postural reactions by infants with Down syndrome. *Developmental Medicine and Child Neurology*, 29, 674–679.

Harris S. R. (1985). Neuromotor development of infants with Down syndrome. *Developmental Medicine and Child Neurology*, 27, 99–100.

Harris, S. R. (1988). Down's Syndrome. *Papers and Abstracts for Professionals*, 11(7), 1–4.

Henderson, S. E. (1985). Motor skill development. In D. Lane & B. Stratford (eds.),

Current Approaches to Down's Syndrome, pp. 187–218. London: Holt, Rinehart & Winston.

Iacoboni, M., Koski, L. M., Brass, M., et al. (2001). Reafferent copies of imitated actions in the right superior temporal cortex. *Proceedings of the National Academy of Sciences of the United States of America*, **98**(24), 13995–13999.

Iarocci, G., Virji-Babul, N., Reebye, P. (2006). The Learn At Play Program (LAPP): merging family, developmental research, early intervention and policy goals for children with Down syndrome. *Journal of Policy and Practice in Intellectual Disabilities*, **3**(1), 11–21.

Jeannerod, M. (1981). Intersegmental coordination during reaching at natural visual objects. In J. Long & A. Baddeley (eds.), *Attention and Performance IX*, pp. 153–168. Hillsdale: Lawrence Erlbaum.

Jeannerod, M. (1984). The timing of nature prehension movements. *Journal of Motor Behavior*, **16**, 235–254.

Jobling, A. & Gavidia-Payne, S. (2002). Early schooling for infants and children with diverse abilities. In A. Ashman & J. Eiken (eds.), *Educating Children with Diverse Abilities*, pp. 116–159. Sydney: Prentice-Hall.

Jobling, A., Virji-Babul, N., Nichols, D. (2006). Children with Down syndrome: discovering the joy of movement. *Journal of Physical Education, Recreation and Dance*, **77**(6), 34–38.

Latash, M. L. (2000). Motor coordination in Down syndrome: the role of adaptive changes. In D. J. Weeks, R. Chua, D. Elliott (eds.), *Perceptual-Motor Behavior in Down Syndrome*, pp. 199–223. Champaign: Human Kinetics.

Leonard, C. T. (1998). *The Neuroscience of Human Movement*. St. Louis: Mosby-Year Book.

Lollar, D. J., Simeonsson, R. J., Nanda, U. (2000). Measures of outcomes for children and youth. *Archives of Physical Medicine and Rehabilitation*, **81**, S46–S52.

Lydic, J. S. & Steele, C. (1979). Assessment of the quality of sitting and gait patterns in children with Down's Syndrome. *Physical Therapy*, **59**, 1489–1494.

MacNeill-Shea, S. H. & Mezzomo, J. M. (1985). Relationship of ankle strength and hypermobility to squatting skills in children with Down syndrome. *Physical Therapy*, **65**, 1658–1661.

Meltzoff, A. N. & Brooks, R. (2008). Self-experience as a mechanism for learning about others: a training study in social cognition. *Developmental Psychology*, **44**(5), 1257–1265.

Parker, A. W. & Bronks, R. (1980). Gait of children with Down syndrome. *Archives of Physical Medicine and Rehabilitation*, **61**, 345–351.

Parker, A. W., Bronks, R., Snyder, C. W., Jr. (1986). Walking patterns in Down's syndrome. *Journal of Mental Deficiency Research*, **30**, 317–330.

Reid, G. & Block, M. E. (1996). Motor development and physical education. In B. Stratford & P. Gunn (eds.), *New Approaches to Down Syndrome*, pp. 309–340. London: Cassell.

Rizzolatti, G. & Craighero, L. (2004). The mirror-neuron system. *Annual Review of Neuroscience*, **27**, 169–192.

Rizzolatti, G., Fadiga, L., Gallese, V., Fogassi, L. (1996). Premotor cortex and the recognition of motor actions. *Cognitive Brain Research*, **3**, 131–141.

Savelsbergh, G., Van Der Kamp, J., Ledebt, A., Planinsek, T. (2000). Information-movement coupling in children with Down syndrome. In D. J. Weeks, R. Chua, D. Elliott (eds.), *Perceptual-Motor Behavior in Down Syndrome*, pp. 251–276. Champaign: Human Kinetics.

Sommerville, J. A., Woodward, A. L., Needham, A. (2005). Action experience alters 3-month-old infants' perception of others' actions. *Cognition*, **96**, B1–B11.

Spiker, D. & Hopmann, M. R. (1997). The effectiveness of early intervention for children with Down syndrome. In M. J. Guralnick (ed.), *The Effectiveness of Early Intervention*, pp. 271–305. Baltimore: Brookes.

Ulrich, B. D. & Ulrich, D. A. (1995). Spontaneous leg movements of infants with Down syndrome and nondisabled infants. *Child Development*, **66**, 1844–1855.

Ulrich, D. A., Ulrich, B. D., Angulo-Kinzler, R. M., Yun, J. (2001). Treadmill training of infants with Down syndrome: evidence-based developmental outcomes. *Pediatrics*, **108**, E84.

Ulrich, B. D., Ulrich, D. A., Collier, D. H. (1992). Alternating stepping patterns: hidden abilities of 11-month-old infants with Down syndrome. *Developmental Medicine and Child Neurology*, **34**, 233–239.

Virji-Babul, N. & Brown, M. (2004). Stepping over obstacles: anticipatory modifications in children with and without Down syndrome. *Experimental Brain Research*, **159**, 487–490.

Virji-Babul, N., Hovorka, R., Jobling, A. (2006). Playground dynamics: perceptual-motor behaviour and peer interactions of young children with Down syndrome. *Journal on Developmental Disabilities*, **12**(1, Suppl 2), 29–42.

Virji-Babul, N., Moiseev, A., Cheung, T., et al. (2008). Changes in mu rhythm during action observation and execution in adults with Down syndrome: implications for action representation. *Neuroscience Letters*, **436**(2), 177–180.

Virji-Babul, N., Moiseev, A., Cheung, T., et al. (2010). Neural mechanisms underlying action observation in adults with Down syndrome. *American Journal of Intellectual and Developmental Disabilities*, **115**, 113–127.

Von Hofsten, C. (1991). Structuring of early reaching movements: a longitudinal study. *Journal of Motor Behavior*, **23**, 280–292.

Wolery, M. (1994). Instructional strategies for teaching children with special needs. In M. Wolery & J. Wilbers (eds.), *Including Children with Special Needs in Early Childhood Programs*, pp. 119–150. Washington, DC: National Association for Education of Young Children.

Memory development and learning

12

Stefano Vicari and Deny Menghini

Introduction

Distinct cognitive profiles among individuals with mental retardation (MR) of different etiologies have recently been documented. Studies from different laboratories, for example, have demonstrated a complex neuropsychological profile in people with Down syndrome (DS), with atypical development in the cognitive and linguistic domains (for a review see Vicari et al., 2004; Vicari, 2006). However, a quite different pattern is often reported in other syndromes such as Williams syndrome (WS). This is another genetic condition, less frequent but equally characterized by MR and typified by a number of severe medical anomalies, such as facial dysmorphology and abnormalities of the cardiovascular system (Bellugi et al., 1999). Differently from DS, WS children often show marked impairment in certain spatial abilities (especially praxic–constructive) and relative preservation of both productive and receptive language, at least concerning the phonological elements (Vicari et al., 2004).

Within the neuropsychological approach to MR, the study of memory and learning is particularly relevant. In fact, altered development of the memory function can seriously interfere with adequate maturation of general intellectual abilities, and thus with the possibility of learning and modifying behavior on the basis of experience.

This chapter is dedicated to reviewing the neuropsychological literature and recent experimental studies on memory and learning development in people with DS, reporting their memory capacities and deficits. Consistent with a neuropsychological approach, distinct memory profiles can be traced to the characteristics of the DS brain development and architecture. Therefore, the possible correlation between memory profiles and brain development will also be presented and discussed.

Short-term memory and Down syndrome

Human memory is a complex cognitive function organized in independent but interactive subcomponents. In agreement with Atkinson and Shiffrin (1971) and Squire (1987), the memory function can first be distinguished in short-term memory (STM) and long-term memory (LTM).

Concerning STM, many previous studies have documented its impairment as measured by digit or word span in individuals with DS compared to groups of mentally age-matched controls (for a review see Vicari & Carlesimo, 2002).

Neurocognitive Rehabilitation of Down Syndrome, eds. Jean-Adolphe Rondal, Juan Perera, and Donna Spiker. Published by Cambridge University Press. © Cambridge University Press 2011.

In an attempt to describe a more accurate model of STM, Baddeley & Hitch (1974) have proposed a tripartite working memory (WM) model. Accordingly, WM is defined as a limited capacity system for the temporary storage of information held for further manipulation (also Baddeley, 1986). WM results from the cooperation of two major systems. The first is a central executive system, a limited-capacity central processor able to temporarily store and process information from many modalities. The second major system of the WM model consists of a number of peripheral slave systems, or limited-capacity systems, which temporarily store and rehearse information belonging to a single modality, when the flow of data surpasses the capacity of the central executive system. The articulatory loop is a two-component system specialized for the temporary storage of verbal material. One component is devoted to the passive maintenance of verbal information in a phonological code (phonological store). The other component (articulatory rehearsal) prevents the decay of material stored in the phonological store by refreshing the memory trace. Moreover, it is involved in the re-coding of visually presented verbal material into a phonological format (Baddeley, 1986).

The articulatory loop model can account for two robust experimental findings in verbal span: the phonological similarity effect and the word-length effect. The first effect refers to the phenomenon that strings formed by phonologically similar words (e.g. *rat, bat, cat, mat*) are more difficult to recall immediately after presentation than strings formed by phonologically dissimilar words (e.g. *fish, girl, bus, hand*). The hypothesis that verbal material is held in an acoustic format in the phonological store and that, as a consequence, acoustically similar words form less distinctive memory traces may explain this finding. The word-length effect refers to the finding that the memory span is longer for strings of short words (e.g. *bus, pig, car, tree*) than for lists of long words (e.g. *banana, elephant, policeman, kangaroo*) (Baddeley & Hitch, 1974). This finding is commonly interpreted as evidence of the contribution of articulatory rehearsal to verbal span because long words take longer to be rehearsed than short words.

The visual spatial sketchpad is the second peripheral slave system and it is specialized for the temporary storage of visual material. Although the functioning of this system has been far less investigated than that of the articulatory loop, there is reason to believe that here there is also an internal fractionation of structure and functioning. Indeed, clinical and experimental data support the hypothesis that temporary memory for visual–object information (such as registering colors and shapes) and for the visuospatial location of objects are processed by different but functionally related subsystems (Logie, 1995; Della Sala & Logie, 2002; Vicari et al., 2003).

Hulme and Mackenzie (1992) reported a reduced contribution of the articulatory loop to the verbal span of persons with DS. Namely, DS people would tend not to repeat the verbal sequences which, as a result, would decay rapidly from the phonological store. At partial variance with Hulme and MacKenzie's results, Jarrold et al. (2000) and Kanno and Ikeda (2002) documented a significant word-length effect in children with DS and mentally age-matched typically developing (TD) children. However, no correlation was found between span extension and speech rate.

These results raise a great deal of perplexity about the mechanisms underlying the word-length effect in the verbal span of individuals with DS and of very young TD children. The non-use of the rehearsal mechanism in very young TD children (forming the control groups in the previously mentioned studies) is also at odds with the hypothesis that defective functioning (or a lack of spontaneous utilization) of the rehearsal mechanism is at the base of the poorer verbal span exhibited by DS individuals.

Involvement of the phonological buffer in the verbal STM deficit of children with DS can be the basis of their difficulties in auditory phonological analysis (Chapman, 1995; Fowler, 1995). In fact, a more general relationship between language development and phonological memory is well demonstrated in children with DS (Laws & Gunn, 2003; Laws, 2004) as well as in TD children (Gathercole & Baddeley, 1993). However, a study by Vicari et al. (2004) provided little support for the hypothesis that defective functioning of the phonological store component of the articulatory loop is responsible for poor verbal span in individuals with DS. Indeed, these authors documented analogous susceptibility to phonological similarity in a word span test in participants with DS and in TD controls.

To date, few data have indicated a malfunctioning central executive system as the origin of poor verbal STM in individuals with DS. In a previous study, Vicari et al. (1995) presented forward digit and spatial (Corsi's block) span tasks and backward digit and spatial span tasks (in which the subject had to repeat the numbers or reproduce the spatial sequence in the reverse order) to groups of individuals with DS, with MR of various etiologies, and to mental age-matched TD children. Results showed a specific performance decay in backward span tasks in individuals with DS compared to both TD children and to persons with MR of various etiologies, thus suggesting that reduced resources of the central executive system are responsible for the particularly poor STM in persons with DS.

In summary, compared to mentally age-matched TD children, individuals with DS show poor verbal STM on span tasks. This deficit seems to be independent of the articulatory difficulty they often present. Instead, greater responsibility should be attributed to a poorly functioning phonological buffer or, even more, to deficits of the central executive system.

There are very few data available on the functioning of the visuospatial sketchpad (the slave system of the WM model devoted to the processing of visual material) in children with MR in general and with DS in particular. Wang & Bellugi (1994) documented a relative advantage for DS participants in visuospatial rather than in verbal span, and similar results were obtained by Jarrold et al. (1999) and by Laws (2002).

Vicari et al. (2005) compared DS, WS, and TD children, matched for mental age, in a visual and spatial span test. The two tests involved studying the same complex, nonverbalizable figures and using the same response modality (pointing to targets on the screen). The crucial experimental variable was that, in one case, the position where the figure appeared on the screen had to be recalled; in the other case, the physical aspect of the figure studied had to be recalled. Results documented that people with DS showed reduced performance in both tests. Instead, individuals with WS exhibited specific difficulties in the visuospatial but not the visual–object WM task. However, while the observed selective deficit in individuals with WS persisted even when perceptual abilities were taken into account, the deficits in individuals with DS were compensated when their scores were adjusted for perceptual levels. Indeed, after covarying for performance level on the visual perceptual tasks, performance of the DS participants and the TD children no longer differed on the WM tasks. These results suggest that WM is not uniformly compromised in DS. Although this has been well established for verbal material, in the visuospatial domain it is far less certain whether impairment in perceptual analysis rather than in memory processes is likely to be responsible for the poor performance of the DS individuals.

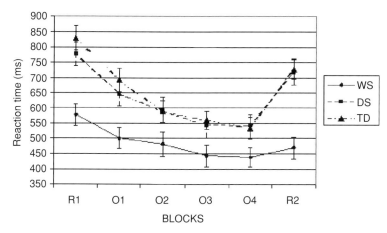

Figure 12.1 Average reaction time performance and standard errors as a function of group and block, ordered (O1, O2, O3, and O4 blocks) vs. random (R1 and R2 blocks) sequences. WS: Williams syndrome; DS: Down syndrome; TD: typically developing. (Reproduced with permission from Vicari et al., 2007.)

Long-term memory in Down syndrome: a diffuse and pervasive impairment?

Verbal and visuospatial LTM have been extensively investigated in persons with MR, and particularly with DS, both in the explicit and in the implicit components (Carlesimo et al., 1997; Nadel, 1999; Vicari & Carlesimo, 2002). Explicit memory concerns intentional recall or recognition of experiences or information. Implicit memory is manifested as a facilitation (that is, an improvement in performance) in perceptual, cognitive, and motor tasks, without any conscious reference to previous experiences. Explicit memory deficits in persons with MR and, particularly, with DS have been extensively documented (Vicari & Carlesimo, 2002). Nevertheless, in the last few years, some experimental data have been reported regarding the possible extension to individuals with MR of the dissociation between explicit and implicit memory processes, so frequently described in brain damaged adults with memory disorders. As for repetition priming, studies investigating facilitation in identifying perceptually degraded pictures or words, induced by the previous exposure to the same material, have consistently reported a comparable priming effect in individuals with MR and in TD children matched for chronological or mental age (for a review see Vicari & Carlesimo, 2002).

Fewer experimental works have been devoted to investigating the ability to learn visuomotor or cognitive skills in individuals with MR, and with DS in particular. Vicari and coworkers documented a difference in the skill learning abilities of DS and WS subjects (Vicari et al., 2000, 2001). Recently, Vicari et al. (2007) directly compared performances obtained by individuals with DS and with WS, and TD persons matched for mental age, in a motor serial reaction time test. As shown in Figure 12.1, Vicari et al. (2007) found a preserved procedural learning in the DS but not in the WS groups, thus confirming a different pattern of implicit learning in the two syndromes of MR individuals.

In comparison with the TD control of comparable mental age, persons with DS usually exhibit peculiar memory patterns (Table 12.1).

Table 12.1 Performances obtained by subjects with Down syndrome and Williams syndrome on different short-term and long-term memory tasks

	DS	WS
STM		
Verbal	−	+
Visuospatial	+	−
LTM		
Explicit	−	+
Verbal	−	+
Visual–object	+	−
Visuospatial	+	+
Implicit	+	−
Repetition priming		
Procedural L.		

DS: Down syndrome; WS: Williams syndrome; STM: short-term memory; LTM: long-term memory; −: impaired; +: relatively preserved.

In STM tasks, people with DS obtain lower performance scores than TD children in processing both verbal and visuospatial material. However, in the visuospatial domain, impairment in perceptual analysis rather than in memory processes is likely responsible for the poor performance of the DS individuals.

In LTM, people with DS exhibit different patterns in explicit and implicit memory domains. Albeit that individuals with DS are usually poorer than the TD mental-age controls in verbal and visuospatial explicit memory tasks, in the implicit memory domain comparable results may be observed between the two groups in repetition priming tasks as well as in procedural learning.

It is worthy of note that the memory profile observed in DS is not shared with other genetic syndromes also characterized by MR. We have, indeed, reported the case of WS that was characterized by relative strengths in verbal and visual STM but impairments in spatial WM (Vicari et al., 2006; Vicari & Carlesimo, 2006). A similar pattern is observed in the explicit LTM domain, whereas an impairment in the ability to learn implicitly new procedures has been reported in adolescents with WS.

Memory, Down syndrome, and brain development

The memory profile in people with DS we described is based on some specific characteristics of anomalous brain development. However, any attempt to identify which neuroanatomical structures are specifically involved in the memory impairment displayed by people with DS is speculative and must be based on qualitative comparisons of their deficits with those displayed by patients with acquired brain lesions.

According to autopsy observations, the brain weight of people with DS is lower than normal and their cerebellum, frontal, and temporal lobes are particularly small (Wisniewski, 1990). Consistent with this, evidence from volumetric magnetic resonance imaging (MRI) studies of individuals with DS suggests reduced overall brain volume, with disproportionately smaller volume in the frontal, temporal (including uncus, amygdala, hippocampus, and parahippocampal gyri) and cerebellar regions (Pinter et al., 2001). By contrast, the brains of people with DS usually show relatively preserved volume of subcortical areas, such as the lenticular nuclei (Bellugi et al., 1999) and posterior (parietal and occipital) cortical gray matter (Pinter et al., 2001).

In the last few years, MRI studies have advanced our understanding of brain anatomy in individuals with genetic syndromes. In particular, a whole-brain, unbiased, objective technique, known as voxel-based morphometry (VBM), has been developed to character-ize brain differences in vivo using MRI images. VBM gives the opportunity to assess differ-ences of brain tissue concentrations or volumes between groups (Ashburner & Friston, 2000; Good et al., 2001). Because it is minimally operator dependent and allows the assessment of regional volumetric effects without an a priori hypothesis about their localization in the brain, VBM is less prone to investigator bias than are predefined volumes-of-interest tech-niques. In particular, the popularity of VBM arises from the opportunity to examine all of the voxels representing the cerebrum, the velocity required to collect data and to analyze results compared to manual methods, and the local specificity for gray or white matter findings that may be lost in large regional volume manual measures.

The VBM technique has recently been employed with individuals with genetic syn-dromes, and it has progressed our understanding of brain anatomy underlying the typical cognitive profile of individuals with MR and, particularly, with DS.

A recent VBM study (White et al., 2003) reported several brain abnormalities in adults with DS compared to age-matched controls, showing both increments and decrements of gray or white matter volume. In particular, concerning the gray matter in DS individuals, a significant decrease in volume in the cerebellum, cingulate gyrus, left medial frontal lobe, right middle/superior temporal gyrus, and left hippocampus was found. Individuals with DS also showed a significant decrease in white matter throughout the inferior brainstem. Conversely, a significant increase in the superior/caudal portion of the brainstem, in the left parahippocampal gyrus, and in the parahippocampal gyri bilaterally was detected.

By applying the VBM method on a group of children and adolescents with DS, Mengh-ini et al., (in press) partially confirmed the previously described VBM study by White et al. (2003). To limit differences in brain development between groups, a sample of children with a restricted age range; namely, 12 children with DS (four girls and eight boys; mean age = 15.5 years, SD = 2.3 years) and 12 age-matched controls (four girls and eight boys; mean age = 15.6 years, SD = 2.2 years) were recruited for the study. Results documented that unlike the controls, children with DS showed a significant local reduction of gray matter density in the left cerebellum, the right hippocampus, the fusiform gyri bilaterally, and the inferior tempo-ral gyri bilaterally. Conversely, they showed a significant increase of gray matter density in the left cerebellum, the right fusiform gyrus, the left and right basal ganglia (putamen, caudate nucleus), the left and right insula, the left and right superior frontal gyrus, the right superior and middle temporal gyrus, and the left and right inferior frontal gyrus (Figure 12.2).

Based on these findings, the neuropsychological profiles described in DS could be because of the differences observed in cortical and subcortical structures. For example, consistent with Fabbro et al. (2002), the reduced performance of people with DS on linguistic tasks may be partially explained as an impairment of the frontocerebellar structures involved in articulation and verbal WM. In other words, the volumetric reduction of frontal and cere-bellar areas in the brains of individuals with DS may determine the reduced efficiency of the cognitive processes usually sustained by the integrity of these cerebral regions, such as speech and phonological WM (at least for the articulatory component). Likewise, reduced LTM capacity, which seems to be the most relevant characteristic of people with DS, may be related to temporal lobe dysfunction and, specifically, to hippocampus dysfunction (Pen-nington et al., 2003). In fact, critical structures in individuals with DS, found to be altered in earlier studies using operator-dependent volumetric MRI techniques (Kesslak et al., 1994;

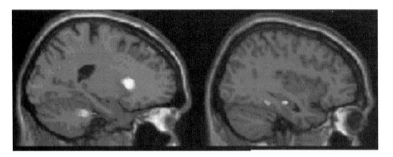

Figure 12.2 Various gray matter areas in which children with Down syndrome had more gray matter density (highlighted; left) than controls, and controls had more gray matter density (highlighted; right) than children with Down syndrome.

Ikeda & Arai, 2002), were the hippocampus and the adjacent medial temporal lobe. However, these results were not always confirmed by automated VBM studies (see Teipel et al., 2004), and the relationship between putative reductions in the hippocampal volume in individuals with DS and specific aspects of their memory phenotype is still unclear. In support of the hypothesis that a reduced hippocampal volume in individuals with DS might explain their episodic memory deficits, hippocampal volumes were reported to be positively correlated with measures of memory function in DS subjects (Krasuski et al., 2002; Teipel et al., 2004). Data in children with DS (Menghini et al., in press) confirmed a hippocampal density reduction in this population group and a general loss of gray matter density in the medial temporal lobe, probably linked with mnesic but also with linguistic difficulties observed in individuals with DS.

Concerning visuospatial abilities, evidence from primates has shown that the extra-striatal cortical areas are organized in two distinct, functionally specialized systems: (1) the dorsal stream (including the structures of the parietal cortex), which is involved in the visual processing of spatial localization; and (2) the ventral stream (including structures of the infer-otemporal cortex) involved in processing information pertaining to the physical characteristics of objects (Mishkin & Ungerleider, 1982). The cortical structures involved in the perceptual processing of stimuli also participate in storage and recovery of the same information (Moscovitch et al., 1995). Concordantly, some experimental data derived from studies on both humans and animals suggest that the maintenance and recovery of information pertaining to spatial position and the physical characteristics of the objects in LTM involve the ventral and dorsal stream in different ways. VBM study on DS (Menghini et al., in press) could contribute to clarifying the dissociation between visual and spatial memory aspects in children with DS. In fact, in order to identify structural brain characteristics potentially accounting for specific clinical features of children with DS, Menghini et al. (in press) used VBM to directly correlate, with no a priori hypothesis on regional changes, brain images and cognitive measures. Toward this aim, an extensive neuropsychological battery was administered to each child with DS, exploring several cognitive domains such as global cognitive functioning, linguistic abilities (lexical production and lexical comprehension), sentence repetition and comprehension, phonological and categorical word fluency, visuomotor and visuospatial abilities, STM abilities (verbal, visual, and spatial STM). Concerning data on memory abilities, significant correlations were found between visual STM measures and the right superior temporal gyrus and the right medial occipital lobe (fusiform gyrus). However, spatial STM measures correlated significantly with the right inferior parietal lobe. Data on STM abilities seemed to confirm the dissociation found in LTM between visual processing and spatial elaboration of the stimuli.

Consistent with the literature and with these written data, we may speculate that people with DS who perform relatively better in visuospatial than in visual–object memory tests might present relatively preserved maturation of the dorsal compared to the ventral component of the visual system. Neuropsychological (Molinari et al., 1997) and neuroimaging data (Van Der Graaf et al., 2004) confirm the critical role of the basal ganglia and the right cerebellum in the implicit learning of visuomotor skills. As reported previously, the brains of individuals with DS exhibit severe cerebellar hypoplasia with normal morphology of basal ganglia. Thus, in view of the normal skill learning displayed by individuals with DS, a prevalent role of basal ganglia development in the normal maturation of procedural memory can be suggested. However, abnormalities in cerebellar areas are still poorly understood. In fact, while some volumetric MRI studies that have measured cerebellar volume in individuals with DS have reported a significant cerebellar reduction (Kesslak et al., 1994; Pinter et al., 2001; Krasuski et al., 2002; White et al., 2003), other studies did not confirm this conclusion (Kesslak et al., 1994; Teipel et al., 2004). Data by Menghini et al. (in press) are consistent with studies that find a cerebellar density reduction in individuals with DS, probably linked to their linguistic difficulties.

In summary, studies of genetic syndromes that describe their individual neuropsychological profiles in relation to specific brain characteristics are still sporadic, and there is no evidence that definitively demonstrates a causal relationship between brain features, cognitive abilities, and behavior in individuals with DS. Other studies directly evaluating the possible correlation between morphovolumetric and spectroscopic indexes of brain functioning and the ability of people with DS to learn visuomotor and cognitive procedures are needed to understand the relative contribution of the basal ganglia and abnormal cerebellar development to the impaired maturation of procedural memory in these people. This is a fascinating challenge with great potential for clarifying the biological nature of behavior and, more specifically, for interpreting the differences observed in the cognitive and LTM functioning of people with DS and, more generally, etiologically well-defined forms of MR.

Conclusions

Memory is usually impaired in people with MR and occurs at different levels of memory articulation. Regarding LTM, differential patterns of impairment are confirmed across different etiological groups of MR individuals. For example, people with DS usually perform worse than TD subjects, matched for mental age on verbal and visuospatial explicit memory tasks, but similarly in the implicit memory domain. It is noteworthy that the memory profile observed in DS is not the same as in persons with WS, who are characterized by relative strength in visual LTM and by impairments in verbal and spatial memory; moreover, impairments in the implicit learning of new procedures.

Findings from the experimental literature reviewed in this chapter can provide invaluable information for educational psychologists and teachers for planning rationally grounded interventions to alleviate the learning difficulties of individuals with DS and to improve their quality of life.

Summary

The neuropsychological approach to mental retardation remarks how the study of memory and learning is of particular relevance. This chapter is dedicated to reviewing the neuropsychological literature and recent experimental studies on memory and learning development in people with Down syndrome (DS), reporting their memory capacities and deficits. Consistently with a neuropsychological approach, distinct memory profiles can be traced to the characteristics of the DS brain development and architecture. Therefore, the possible correlation between memory profiles and brain development are also presented and discussed.

References

Ashburner, J. & Friston, K. J. (2000). Voxel-based morphometry: the methods. *NeuroImage*, **11**, 805–821.

Atkinson, R. C. & Shiffrin, R. M. (1971). The control of short-term memory. *Scientific American*, **225**, 82–90.

Baddeley, A. D. (1986). *Working Memory*. London: Oxford University Press.

Baddeley, A .D. & Hitch, G. (1974). Working memory. In G. Bower (ed.), *The Psychology of Learning and Motivation*, Vol. 8, pp. 47–90. New York: Holt, Rinehart & Winston.

Bellugi, U., Mills, D., Jerningan, T., Hickok, G., Galaburda, A. (1999). Linking cognition, brain structure, and brain function in Williams syndrome. In H. Tager-Flusberg ed.), *Neurodevelopmental Disorders*, pp. 111–136. Cambridge: MIT Press.

Carlesimo, G. A., Marotta, L., Vicari, S. (1997). Long-term memory in mental retardation: evidence for a specific impairment in subjects with Down's syndrome. *Neuropsychologia*, **35**, 71–79.

Chapman, R. S. (1995). Language development in children and adolescents with Down syndrome. In P. Fletcher & B. MacWinney (eds.), *The Handbook of Child Language*, pp. 641–663. Oxford: Blackwell.

Della Sala, S. & Logie, R. H. (2002). Neuropsychological impairments of visual and spatial working memory. In A. Baddeley, B. Wilson, M. Kopelman (eds.), *Handbook of Memory Disorders*, pp. 271 –292. Chichester: Wiley.

Fabbro, F., Alberti, A., Gagliardi, C., Borgatti, R. (2002). Differences in native and foreign language repetition task between subjects with Williams and Down syndromes. *Journal of Neurolinguistics*, **15**, 1–10.

Fowler, A. E. (1995). Linguistic variability in persons with Down syndrome. In L. Nadel & D. Rosenthal (eds.), *Down Syndrome: Living and Learning in the Community*, pp. 121–131. New York: Wiley-Liss.

Gathercole, S. E. & Baddeley, A. D. (1993). *Working Memory and Language*. Hove: Erlbaum.

Good, C. D., Johnsrude, I., Ashburner, J., et al. (2001). A voxel-based morphometric study of ageing in 465 normal adult human brains. *NeuroImage*, **14**, 21–36.

Hulme, C. & Mackenzie, S. (1992). *Working Memory and Severe Learning Difficulties*. Hove: Erlbaum.

Ikeda, M. & Arai, Y. (2002). Longitudinal changes in brain CT scans and development of dementia in Down's syndrome. *European Neurology*, **47**, 205–208.

Jarrold, C., Baddeley, A. D., Hewes, A. K. (1999). Genetically dissociated components of working memory: evidence from Down and Williams syndrome. *Neuropsychologia*, **37**, 637–651.

Jarrold, C., Baddeley, A. D., Hewes, A. K. (2000). Verbal short-term memory deficits in Down syndrome: a consequence of problems in rehearsal? *Journal of Child Psychology and Psychiatry*, **40**(2), 233–244.

Kanno, K. & Ikeda, Y. (2002). Word-length effect in verbal short-term memory in individuals with Down's syndrome. *Journal of Intellectual Disability Research*, **46**, 613–618.

Kesslak, J. P., Nagata, B. S., Lott, I., Nalcioglu, O. (1994). MRI analysis of age-related changes in the brains of individuals with DS. *Neurology*, **44**, 1039–1045.

Krasuski, J. S., Alexander, G. E., Horowitz, B., Rapoport, S. I., Shapiro, M. B. (2002). Relation of medial temporal volumes to age and memory function in non-demented adults with Down's syndrome: implications for the prodromal phase of Alzheimer's disease. *American Journal of Psychiatry*, **159**, 74–81.

Laws, G. (2002). Working memory in children and adolescents with Down syndrome: evidence from a colour memory experiment. *Journal of Child Psychology and Psychiatry*, **43**, 353–364.

Laws, G. (2004). Contributions of phonological memory, language comprehension and hearing to the expressive language of adolescents and young adults with Down syndrome. *Journal of Child Psychology and Psychiatry*, **45**, 1–11.

Laws, G. & Gunn, D. (2003). Phonological memory as a predictor of language comprehension in Down syndrome: a five-year follow-up study. *Journal of Child Psychology and Psychiatry*, **44**, 1–11.

Logie, R. H. (1995). *Visuo-spatial Working Memory*. Hove: Erlbaum.

Menghini, D., Costanzo, F., & Vicari, S. (in press). Relationship between brain and cognitive processes in Down syndrome. *Behavior Genetics*. DOI 10.1007/s10519-011-9448-3.

Mishkin, M. & Ungerleider, L. G. (1982). Contribution of striate inputs to the visuospatial functions of parieto-preoccipital cortex in monkeys. *Behavioral Brain Research*, **6**, 57–77.

Molinari, M., Leggio, M. G., Solida, A., et al. (1997). Cerebellum and procedural learning: evidence from focal cerebellar lesions. *Brain*, **120**, 1753–1762.

Moscovitch, C., Kapur, S., Kohler, S., Houle, S. (1995). Distinct neural correlates of visual long-term memory for spatial location and object identity: a positron emission tomography study in humans. *Proceedings of the National Academy of Science of the United States of America*, **92**, 3721–3725.

Nadel, L. (1999). Learning and memory in Down syndrome. In J. A. Rondal, J. Perera, L. Nadel (eds.), *Down Syndrome: A Review of Current Knowledge*, pp. 133–142. London: Whurr.

Pennington, B. F., Moon J., Edgin, J., Stedron, J., Nadel, L. (2003). The neuropsychology of

Down syndrome: evidence for hippocampal dysfunction. *Child Development*, **74**, 75–93.

Pinter, J. D., Eliez, S., Schmitt, J. E., Capone, G. T., Reiss, A. L. (2001). Neuroanatomy of Down's syndrome: a high-resolution MRI study. *American Journal of Psychiatry*, **158**, 1659–1665.

Squire, L. R. (1987). *Memory and Brain*. Oxford: Oxford University Press.

Teipel, S. J., Alexander, G. E., Schapiro, M. B., et al. (2004). Age-related cortical grey matter reductions in nondemented Down's syndrome adults determined by MRI with voxel-based morphometry. *Brain*, **127**, 811–824.

Van Der Graaf, F. H., De Jong, B. M., Maguire, R. P., Meiners L. C., Leenders K. L. (2004). Cerebral activation related to skills practice in a double serial reaction time task: striatal involvement in random-order sequence learning. *Brain Research and Cognitive Brain Research*, **20**, 120–131.

Vicari, S. (2006). Motor development and neuropsychological patterns in persons with Down syndrome. *Behavior Genetics*, **36**, 355–364.

Vicari, S., Bates, E., Caselli, M. C., et al. (2004). Neuropsychological profile of Italians with Williams syndrome: an example of a dissociation between language and cognition? *Journal of the International Neuropsychological Society*, **10**, 862–876.

Vicari, S., Bellucci, S., Carlesimo, G. A. (2000). Implicit and explicit memory: a functional dissociation in persons with Down syndrome. *Neuropsychologia*, **38**, 240–251.

Vicari, S., Bellucci, S., Carlesimo, G. A. (2001). Procedural learning deficit in children with Williams syndrome. *Neuropsychologia*, **39**, 665–677.

Vicari, S., Bellucci, S., Carlesimo, G. A. (2003). Visual and spatial working memory dissociation: evidence from a genetic syndrome. *Developmental Medicine and Child Neurology*, **45**, 269–273.

Vicari, S., Bellucci, S., Carlesimo, G. A. (2005). Visual and spatial long-term memory: differential pattern of impairments in Williams and Down syndromes.

Developmental Medicine and Child Neurology, **47**, 305–311.

Vicari, S., Bellucci, S., Carlesimo, G. A. (2006). Evidence from two genetic syndromes for the independence of spatial and visual working memory. *Developmental Medicine and Child Neurology,* **48**, 126–131.

Vicari, S. & Carlesimo, G. A. (2002). Children with intellectual disabilities. In A. Baddeley, B. Wilson, M. Kopelman (eds.), *Handbook of Memory Disorders,* pp. 501–518. Chichester: Wiley.

Vicari, S. & Carlesimo, G. A. (2006). Short-term memory deficits are not uniform in Down and Williams syndromes. *Neuropsychological review,* **16**, 87–94.

Vicari, S., Carlesimo, G. A., Caltagirone, C. (1995). Short-term memory in persons with intellectual disabilities and Down syndrome. *Journal of Intellectual Disability Research,* **39**, 532–537.

Vicari, S., Verucci, L., Carlesimo, G. A. (2007). Implicit memory is independent from IQ and age but not from etiology: evidence from Down and Williams syndromes. *Journal of Intellectual Disability Research,* **51**, 932–941.

Wang, P. P. & Bellugi, U. (1994). Evidence from two genetic syndromes for dissociation between verbal and visual-spatial short-term memory. *Journal of Clinical Experimental Neuropsychology,* **16**, 317–322.

Wisniewski, K. E. (1990). Down syndrome children often have brain with maturation delay, retardation of growth, and cortical digenesis. *American Journal of Medical Genetics,* **7**, 274–281.

White, N. S., Alkire, M. T., Haier, R. J. (2003). A voxel-based morphometric study of nondemented adults with Down syndrome. *NeuroImage,* **20**, 393–403.

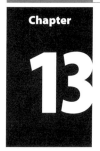

Chapter

13

Prelinguistic and early development, stimulation, and training in children with Down syndrome

Jean-Adolphe Rondal

Language before birth

Language development in typically developing children begins three months before birth. By that time, the auditory system of the fetus/baby is already functional. It is tuned to the speech frequencies (400 to 4000 cycles per second). This is a unique feature of human ontogenesis corresponding to a species-specific predisposition for speech. During the waking periods, every acoustical stimulus exceeding 60 decibels is normally received by the baby's auditory apparatus and treated by the brain. The partial loss of intensity is owing to an energy absorption by the aquatic milieu surrounding the baby and the fact that her/his middle ear is filled with amniotic liquid. As a likely consequence of this exposure, the typically developing baby at birth demonstrates an ability to recognize the mother's voice and individuate it from other voices. This ability is purely prosodic. It relies on the unique tonal and rhythmic characteristics of the mother's voice. This is objectified using the techniques of cognitive–behavioral investigation in neonates (De Boysson-Bardies, 1996). Beyond the particular mother's voice (and through it), typically developing neonates demonstrate an ability to recognize the maternal language (again through its rhythmic characteristics); that is, they can differentiate between the one language that they have been exposed to in utero and other languages (Nazzi et al., 1998).

Young typically developing babies can also differentiate accentuated syllables from non-accentuated ones (Jusczyk et al., 1993). They recognize varied sequences of syllables (Saffran et al., 1996; Marcus et al., 1999). Typically developing neonates can differentiate between functional words in English (i.e. prepositions, articles, auxiliaries, pronouns, conjunctions) and content words (verbs, nouns, adjectives, adverbs), relying on prosodic information (the first category is less accentuated and tends to be shorter in length as well as poorer in mean number of vowels; Shi et al., 1999).

Lastly, typically developing neonates have an inborn ability to discriminate between all possible pairs of sounds present in human speech. This capacity gradually recedes during the first year of life owing to a progressive specialization in the sounds (future phonemes) of the community language (Eimas, 1996).

These abilities and prelanguage knowledge supply a valid point of departure for cracking the language code of the community.

Neurocognitive Rehabilitation of Down Syndrome, eds. Jean-Adolphe Rondal, Juan Perera, and Donna Spiker. Published by Cambridge University Press. © Cambridge University Press 2011.

We know almost nothing about the corresponding abilities in infants and children with Down syndrome (DS). Not knowing when and how exactly prelanguage development starts in babies with DS makes it more difficult to define and elaborate very early intervention programs that may be highly desirable on several grounds (e.g. brain plasticity, short- and middle-term efficiency). The kind of research needed to answer this question should rank high on our agendas for there are reasons to suspect that infants with DS may not be born with the same beginning knowledge regarding the prosodic properties of maternal language as typically developing newborns.

Preliminary data indicate that babies with DS exhibit patterns of attention and habituation to speech sounds that differ from typically developing babies; for instance, longer responses to complex auditory stimuli, and that the former babies are more easily distracted from such stimuli (Tristao & Feitosa, 2000). Investigation with event-related brain potentials and reaction times reveal that children with DS process complex auditory information more slowly than typically developing chronological age- and even mental age-matched pairs (Eilers et al., 1985).

Aberrant lateralization of auditory processing (using brainstem evoked responses) is observed in some individuals with DS (Rondal, 1995). Reversed ear advantages for verbal material in a proportion of children and adults with DS have been reported (Elliott et al., 1987; Rondal, 1995). These indications add to the well-documented auditory transmission and, in some cases, neurosensory deficit in at least 25% of children with DS (Rasore Quartino, 2007).

If this is so, then early prelanguage intervention with babies with DS is in order. It should consist in intensifying the natural verbal and vocal interaction with the baby, quantitatively (at least half-an-hour a day) and qualitatively (slowing down the pace of speech addressed to the baby without altering the normal prosody, except for a higher pitch which is known to act as an attention getter). More on the vanguard side but realistic pending appropriate research, it might prove interesting to increase the intensity level of the mother's voice for several hours a day during the lasts three months of pregnancy in a plausible attempt to sensitize the fetus/baby to the prosodic parameters of maternal speech and language.

Prelanguage in the first year

The typical course of babbling (indiscriminate – in the sense that one cannot recognize any clear vowel or consonant, vocalic, syllabic, reduplicated, and variegated) is observed in infants with DS albeit with some delays. Reduplicated babbling (productions like *bababa*, *papapa*, *tatata*) is a distinct precursor of conventional speech; it is particularly retarded in infants with DS. The same is true for another important prelinguistic aspect, interactive or intermittent babbling, also called prelinguistic phrasing. The infant terminates his/her vocal production after roughly three seconds, waiting for an answer from the interlocutor. Infants with DS tend to vocalize longer (an average of five seconds) with shorter phrase intervals, thus leaving less time for the interlocutor to intervene (hence a higher frequency of vocal clashes between mothers and their infants with DS [Berger & Cunningham, 1983]).

Two other important prelinguistic aspects, also delayed in infants with DS, are preword production and symbolic play.

Prewords are nonconventional words invented or borrowed by the child to refer to a familiar object or event (e.g. *brm-brm* referring to a truck or a plane regularly passing by).

They mark the beginning of symbolic representation and lexical development. The child has understood that a sound or sequence of sounds can be used to signify (that is stand for or represent) an object or an event: symbolic play such as pretending to sleep by putting one's head on a pillow or a flat surface, making a doll eat, sleeping, sliding; using an object to represent another one or an event by moving a piece of wood to indicate a car moving along a street, for instance. Symbolic play is of the same nature as lexical representation. It is a precursor and/or a correlate of early lexical development.

Prelanguage intervention

All vocal productions and the various phases of babbling should be strongly encouraged and socially reinforced in order to promote prelinguistic abilities as a precursor of early linguistic development. Interactive babbling must receive particular attention and be encouraged by having the adult partner frequently addressing the child vocally or verbally for a few seconds at a time, then stopping to leave a four- or five-second interval available to the child for responding.

Prewords are to be welcomed and repeated (child–adult; adult–child), moving gradually toward conventional wording. Symbolic play should also be demonstrated and encouraged in play sessions as a way to increase the symbolic sensitivity of the child with DS. In general, three types of parental responses to the children's attempts at communicating have been found to facilitate later language development (Yoder & Warren, 2001). They are: compliance (with the presumed intentional meaning and communication motive of the child), responding, and linguistic mapping (the adult expressing verbally what the child's nonverbal communication appears to convey).

Orofacial physical therapy

In cases of serious hypotony of the orofacial structures (with buccal malocclusion and tongue protrusion), palatal plate therapy may be recommended as early as the first year of life (Castillo-Morales, 1991). Research shows that after four years of this type of therapy, the orofacial functions had improved significantly in children with DS and that the gains remain after 12 months without the plate. De Andrade et al. (1998) had the idea of tying the original plate to a standard pacifier. This allows securing it and using it for longer periods of time including during sleep.

When the volume of the oral cavity is too reduced, it is possible to carry out functional maxillary expansion. De Andrade et al. (2008) report stable benefits over time in a group of children with DS aged between 4 and 12 years, compared with a control group, among which are an increase in nasal volume, a reduction of upper airway obstruction, and esthetical improvement.

Parents sometimes ask whether it is advisable to resort to tongue surgery in order to improve articulation in children with DS. Such a strategy had indeed been recommended years ago by physicians and surgeons. My opinion is that one should dispense with this sort of treatment except perhaps in very rare cases that combine a short buccal cavity and extreme macroglossia. The functional techniques available nowadays for improving oral praxis should be enough in almost all cases for improving articulation and speech intelligibility.

Lexical development and intervention

Vocabulary development is markedly delayed in children with DS (Rondal & Edwards, 1997). The reasons are:

1 Difficulties in perceiving and producing the sounds and canonical sequences of speech sounds (phonemes) that constitute the word envelopes; for example, lasting problems with later-acquired consonants (fricatives), clusters of consonants, final consonant deletion, and word final vocalization (Stoel-Gammon, 2001).

2 Limitations of short-term memory rendering the task of associating form and meaning more difficult.

3 Particular difficulties in identifying the referents of the words. This is a challenging task, even for the typically developing child, given that any sign can refer to a number of dimensions of the objects or events (form, function, shape, color, number, constituent parts, etc.), and that in customary verbal exchanges no cue is usually given to the learning child of which particular aspect is being referred to.

Regarding speech perception (word identification) and production (articulation and co-articulation), specialized training, which needs to be conducted by a speech pathologist, is in order. These specialists know of the typical sequences of articulatory development, how to train them in an orderly way (Stoel-Gammon, 2001), as well as the ways to improve the orofacial praxis through appropriate intervention.

Short-term memory training should be part of all intervention programs with children with DS. Any complex learning requires efficient short-term and longer-term memory processes. The technology now exists for boosting short-term memory development in children with intellectual disabilities. It has been successfully tested with children with DS (Conners, 2001). It is possible to procure developmental gains of more than one point over a few months, working a couple of hours a week and using some simple techniques of repetition of series of stimuli increasing in number and complexity.

As to the identification of the referents to which the words relate and the construction of meaning, recent research has documented a list of specific strategies used by typically developing children to proceed in early referential development (Mervis & Becerra, 2001). The major ones are:

• whole object (a new name encountered refers to a whole object and not to one of its parts)
• exclusivity (one name, one object category)
• function
• form (shape)
• stability over time and space
• new name category without a name.

When taught these strategies (which they do not seem to use spontaneously), children with DS exhibit speedier progress in referential development (Mervis & Becerra, 2001). Demonstrating these strategies to the child with intellectual disability appears to be a powerful intervention tool for boosting early lexical acquisition.

Another interesting tool for assisting in early lexical development is the simultaneous use with the child of the word plus a specific gesture when referring to a familiar object or event. The gestures may be borrowed from a dictionary of sign language for the deaf. They share the same referents and are signified with the words, but are of the gross motor type (as opposed to finer motor type for the many subtle articulatory and co-articulatory movements) and pertain to the visual modality (better preserved in persons with DS). The gestures have the property of gradually drawing the child toward expressing the verbal form of the corresponding words as well (Powell & Clibbens, 2001). When the latter is acquired, the gestures quickly fade away.

Grammatical development

When able to produce approximately 50 words, the typically developing child begins combining them, two or three at a time, in short utterances. The individual elements are initially separated by a short pause. Slightly later, they come to be uttered within a unique prosodic envelope. The same development can be observed in children with DS but with a delay that may amount to several months, one year, or more in some cases.

Syntax is a tool for organizing the expression of complex meanings or semantic relations. The basic ones known to the typically developing child around 18 months (later in the child with DS) are:

- possession
- time relationships (proximal sequential)
- space relationships (proximity)
- presence, absence, return, disappearance of an object or a person
- acknowledgment, denial, acceptance, refusal of a fact, event, or proposal
- accompaniment
- transitivity (an effect transferred from an agent onto a patient – animate or inanimate).

It follows that the first thing to do in order to boost early syntactic development is to demonstrate, repeat, and stress the various events and episodes in ordinary life and play situations that illustrate basic semantic relationships; presenting the child simultaneously with short sequences of words that encode the participating elements in the events referred to. One should be attentive to regularly reinforce and encourage all attempts by the child, including the most primitive ones, at combining two words together in utterances relevant to the context and the action under way. The length of the utterances modeled to the child can be gradually increased. They need to always be organized according to the canonical sequential patterns of the particular tongue.

Children with DS do not usually encounter serious difficulties in reproducing the canonical patterns of the community language. They have problems, however, with several categories of words (articles, prepositions, pronouns, conjunctions, auxiliaries). These words tend to be shorter, less accentuated, poorer in vowels, therefore less perceptually salient. They bear less semantic weight than the content words (nouns, main verbs, adjective, and adverbs). These characteristics make them all the more difficult to isolate in the speech stream.

The same is true, even more, for the inflexional morphemes located at the end of the nouns and verbs generally. These morphemes express semantic indications such as number, gender, person, time, and aspect (e.g. duration or completion of an action).

These formal structures can be modeled with a particular stress, frequently repeated, and carefully reinforced as soon as the child attempts to produce them. A simple expansion technique can be useful. It consists in repeating a grammatically incorrect production by the child, adding the missing elements (one at a time, preferentially).

Exposing the child with DS to learning to read earlier than is usually the case (e.g. as soon as the chronological age of four years) can also help in stabilizing some language structures (e.g. prepositions, conjunctions, pronouns, and grammatical morphemes; Buckley, 2001). Written language presentation allows for a longer exposure to the forms than the more passing speech, favoring notice and memorization.

Conclusions

A large number of useful things can and should be done in early and very early language (prelanguage) intervention with the child with DS. Congenital genetic syndromes, in spite of their gravity, offer the opportunity to intervene efficiently almost from the beginning. Given the highly cumulative nature of language development, this gives the opportunity to markedly reduce the important delays that plague these conditions in so many individual cases.

Summary

Language development in the typically developing child begins on a prosodic basis three months before birth. The typical neonate is already able to recognize her/his mother's voice and language from birth. This confers a potent advantage in early language acquisition to the extent that the neonate is already familiar with the communicative system to attend. Although we know very little about the same development in babies with DS, it is possible to recommend a number of steps and strategies for optimizing early language sensitization in these babies. This chapter also deals with early lexical and grammatical development including concrete ways to improve these acquisitions through systematic and cumulative intervention.

References

Berger, J. & Cunningham, C. (1983). The development of early vocal behaviours and interaction in Down's syndrome and non-handicapped infant mother. *Developmental Psychology*, **19**, 322–331.

Buckley, S. (2001). Literacy and language. In J. A. Rondal & S. Buckley (eds.), *Speech and Language Intervention in Down Syndrome*, pp. 132–153. London: Whurr.

Conners, F. (2001). Phonological working memory difficulty and related interventions. In J. A. Rondal & S. Buckley (eds.), *Speech and Language Intervention in Down Syndrome*, pp. 31–48. London: Whurr.

Castillo-Morales, R. (1991). *Die orofaziale Regulationstherapie*. Munich: Pflaum.

De Andrade, D., Macho, V., Loura, C., Costa, R., Palha, M. (2008). Effects of rapid maxillary expansion in children with Down syndrome. Communication at the Seventh International Congress on *Early Intervention in Down Syndrome and Related Genetic Conditions.* Palma de Mallorca, Spain (unpublished).

De Andrade, D., Tavares, B., Rebelo, P., Palha, M., Tavares, M. (1998). Placa modificada para tratamento de hipotonia oro-muscular em crianças com i dade compreendida entre os 2 meses e os 2 anos. *Ortodontia*, **3**, 111–117.

De Boysson-Bardies, B. (1996). *Comment la parole vient aux enfants*. Paris: Jacob.

Eilers, R., Oller, D., Bull, D., Gavin, W. (1985). Linguistic experience and infant perception. *Journal of Child Language*, **11**, 467–475.

Eimas, P. (1996). The perception and representation of speech by infants. In J. Morgan & K. Demuth (eds.), *Signal of Syntax*, pp. 25–39. Mahwah: Erlbaum.

Elliott, D., Weeks, D., Elliott, C. (1987). Cerebral specialization in individuals with Down's syndrome. *American Journal on Mental Retardation*, **92**, 263–271.

Jusczyk, P., Cutler, L., Redanz, N. (1993). Infants' preferences for the predominant stress patterns of English words. *Child Development*, **64**, 675–687.

Marcus, G., Vijayan, S., Bandi Rao, S., Vishton, P. (1999). Rule learning by seven-month-old infants. *Science*, **283**, 77–80.

Mervis, C. & Becerra, A. (2001). Lexical development and intervention. In J. A. Rondal & S. Buckley (eds.), *Speech and Language Intervention in Down Syndrome*, pp. 63–85. London: Whurr.

Nazzi, T., Bertoncini, J., Mehler, J. (1998). Language discrimination by newborns: towards an understanding of the role of rhythm. *Journal of Experimental Psychology: Human Perception and Performance*, **24**, 1–11.

Powell, G. & Clibbens, J. (2001). Augmentative communication. In J. A. Rondal & S. Buckley (eds.), *Speech and Language Intervention in Down Syndrome*, pp. 116–131. London: Whurr.

Rondal, J. A. (1995). *Exceptional Language Development in Down Syndrome. Implications for the Cognition-Language Relationship*. New York: Cambridge University Press.

Rondal, J. A. & Edwards, S. (1997). *Language in Mental Retardation*. London: Whurr

Rasore Quartino, A. (2007). Medical therapies in the life span. In J. A. Rondal & A. Rasore Quartino (eds.), *Therapies and Rehabilitation in Down Syndrome*, pp. 43–62. Chichester: Wiley.

Saffran, J., Aslin, R., Newport, E. (1996). Statistical learning by 8-month-old infants. *Science*, **274**, 1926–1928.

Shi, R., Werker, J., Morgan, J. (1999). Newborn infants' sensitivity to perceptual cues to lexical and grammatical words. *Cognition*, **72**, B11–B21.

Stoel-Gammon, C. (2001). Speech acquisition and approaches to intervention. In J. A. Rondal & S. Buckley (eds.), *Speech and Language Intervention in Down Syndrome*, pp. 49–62. London: Whurr.

Tristao, R. & Feitosa, M. (2000). Percepçao auditiva e implicacôes para o desenvolvimento global e de linguagem en crianças com sindrome de Down. *Arquivos Brasileiros de Psicologia*, **52**, 118–142.

Yoder, P. & Warren, S. (2001). Relative treatment effects of two prelinguistic communication interventions on language development in toddlers with developmental delays vary by maternal characteristics. *Journal of Speech, Language, and Hearing Research*, **44**, 224–237.

Chapter

14

Speech perception, stimulation, and phonological development

Michèle Pettinato

Children with Down syndrome (DS) have poorer speech abilities than would be predicted on the basis of their cognitive functioning. This delay may be a result of poor control of articulators and decreased oral–motor skills or hearing difficulties, especially in the first years of life. How can we investigate the relative importance of these factors? It may be interesting to consider the development of phonological abilities in children with cochlear implants, as these children have difficulties with hearing, but do not also have issues with oral–motor skills. The aim of this chapter is to reevaluate the notion that speech and phonological difficulties in children with DS should be mainly conceived of in terms of speech production difficulties. Instead, the comparison with children with cochlear implants reveals that auditory deprivation within the first years of life may lead to a highly similar profile of speech processing deficits.

Phonological difficulties in children with Down syndrome

An uneven profile

In individuals with learning difficulties, there is a delay in the development of phonology, which is commensurate with the level of development in nonverbal mental age (Smith & Stoel-Gammon, 1983; Sommers et al., 1988; Dodd & Leahy, 1989). For children with DS, phonological abilities are below the level predicted on mental age alone (Abbeduto et al., 2001; Dodd & Thompson, 2001). Roberts et al. (2005) compared the phonological skills of boys with fragile-X syndrome and boys with DS. These syndromes were compared because learning difficulties and poor intelligibility are common to both groups, and the question therefore was whether they shared the same profile of phonological impairment. The two groups were matched on nonverbal mental age to a group of younger, typically developing boys. Only the group with DS differed significantly from the typically developing control group on number and types of errors, confirming that while phonology was in line with cognitive development for boys with fragile-X syndrome, additional difficulties were present in boys with DS.

Inconsistency and non-developmental errors

The reasons for this uneven profile between cognitive and phonological development are not entirely clear. Several authors have suggested that phonological development in children

Neurocognitive Rehabilitation of Down Syndrome, eds. Jean-Adolphe Rondal, Juan Perera, and Donna Spiker. Published by Cambridge University Press. © Cambridge University Press 2011.

with DS may not only be delayed, but also follow a different path from typical development. Dodd and colleagues point to the high degree of inconsistency in the phonological system of children with DS: in typical development and in delayed phonology (i.e. children who are acquiring phonology at a slower rate, often because of learning difficulties), phonological errors are highly consistent; thus, if the child mispronounces *fish* as *fis*, the error pattern will be the same every time the word is produced. In children with DS, errors are less predictable and often vary on different occasions; hence *fish* may be produced as *fi*, *fis*, or *ish* (Dodd & Thompson, 2001; Dodd et al., 2002; Dodd, 2005). Another aspect of the speech of children with DS, which has been described by several authors, is the high number of non-developmental errors in their mispronunciations (Dodd & Leahy, 1989; So & Dodd, 1994; Bray et al., 1995; Hesselwood et al., 1995; Dodd & Thompson, 2001; Timmins et al., 2007). These are errors that are not usually encountered in typical development; for example, producing *s* by sucking air in rather than letting it escape. Moreover, using electropalatography,[1] Timmins et al. (2007) identified a number of atypical articulatory patterns for phonemes, which had been classified as correct during perceptual analyses. Finally, Smith and Stoel-Gammon (1983) described not only a higher occurrence for phonological processes such as fronting and stopping[2] in children with DS, but also that these resolved at a much slower pace than in typically developing children of a similar cognitive level. For example, between the ages of 18 and 36 months, there was a 38% decrease for a given phonological process in typically developing infants. In contrast, when children with DS had reached a similar cognitive level, the same process only decreased at a rate of 3% during a longer period between the ages of three and six years.

Possible causes of phonological difficulties

Speech production

Explanations for these phenomena have mainly been based on the idea of production difficulties; Dodd and colleagues have suggested that children with DS struggle to assemble phonological plans for producing words at a cognitive level (Dodd & Thompson, 2001; Dodd et al., 2002; Dodd, 2005); thus, although the issue is within the production of speech, it is not based directly on articulation, but on the planning of articulation. Other authors have placed more emphasis on difficulties in the oral–motor praxis itself and have pointed to the presence of symptoms of apraxia of speech (Kumin & Adams, 2000; Kumin, 2006; Timmins et al., 2007). The work of Bray and Heselwood unifies these two approaches by pointing out that although there are obvious difficulties with the control of the articulators necessary for speech in children with DS, the occurrence of such difficulties is influenced by higher-level phonological planning (Bray et al., 1995; Heselwood et al., 1995). These views all focus on different aspects of the speech production chain, and indeed the majority of interventions have addressed speech production difficulties (Dodd & Thompson, 2001; Dodd, 2005; Kumin 2006).

---

[1] Electropalatography involves the participant wearing an artificial palate with embedded electrodes. These register contact with the tongue during articulation and display this information on a computer screen.
[2] Fronting means articulating sounds that are normally at the back of the mouth at the front of the mouth, for example, *key -> tea*; stopping refers to sounds such as *s*, *f*, and *sh*, where the air normally escapes the mouth, being articulated with a complete obstruction, for example, *sing -> ting*.

Speech perception

While there is clearly a significant role for speech production difficulties, the presence of hearing problems in children with DS should not be underestimated as a contributing factor to poor phonological abilities. The majority of children have some form of hearing loss, usually because of glue ear but also owing to sensorineural losses (Roizen et al., 1993; Marcell, 1995). In infants with DS, Jiang et al. (1990) report evidence of either delayed or atypical auditory system development. It is not exactly clear whether this is the consequence of slower brain maturation, or whether this represents a true difference from typical brain development. However, it is possible that consequently the auditory abilities of infants with DS are somewhat diminished when compared to those of typically developing infants of a similar age. In older individuals with DS, neuroanatomical studies have found that cell columns were further apart and cell density was decreased in the areas responsible for auditory processing (Schmidt-Sidor et al., 1990; Golden & Hyman, 1994; Kemper, 1988; Buxhoeveden et al., 2002). However, this may not be directly the result of trisomy 21 but rather of less adequate auditory stimulation early on, possibly because of glue ear. Although this is an area that is still little understood, the presence of glue ear and sensory-neural losses in many children suggests that auditory input may be less optimal for a lot of infants and children with DS.

The impact such early auditory deprivation may have had on the phonological abilities of children with DS is not easy to demonstrate, as concurrent learning difficulties and a degree of oral–motor problems in almost all children make it hard to tease apart causalities. Nevertheless, the question is far from trivial, as psycholinguists and speech scientists think that early exposure to speech sounds is crucial for the subsequent development of speech and language (Morgan & Demuth, 1996).

The importance of early speech perception in typical development

Within the first year of life, typically developing infants acquire an acute sensitivity to the phonological and acoustic features of their native language. As early as four months, infants show a preference for the most common stress pattern in the words of the surrounding language (Mattys et al., 1999; Weber et al., 2004) (stress refers to the most prominent syllable in a word; for example, in *banana* it is the second syllable, but for *daffodil* it is the first) and by six months, infants seem to have established what the vowels of their native language are (Kuhl et al., 1992). For consonants, this process is thought to be accomplished by one year (Werker & Tees, 1984, 2005). Infants are also building up an awareness of the most common ways in which sounds occur together (the technical term for this is phonotactics); for example, the fact that in English, *bl* is a frequent combination, whereas *lb* is not (Friederici & Wessels, 1993).

Infants face a difficult task when learning the words of their language: how can they recognize words in fluent speech, when there are no clear acoustic cues to word boundaries and most utterances consist of several words (think of the experience of listening to an unfamiliar language)? However, knowledge of the sounds of their native language and how they can combine helps infants begin to recognize separate units in the continuous stream of speech. For example, because the majority of English words start with a stressed syllable, a good strategy for determining word boundaries would be to assume the start of a new word when hearing a stressed syllable. By nine months of age, infants indeed seem to use this strategy (Mattys et al., 1999). Friederici and Wessels (1993) showed that infants also used frequent phonotactic patterns to recognize words in fluent speech.

These studies indicate that infants are learning about and performing quite complex analyses on the sound structure of their native language long before they begin to utter their first words. It seems that this exposure to speech and the intensive analysis of its sound patterns is necessary for later more complex language learning. In an important study, Newman et al. (2006) retrospectively compared the performance of children who, at two years of age, had high versus low vocabularies. These children had all taken part in a variety of speech perception tasks during the first year of their lives. The performance on speech segmentation tasks (i.e. the ability to use phonological cues such as stress or phonotactics for recognizing words in continuous speech) of the two groups differed significantly, in that the group who later had small vocabularies had also performed significantly worse on speech segmentation tasks during the first year than the children who would go on to develop large vocabularies at two years of age. A second study was carried out between the ages of four and six years, and again children who obtained higher measures on a variety of language tests had also performed significantly better on speech segmentation tasks as babies. As better segmentation and higher language scores could simply have been a consequence of overall better cognitive abilities in this group, the researchers also assessed the two groups of children on non-linguistic cognitive abilities. The groups did not differ on measures of cognitive development, and it was concluded that the relationship between segmentation skills and later language development was not based on general cognitive abilities, but seemed to be the result of a specific ability to recognize regularities in speech patterns and to use this to learn language.

Surprisingly, very little is known about how speech discrimination and segmentation abilities develop in infants with DS and how they may relate to the difficulties with language development. The studies that have been carried out assessing speech processing in infants with DS are not fully conclusive. Nevertheless, their importance lies in showing that the same methodologies that have been used with typically developing infants, that is, essentially operant-conditioning techniques such as the head-turn paradigm, can also be be used with infants with DS (Eilers et al., 1985; Tristao & Feitosa, 2002).

The impact of early auditory deprivation – the case of children with cochlear implants

In the absence of information on infants with DS, it may be informative to look at another clinical population where the perception of speech is disrupted early in development. This is the case for children who were born profoundly deaf and who have received cochlear implants. Although the cochlear implant provides auditory stimulation, this does not fully restore normal hearing. Cochlear implants can have a maximum of 22 to 24 channels, so all sounds have to be broken down and processed as having a maximum of 22 or 24 frequencies, whereas the normally hearing ear can distinguish many hundreds of different frequencies. Therefore, these children are not only deprived of sound stimulation from birth, but once the implant has been fitted, the auditory input continues to be less optimal. Nevertheless, it is important to note that some children with cochlear implants do achieve age-appropriate language levels (Cleary et al., 2001; Crosson & Geers, 2001; Nicholas & Geers, 2006). Although it would be premature to draw direct parallels between the two clinical populations, there are some surprising similarities in their language development.

Phonological difficulties

Like children with DS, children with cochlear implants are considerably delayed in their language acquisition (Crosson & Geers, 2001; Nicholas & Geers, 2006). This includes difficulties with articulation and intelligibility (Burkholder & Pisoni, 2003; Dillon et al., 2004), even though there is no reason to expect prior difficulties with oral–motor skills in children with cochlear implants. Researchers also report greater variability in sound productions than in typically developing children (Hide et al., 2007), and this inconsistency in production has been described as a key feature of the speech of children with DS (Dodd & Thompson, 2001; Dodd, 2005). Crucially, early auditory deprivation may lead to articulation problems that might look like insufficient oral–motor skills on the surface, but are actually grounded in auditory difficulties. Kent and Vorperian (2007) discuss how, in order to acquire speech, children need to be able to link their own speech productions to the corresponding sounds produced by those around them. This process seems necessary to establish precise and automatic articulatory targets.[3]

Early auditory deprivation and higher-level speech processing abilities

The two groups not only have problems with producing clear speech, but they also have difficulties with retaining speech in short-term memory, also known as phonological short-term memory (Jarrold et al., 2002; Burkholder & Pisoni, 2003). For most phonological short-term memory assessments, participants are asked to repeat either numbers or words; therefore, accurate perception and good speech are necessary to complete these tasks. Because hearing and speech are areas of weakness for both groups of children, a number of studies have tried to establish their role in phonological short-term memory problems. Both groups of children seem to have phonological short-term memory problems that go beyond a mere difficulty in reproducing the words they have been asked to remember: when tasks did not require a verbal response and children could point to pictures or written words of the items they were asked to remember instead, impaired phonological short-term memory was still present (Cleary et al., 2001; Jarrold et al., 2002). Similarly, presenting the items to remember as pictures or written text so that hearing difficulties could be discounted did not improve phonological short-term memory performance in either group (Cleary et al., 2001; Jarrold et al., 2002). Therefore, it has been suggested that for both groups there is a specific difficulty with retaining, scanning, and retrieving speech in short-term memory, which is independent of the immediate effects of hearing or speech problems. In addition, recent work by Jarrold and colleagues has indicated that for children with DS, phonological short-term memory problems are possibly compounded by less adequate phonological representations (Brock & Jarrold, 2004; Jarrold et al., 2009).

The studies with children with cochlear implants indicate that the lack of early experience of speech sounds not only significantly affects the development of speech, but also feeds into more abstract abilities such as being able to process speech in short-term memory. By analogy, some of the problems with the development of phonology and later phonological short-term memory deficit in children with DS may, in part, be a result of the disruption of early perception of speech sounds (Jiang et al., 1990). Presently, it is only possible to speculate on this issue, but as the studies on speech perception in infants with DS have shown that the

---

[3] The reader is referred to Kent & Vorperian (2007) for an in-depth discussion of the interplay between perception and production in speech development.

same methodologies can be used with this population, it is hoped that future investigations will begin to address this gap in our knowledge.

As there are strong indications that lack of or less optimal exposure to early speech sounds has a detrimental effect on later language development, an important question is whether there are interventions that may be applied to counter or diminish this effect. Again a comparison with the literature on cochlear implants may be appropriate.

Questions to consider for intervention

Children with cochlear implants vary in how they communicate. They can be divided into two groups: those who use speech as their main mode of communication and those who use a mixture of signs, lip-reading, and speech, also known as total communication (Burkholder & Pisoni, 2003). Some studies (Cleary et al., 2001; Burkholder & Pisoni, 2003) have found that the mode of communication has a strong influence on speech and short-term memory abilities. Children who used speech as their main means of communication had clearer speech, spoke faster, and had better phonological short-term memory than children who used total communication (Cleary et al., 2001; Burkholder & Pisoni, 2003). The authors of these studies have commented that amount of experience with speech sounds seems to be the determining factor, irrespective of whether this is through the auditory modality or indirectly through visual and proprioceptive cues to speech sounds (i.e. feeling where and how in the mouth sounds are produced) (Cleary et al., 2001; Burkholder & Pisoni, 2003). In terms of early interventions, this would mean that the actual practice of speech sounds should be encouraged as much as possible. However, it is important to note that other studies with children with cochlear implants contend that age of implantation, rather than communication mode, has a stronger influence on language and speech outcomes (Connor et al., 2000; Nicholas & Geers, 2006). If this view is correct, early interventions should place greater emphasis on the auditory modality. Irrespective of the extent to which visual and proprioceptive cues can lessen the effect of auditory deprivation, both opinions emphasize the importance of early exposure to speech sounds. Intervention methods for children with DS should therefore encompass both listening activities to encourage speech discrimination and the practice of speech sounds and speaking.

In conclusion, the phonological delay of children with DS may not only be based on speech output difficulties, such as assembling phonological representations for articulation and executing this, but may also be a sequel to disrupted perception of speech sounds in infancy. Early interventions need to address such difficulties, as lower-level speech abilities feed into more abstract language processing. Whether oral practice of speech sounds can compensate for this lack of early stimulation is not entirely clear, and it is recommended that intervention methods address both the production and perception of speech. Future investigations of speech perception and processing abilities in infants with DS should yield a more detailed profile of the abilities and needs of this population and should enable us to draw up more targeted and therefore more effective methods for encouraging speech and language development.

Summary

This chapter discusses the profile of phonological difficulties in children with DS. Traditional explanations that mainly rely on speech production difficulties are considered, and it is suggested that, given the literature on hearing difficulties in this population, it may be timely to explore the impact of early auditory problems on later speech processing abilities. To this end, the importance of early speech perception for typical language development is illustrated, and a review of the literature on children with cochlear implants is presented. It is argued that these two populations show a strikingly similar profile of phonological impairment in spite of different etiologies, and that the speech problems of children with DS may equally be a result of auditory deprivation. It is proposed that early interventions need to place more emphasis on speech discrimination.

References

Abbeduto, A., Pavetto, M., Kesin, E., et al. (2001). The linguistic and cognitive profile of Down syndrome: evidence from a comparison with fragile X syndrome. *Down Syndrome Research and Practice*, 7, 9–15.

Bray, M., Heselwood, B., Crookston, I. (1995). Down' s syndrome: linguistic analysis of a complex language difficulty. In M. Perkins & S. Howard (eds.), *Case Studies in Clinical Linguistics*, pp. 123–145. London: Whurr.

Brock, J. & Jarrold, C. (2004). Language influences on verbal short-term memory performance in Down syndrome: item and order recognition. *Journal of Speech, Language, and Hearing Research*, 47(6), 1334–1346.

Burkholder, R. A. & Pisoni, D. B. (2003). Speech timing and working memory in profoundly deaf children after cochlear implantation. *Journal of Experimental Child Psychology*, 85(1), 63–88.

Buxhoeveden, D., Fobbs, A., Roy, E., Casanova, M. (2002). Quantitative comparison of radial cell columns in children with Down's syndrome and controls. *Journal of Intellectual Disability Research*, 46(1), 76–81.

Cleary, M., Pisoni, D. B., Geers, A. (2001). Some measures of verbal and spatial working memory in eight- and nine-year-old hearing-impaired children with cochlear implants. *Ear and Hearing*, 22, 395–411.

Connor, C. M., Hieber, S., Arts, H. A., Zwolan, T. A. (2000). Speech, vocabulary, and the education of children using cochlear implants: oral or total communication? *Journal of Speech, Language, and Hearing Research*, 43(5), 1185–1204.

Crosson, J. & Geers, A. (2001). Analysis of narrative ability in children with cochlear implants. *Ear and Hearing*, 22(5), 381–394.

Dillon, C. M., Cleary, M., Pisoni, D. B., Carter, A. K. (2004). Imitation of nonwords by hearing-impaired children with cochlear implants: segmental analyses. *Clinical Linguistics & Phonetics*, 18(1), 39–55.

Dodd, B. J. (2005). *Differential Diagnosis and Treatment of Children with Speech Disorder*. London: Whurr.

Dodd, B. J., Hua, Z., Crosbie, S., Holm, A., Ozanne, A. (2002). *Diagnostic Evaluation of Articulation and Phonology*. London: The Psychological Corporation.

Dodd, B. J. & Leahy, P. (1989). Phonological disorders and mental handicap. In M. Beveridge, G. Conti-Ramsden, I. Leudar (eds.), *Language and Communication in Mentally Handicapped People*. London: Chapman and Hall.

Dodd, B. J. & Thompson, L. (2001). Speech disorder in children with Down's syndrome. *Journal of Intellectual Disability Research*, 45(4), 308–316.

Eilers, R., Bull, D., Oller, D., Lewis, D. (1985). The discrimination of rapid spectral speech cues by Down syndrome and normally developing infants. In S. Harel & N. Anastasiouw (eds.), *The At-risk Infant. Psycho/Social/Medical Aspects*, pp. 115–132. Baltimore: Brookes.

Friederici, A. D. & Wessels, J. M. (1993). Phonotactic knowledge of word boundaries and its use in infant speech perception. *Perception and Psychophysics*, 54(3), 287–295.

Golden, J. A. & Hyman, B. T. (1994). Development of the superior temporal neocortex is anomalous in trisomy 21. *Journal of Neuropathology and Experimental Neurology*, 53(5), 513–520.

Heselwood, B., Bray, M., Crookston, I. (1995). Juncture, rhythm and planning in the speech of an adult with Down's syndrome. *Clinical Linguistics & Phonetics*, **9**(2), 121–137.

Hide, O., Gillis, S., Govaerts, P. (2007). Suprasegmental aspects of pre-lexical speech in cochlear implanted children. *Proceedings of Interspeech 2007*: Eighth Annual Conference of the International Speech Communication Association, Antwerp, pp. 638–641.

Jarrold, C., Baddeley, A. D., Phillips, C. E. (2002). Verbal short-term memory in Down syndrome: a problem of memory, audition, or speech? *Journal of Speech, Language, and Hearing Research*, **45**(3), 531–544.

Jarrold, C., Thorn, A. S. C., Stephens, E. (2009). The relationships among verbal short-term memory, phonological awareness, and new word learning: evidence from typical development and Down syndrome. *Journal of Experimental Child Psychology*, **102**(2), 196–218.

Jiang, Z. D., Wu, Y. Y., Liu, X. Y. (1990). Early development of brainstem auditory evoked potentials in Down's syndrome. *Early Human Development*, **23**(1), 41–51.

Kemper, T. (1988). Neuropathology of Down syndrome. In L. Nadel (ed.), *The Psychobiology of Down Syndrome*, pp. 269–289. Cambridge: MIT Press.

Kent, R. D. & Vorperian, H. K. (2007). In the mouths of babes: anatomic, motor, and sensory foundations of speech development in children. In R. Paul (ed.), *Language Disorders from a Developmental Perspective: Essays in Honor of Robin S. Chapman*, pp. 55–81. Mahwah: Lawrence Erlbaum Associates Publishers.

Kuhl, P. K., Williams, K. A., Lacerda, F., Stevens, K. N., Lindblom, B. (1992). Linguistic experience alters phonetic perception in infants by 6 months of age. *Science*, **255**, 606–608.

Kumin, L. (2006). Speech intelligibility and childhood verbal apraxia in children with Down syndrome. *Down Syndrome Research and Practice*, **10**, 10–22.

Kumin, L. & Adams, J. (2000). Developmental apraxia of speech and intelligibility in children with Down syndrome. *Down Syndrome Quarterly*, **5**(3), 1–7.

Marcell, M. M. (1995). Relationships between hearing and auditory cognition in Down's syndrome youth. *Down Syndrome Research and Practice*, **3**(3), 75–91.

Mattys, S., Jusczyk, P. W., Morgan, J. L. (1999). Phonotactic and prosodic effects on word segmentation in infants. *Cognitive Psychology*, **38**, 465–494.

Morgan, J. L. & Demuth, K. (1996). *Signal to Syntax: Bootstrapping from Speech to Grammar in Early Acquisition*. Mahwah: Erlbaum Associates.

Newman, R., Ratner, N. B., Jusczyk, A. M., Jusczyk, P. W., Dow, K. A. (2006). Infants' early ability to segment the conversational speech signal predicts later language development: a retrospective analysis. *Developmental Psychology*, **42**(4), 643–655.

Nicholas, J. G. & Geers, A. (2006). Effects of early auditory experience on the spoken language of deaf children at 3 years of age. *Ear and Hearing*, **27**(3), 286–298.

Roberts, J., Long, S., Malkin, C., et al. (2005). A comparison of phonological skills of boys with fragile X syndrome and Down syndrome. *Journal of Speech, Language and Hearing Research*, **48**(5), 980–995.

Roizen, N. J., Wolters, C., Nicol ,T., Blondis, T. A. (1993). Hearing loss in children with Down syndrome. *Journal of Pediatrics*, **123**, 9–12.

Schmidt-Sidor, B., Wisniewski, K. E., Shepard, T. H., Sersen, E. A. (1990). Brain growth in Down syndrome subjects 15 to 22 weeks of gestational age and birth to 60 months. *Clinical Neuropathology*, **9**(4), 181–190.

Smith, B. L. & Stoel-Gammon, C. (1983). A longitudinal study of the development of stop consonant production in normal and Down's syndrome children. *Journal of Speech and Hearing Disorders*, **48**, 114–118.

So, L. K. H. & Dodd, B. J. (1994). Downs syndrome and the acquisition of phonology by Cantonese-speaking children. *Journal of Intellectual Disability Research*, **38**, 501–517.

Sommers, R. K., Patterson, J. P., Wildgen, P. L. (1988). Phonology of Down syndrome speakers, ages 13–22. *Journal of Childhood Communication Disorders*, **12**(1), 65–91.

Timmins, C., Hardcastle, W. J., Wood, S., McCann, J., Wishart, J. (2007). Variability in fricative production of young people with Down's syndrome: an EPG analysis. In J. Trouvain & W. J. Barry (eds.), *Proceedings of the 16th International Congress of the ICPhS*, pp. 1981–1984.

Tristao, R. & Feitosa, M. (2002). Use of visual habituation paradigm to investigate speech perception in Down syndrome infants. *Proceedings of the International Society for Psychophysics*, **18**, 552–557.

Weber, C., Hahne, A., Friedrich, M., Friederici, A. D. (2004). Discrimination of word stress in early infant perception: electrophysiological evidence. *Cognitive Brain Research*, **18**, 149–161.

Werker, J. F. & Tees, R. C. (1984). Cross-language speech perception: evidence for perceptual reorganization during the first year of life. *Infant Behaviour and Development*, **7**, 49–63.

Werker, J. F. & Tees, R. C. (2005). Speech perception as a window for understanding plasticity and commitment in language systems of the brain. *Developmental Psychobiology*, **46**(3), 233–251.

Chapter

15

Goal-directedness as a target for early intervention in Down syndrome

Deborah Fidler, Susan L. Hepburn, Diane Osaki

Goal-directedness as a target for early intervention in Down syndrome

In discussing the notion of temperament, Wachs (1999) proposes that it is best viewed as a fuzzy set or a hybrid class. He explains that behaviors that are considered to be at the core of the notion of temperament are also considered integral to other areas of development. Wachs (1999) identifies temperament components such as attention skills and goal-directed behavior as critical to many of the leading theories of temperament, but he also notes that attention and goal-directed behavior are discussed as foundational to conceptualizations of other domains of development, such as cognitive development and motivation orientation.

The notion of temperament as a fuzzy set may be of particular interest to research on the emergence of the Down syndrome (DS) behavioral phenotype, and is of great clinical relevance for individuals with DS as well. This is because the early development of goal-directed behavior, one of the two overlapping constructs identified by Wachs (1999), may follow an atypical course in DS (Fidler, 2006). The fact that goal-directed behavior may be foundational to several different developmental domains means that atypical development in this area may have far reaching downstream effects in many different areas of functioning.

While work to uncover the developmental pathway is still quite preliminary, there is evidence that individuals with DS may show a disruption in the development of goal-directed behavior, manifested in the form of difficulties with problem solving and instrumental thinking throughout childhood. A handful of studies have demonstrated that children with DS have difficulty in the area of instrumental problem solving and purposeful behavior with objects (Pitcairn & Wishart, 1994; Ruskin et al., 1994; Kasari & Freeman, 2001; Fidler et al., 2005). Children with DS take longer to complete instrumental problem solving tasks, are more likely to abandon instrumental problem solving tasks, and perform more poorly than developmentally matched children on instrumental problem solving tasks (Pitcairn & Wishart, 1994; Kasari & Freeman, 2001; Fidler et al., 2005). These poor instrumental thinking skills impact on academic performance, as older children with DS (9–13 years of age) show fewer self-corrections than their typically developing classmates on mathematical exercises (Gelman & Cohen, 1988). Researchers have also described cognitive avoidant behaviors as a unique feature in the performance of children with DS on developmental assessments (Wishart, 1996).

Neurocognitive Rehabilitation of Down Syndrome, eds. Jean-Adolphe Rondal, Juan Perera, and Donna Spiker. Published by Cambridge University Press. © Cambridge University Press 2011.

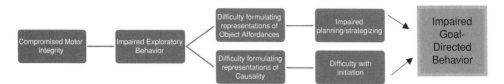

Figure 15.1 Hypothetical model of the impact of motor impairments on goal-directed behavior in Down syndrome.

In this chapter, we examine one set of factors that may contribute to the atypical development of goal-directed behavior in young children with DS. Specifically, we explore a hypothetical model of the cascading effects of motor impairments onto early exploratory experiences and early cognitive representations. We specifically review the literature on the critical role of early exploratory motor behavior in the formulation of representations of: (1) object affordances; and (2) causality in typically developing children. We then identify how a disruption in this pathway may contribute to impairments in the formulation of these representations and may impact on the goal-directed behavior outcomes observed in DS. We conclude the chapter with a discussion of intervention techniques that target aspects of this trajectory. It is important to note that we emphasize the hypothetical nature of this trajectory now, and we suggest that there may be numerous additional pathways and developmental factors that influence outcomes with respect to goal-directed behavior in this population (Figure 15.1).

Motor exploration, cognitive representations, and goal-directed behavior

Belsky and Most (1981) describe the development of infant engagement with the physical world as moving from an undifferentiated stage that involves mouthing and simple manipulation of objects without any specificity to the object being explored, to a more differentiated stage where the child's behavior becomes "more tailored to fit the specific features of the object" (p. 631). There is an important refining process that takes place in exploratory behavior that moves from global, undifferentiated acts on any object encountered to selecting more specific actions to be executed on specific objects. This process ultimately leads to the third phase of engagement, which moves beyond the discovery process and involves using an object purposefully, in goal-directed ways, based on preexisting knowledge about that object (Belsky & Most, 1981).

Early motor exploration

What propels this process? What makes it possible for an infant to move from undifferentiated exploration to purposeful, goal-directed behavior? Gibson (1988) argues for the importance of early integrity of the motor system in facilitating this process, and this notion has since been widely accepted (Rochat, 1989; Needham et al., 2002). Motor exploration begins as early as two to three months in typically developing infants, where the mouth is the main modality for exploration. At four to five months, a major shift takes place that involves the use of hands in new ways to facilitate exploration. Reaching and grasping become more prevalent, which makes closer visual inspection of objects possible (Rochat, 1989). Advances in hand and finger use, such as hand transfer of objects and the development of fingering (grasping an object with one hand while the other hand scans the object with the fingertips), also become pronounced at five months in typically developing infants (Rochat, 1989). As arm and hand strength increase during the first five months of life, an infant is able to grasp an object for longer periods of time, which extends the period of time in which an infant can explore an object (Needham et al., 2002). Ambulation in the form of pivoting, crawling, cruising, and walking emerges after seven or eight months in typically developing infants, and makes it possible for an infant to discover new information about his/her natural environment.

Cognitive consequences of motor exploration

Thus, early motor milestones, especially in the form of hand use and ambulation, facilitate the onset of exploratory capacities in typically developing infants. Once early motor exploration is underway, the effects on development are far-reaching. Rochat (1989) notes, "the emergence of these manual behaviors is a developmental milestone, because they provide the young infant with novel means for action for potential discoveries of objects' properties and their affordances" (p. 876). In other words, by engaging in object exploration with the hands, an infant presents him/herself with countless opportunities to learn about the objects that he/she is exploring.

Similarly, Gibson (1988) states that, "As the hands become active and controllable, a whole new set of affordances is opened up for the baby's discovery; things can be displaced, banged, shaken, squeezed, and thrown – actions that have informative consequences about an object's properties" (p. 20). Gibson is interested in the fact that improved hand use makes it possible to perform new actions, such as shaking and squeezing objects. The importance of these new behaviors lies in the fact that these exploratory behaviors "have informative consequences about an object's properties" (p. 20). The outcomes of these motor acts on an object teach an infant about the object. What begins as a motor exploration (i.e. an infant attempting to manipulate an object in a novel way) leads to a cognitive advance (i.e. a new representation of the nature of the object being explored).

To capture this process in a laboratory setting, Needham (2000) examined the relationship between early exploratory behavior and an infant's ability to interpret two objects (a cylinder and a box) as separate from one another when placed next to one another in a display. In a laboratory setting, three-and-a-half-month-old infants were shown an expected event (the move apart condition where a hand pushes the cylinder and the box stays in place) and an unexpected event (the move together condition where a hand pushes the cylinder and the box moves as well). She found that infants who were categorized as more active explorers (as measured by the amount of holding objects, oral exploration, visual exploration, and changes of exploration modality) showed more pronounced dishabituation to the unexpected move together event than they showed in their response to the expected move apart event. In contrast, the infants who were categorized as less active explorers showed no meaningful differences between their dishabituation responses to the two events. To explain this phenomenon, Needham (2000) hypothesized that "infants who explore objects more actively gather more extensive information about the objects they hold, and these self-produced observations about objects and their features may be especially helpful in learning to interpret these features" (p. 152). In other words, it was through active motor exploration that infants came to construct a basic representation of object features, such as boundaries. Those infants who had more exploration experience by three-and-a-half months had gained a more sophisticated representation of the nature of object boundaries.

Thus, there is evidence that motor exploration of objects and the physical environment impacts object awareness and cognitive representation of object properties in typically developing infants. Given the early gross and fine motor delays observed in infants with DS, these findings suggest that there may be developmental consequences of motor delays that extend beyond the motor system, and may involve the development of cognitive representations of objects and events in the physical world. In the next section, we examine more deeply the critical role of infant motor exploration in facilitating the development of two types of cognitive representations: (1) object affordances; and (2) causality. The atypical development of these constructs in DS, which will be explored later in this chapter, may be significant in that it may predispose children with DS to difficulties with self-regulatory behaviors such as planning and initiation (learning how to be a cause of events; Carlson, 2003) when facing instrumental tasks.

Object affordances

In typical development, as infants and then toddlers explore objects in their environments, they begin to identify the specific features of an object that make it possible to perform specific actions on that object. For example, the handle on a teacup affords a child the opportunity to grasp it with their fingers around the handle and then raise the cup. The stability of a coffee table affords a toddler the opportunity to grasp the table and support his/her weight as he/she pulls him/herself up to stand. These properties of an object that make it possible to act on the object in a particular manner are called object affordances (Gibson, 1988). Many different properties of objects can be represented as affordances – dimensions of shape, weight, size, and texture can each contribute to the possible actions that one can engage in with an object.

Rochat (1987, 1989) found evidence that these representations of object affordances begin to form in the earliest months of life, and they develop in close connection with motor exploratory behavior. In one study, Rochat (1987) found that newborn infants show differential manual and oral behavior when presented with a cylinder made out of Lucite and when presented with a cylinder of the same shape made out of foam. When presented to an infant's hand, typically developing newborns spent an average of 37 seconds squeezing the hard cylinder but only three seconds squeezing the soft cylinder. In contrast, when the objects were presented to an infant's mouth, typically developing newborns spent an average of 135 seconds sucking the soft cylinder and 89 seconds sucking the hard cylinder. In the earliest moments of life, the newborn's behavior was object-dependent and the type of exploratory behavior evidenced was modality specific. Rochat (1987) describes that early in life, infants form representations regarding the suckability of an object that is explored orally and the graspability of an object that is being explored manually. Increased sucking of a soft object demonstrates that the newborns represented the physical properties of the soft object and were organizing their future behavior with respect to that representation. Similarly, increased squeezing of the hard object in the manual condition suggests that the infants had represented features of the hard object and were organizing their behavior with respect to that representation as well.

As development progresses in the first few months of life, infants continue to engage in this process of formulating representations of object affordances. In another study, four-month-old infants used one set of exploratory manual acts when exploring one object (a ring-shaped rubber teether) and another set of manual acts when exploring another object (red sphere attached to a wooden rod; Rochat, 1989). Rochat (1989) describes that, "within seconds of interaction with a novel object, young infants display manual actions that are appropriate to potentially maximize the affordances of the object" (p. 882).

These skills continue to become refined in 6- to 10-month-old infants, who adapt the manual exploratory behavior they demonstrate, based on the type of surface they are exploring (liquid, discontinuous, flexible, or rigid) and other dimensions as well (Bourgeois et al., 2005). Age effects have been found for behaviors such as squeezing, as 10-month-old infants will squeeze soft objects more than hard objects. To describe the nature of the relationship between motor exploration and the representation of object affordances, Bourgeois et al. (2005) note that "infants are exploiting the material properties of surfaces in their immediate world. By pressing the flexible surface, infants are gaining additional information about its pliability. By rubbing and slapping their hands across the liquid surface, infants are gaining information about the surface's wetness and responsiveness to movement. By picking at the netting surface, infants are gaining additional information about its discontinuous quality" (p. 247). Motor acts of exploration, such as pressing, rubbing, and slapping, are teaching the child about the nature of objects and object affordances in the physical world.

Beyond manual exploration, there is evidence that the achievement of ambulation milestones facilitates the representation of affordances regarding surfaces on which an infant crawls and walks. Campos et al. (1992) exposed precrawling and crawling infants to the visual cliff and found physiological fear responses in the crawling infants that were not observed in the precrawling infants. This suggests that precrawling infants had not yet formulated a representation of the stability afforded by a solid surface, while the crawling infants had formulated these representations. In order to test whether it was the experience of self-ambulation that triggered the onset of fear of heights, Campos et al. (1992) conducted a study of only precrawling infants, half of whom were placed daily in a walker that enabled them to move themselves around their environment with their legs while supported by a harness seat. When subsequently exposed to the visual cliff, the precrawling infants who were given exposure to a walker showed physiological fear responses, while the precrawling infants with no walker experience did not.

Relevance for development in Down syndrome

Taken together, these findings suggest that manual and ambulatory exploration facilitate the development of representations of object affordances. The ability to identify how an object can be used (what opportunities it affords) is a critical skill for the development of early tool use and other aspects of planning/problem solving (Fontenelle et al., 2007). As Lockman (2000) notes, "the origins of tool use in humans can be found during much of the first year of life, in the perception–action routines that infants repeatedly display as they explore their environments" (p. 137). He explains that, "tool use may arise from infants' instrumental attempts to relate objects to other objects and surfaces in the world. This involves detecting affordances based on information that is directly perceptible" (p. 138). Disruption in the ability to represent object affordances undoubtedly has a direct impact on the ability of a child to plan and strategize with objects (use objects as tools) in their environment in goal-directed ways. This may be a critical challenge in young children with DS who, because of motor delays and attenuated motor exploration, may not be formulating representations of object affordances in a fluid manner. Difficulty formulating these representations may be one of the main causes of the difficulty with planning observed on instrumental problem solving tasks in laboratory studies in this population (see Fidler et al., 2005).

Causality

In addition to facilitating representations of object affordances, early motor experience also facilitates the development of representations of cause-and-effect. The development of representations of causality begins in the first year of life, when infants as young as six months show greater interest (dishabituation) when observing an actor who changes their goal (reaching for one object and then reaching for another object) than when they observe changes in the location of the goal object and other similar properties (Woodward, 1998). However, only recently researchers have begun to better understand the critical role of exploratory motor experience in the formation of the representations of causality in infancy. Sommerville (2007) argues that "infants' experience of their own actions and the consequences that these actions have on the world play an important role in their developing understanding of causal relations" (p. 48). When infants act on the world with a motor action (banging a toy on a surface; pulling on the string of a toy), they begin to pair the outcome of their action with the action they produced. From this process, infants begin to formulate hypotheses about cause-and-effect in the physical world.

In a laboratory study, Somerville and colleagues carefully isolated the role of motor experience in facilitating the development of the causal or means–end associations. In one study, three-month-old infants were randomly assigned either to a motor action-first or a watch-first condition (Sommerville et al., 2008). In the motor action-first condition, infants wore sticky mittens that had Velcro covering their palms, and they played with toys that had edges that were covered with the other side of the Velcro. This experience simulates reaching and grasping before these behaviors typically emerge. Infants in the watch-first group were exposed to a habituation/dishabituation display that involved detecting goal-directed reaching. Findings from the study showed that infants in the motor action-first group detected changes in goal-directed reaching significantly more than infants in the watch-first group. By being given the opportunity to experience a motor sequence (facilitated by artificial means) earlier than it would be observed developmentally, infants in the action-first group had quickly represented an understanding of goal-directed reaching and were able to detect the presence of this behavior in a way that infants without the motor experience were unable to detect.

Thus, exposure to motor experience facilitates the development of causal thinking. Motor experience may also facilitate the development of motor goal-directed behavior in infancy; that is, motor experience may help infants not only represent cause-and-effect, but also begin to use cause-and-effect relationships in order to perform real world strategizing. In one study, Bojczyk and Corbetta (2004) exposed infants, starting at six months, to a problem solving task that involves retrieving a desired object from an opaque box. Infants were given a chance to engage weekly with the problem solving task in an exploratory manner, until they successfully retrieved the desired object. Results showed that this motor practice experience facilitated the successful retrieval of the object sooner than was observed in infants with one-time exposure to the task.

In order to explain this effect, the authors suggest that the exploratory experiences likely facilitated a continuous adaptive process that involved a dynamic process of information acquisition from the environment. They state that "each encounter with the task provided novel motor and cognitive experience to the child, which in turn contributed to the modification of the infants' underlying cognitive and perceptual–motor repertoire" (p. 63). At first, infants showed many exploratory behaviors such as scratching, banging, and pushing the box. When, by chance, their actions led to the result of an open box, the infants then attempted to recreate that outcome by pushing the box forward and upward. When infants discovered how to open the lid, they began motor attempts to retrieve the toy from inside the box (Bojczyk & Corbetta, 2004). This characterization of the gradual shaping of strategies across many exploratory sessions likely captures the dynamic interplay between engaging in exploratory motor behavior and organizing one's behavior in order to cause an outcome. Over time, the infants moved from global exploration in the form of random banging and scratching to the specific actions that led to opening the box and obtaining the toy inside.

Relevance for development in Down syndrome

These studies not only demonstrate that exploratory behavior facilitates a cognitive representation of cause-and-effect, but also suggest that this ability to represent cause-and-effect becomes a critical aspect of goal-directedness and begin to be the cause of actions that will lead to a desired effect. Specifically, it appears that within motor exploration opportunities, typically developing infants engage in a dynamic process that may start in a more undifferentiated way, but the exploratory process leads to associations between behaviors an infant produces and the effects of those behaviors, which then leads to more purposeful and organized behavior patterns. We emphasize that young children with DS experience a disruption in the early exploratory processes that results from compromised integrity of the motor system. Infants with DS may, as a result, lack the dynamic experience of discovering patterns of cause-and-effect that result from acting on objects with their hands in exploratory ways. As a result, they may miss critical opportunities where they can gradually shift from exploration to more intentional causal initiations with objects.

Taken together, the literature on typically developing infants suggests that motor activity in the form of prehension and ambulation plays a critical role in facilitating exploratory behavior in the first year of life. This motor exploration in turn plays a critical role in the formulation of cognitive representations of both object affordances and causality. In particular, typically developing infants seem to be learning how to use objects in effective ways (object affordances) and how to link action and outcome (causality) in the context of these exploratory behaviors. In the next section, we link these early developmental processes to early development in infants with DS and examine the potential relevance of these findings for the development of goal-directed behavior in this population.

Goal-directedness and development in Down syndrome

Given the evidence for the role of early motor exploration in the formation of cognitive representations in typically developing infants, we now examine the relevance of these findings for early development in DS. Can this pathway in typically developing infants shed light on emerging phenotypic patterns of strength and weakness that have been described in this population? One aspect of the DS behavioral phenotype that has been well characterized involves gross and fine motor delays. Motor delays have been widely documented in early development in DS (Chen & Woolley, 1978; Dunst, 1988), including the presence of abnormal movement patterns, hypotonia, and hyperflexibility (Harris & Shea, 1991). Delays in the emergence and termination of reflexes provide further evidence of impairment in the integrity of the motor system in this population (Block, 1991; Harris & Shea, 1991).

We argue that these early motor impairments in DS may have cascading effects on the development of goal-directedness in this population. Atypical motor exploration is clearly evident by nine months in infants with DS (MacTurk et al., 1985). When compared to mental age-matched typically developing six-month-old infants, nine-month-old infants with DS show significantly fewer instances of exploratory behaviors such as banging, shaking, hitting, dropping, and examining objects (MacTurk et al., 1985). In contrast, they spend significantly more time than their mental age-matched counterparts looking at objects (without holding them). Based on the discussion presented in the previous section, it is clear that this atypical pattern of exploratory behavior can potentially disrupt the formation of critical cognitive representations. A lack of manual and ambulatory exploration may disrupt the typical process of learning about object affordances, as well as the pairing of actions on objects with outcomes, which leads to representations of causality. Indeed, it has been demonstrated that infants with DS show impaired ability to detect causal relationships at nine months, as they show difficulty representing the causal relationship between an arm movement and a reinforcing outcome (Ohr & Fagen, 1994).

Implications for goal-directed behavior

Most critically, we argue here that atypical development of representations of object affordances and causality may specifically impair the ability of a young child with DS to organize their behavior into regulated, goal-directed patterns. Because young children with DS are not building rich understandings of what features of objects enable them to use the object in effective ways, when they encounter objects in the physical world, they may be less effective at organizing their actions on objects in ways that help them reach desired end states. In other words, a disruption in the representation of object affordances may directly impact on the development of planning skills in this population. This difficulty with planning may already be observed early in development, as toddlers with DS demonstrate difficulty with praxis tasks such as putting a necklace in a cup, putting coins in a bank, and pulling on a pull toy (Fidler et al., 2005). Later in development, this planning deficit may continue to manifest itself in more complex ways, as the demands involved in planning require multiple steps and more abstract strategizing.

Disruptions in the formation of representations of causality may also have far-reaching downstream effects in this population. In particular, we hypothesize that difficulties with detecting causality may impact on the development of the ability to identify one's own behavior as the cause of specific outcomes, which then may impact on the development of initiation skills in this population. If the ability to link cause-and-effect is impaired, then young children with DS may have difficulty organizing their own behavior in such a way that they can be a cause of specific outcomes (Carlson, 2003). This difficulty with initiation has a direct impact on goal-directed behavior, as acting in goal-directed ways is fundamentally dependent on one's ability to see oneself as a causal agent.

Although this account of cascading effects will require empirical validation from longitudinal studies, its predictions are in line with the literature on early development in DS: (1) infants with DS show pronounced motor delays (Block, 1991; Harris & Shea, 1991); (2) infants with DS show attenuated exploratory motor behavior (MacTurk et al., 1985);

(3) toddlers with DS show difficulties with early praxis skills (Fidler et al., 2005), which involve manipulating objects based on their affordances; (4) infants with DS show difficulties with detection of causal relationships (Ohr & Fagen, 1994); and (5) there is strong evidence for attenuated goal-directedness in individuals with DS.

While longitudinal empirical investigation of the development of this pathway is necessary, we offer this hypothesized pathway as a framework to begin to understand the dynamic process of self-organization that takes place in the emergence of the DS behavioral phenotype. This framework takes into account the specific constraints that are built into the atypically developing system in DS from the earliest stages, and describes how these constraints set into motion a cascading pathway that ultimately leads to an area of pronounced weakness, in this case goal-directed behavior. As such, this hypothesized model is in line with the dynamic systems perspective that recognizes the dynamic process of self-organization that leads to various patterns of outcomes throughout development.

Clinical interpretation and intervention implications

Although speculation regarding appropriate intervention approaches is potentially premature, in this section we present examples of intervention approaches that may strengthen the construct of goal-directed behavior in DS. From a clinical perspective, goal-directedness is involved in several dimensions that are observable in real-world settings, such as home and school environments. Persistence, mastery motivation, goal-directedness, causality, agency are all terms that can be applied to understanding how an individual perceives his or her competence in impacting on the environment or responding to task demands (Barrett & Morgan, 1995; Berk, 2001; Piaget, 2001; Zelazo & Cunningham, 2007). Although the terminology differs depending upon one's theoretical orientation, there is consensus across conceptual fields on the following concepts:

1 Development is facilitated by a child's ability to tolerate and seek developmentally appropriate challenges (Piaget & Inhelder, 1987).
2 Children who do not perceive themselves as competent, independent agents of action tend to develop a prompt-dependent style, thus passively recruiting others to manage their challenges, resulting in missed learning opportunities and a reification of the child's (and possibly parent's) conception that he/she is not capable (Baer & Pinkston, 1997; Bandura, 1997).
3 Without the benefit of active practice, mastery of skills slows, thus leading to fewer and fewer experiences of competence for the child (Barrett & Morgan, 1995).
4 A lack of experience tolerating and managing frustration (i.e. negative affect that arises from the experience of meeting an obstacle in pursuit of a goal) results in the lack of development of self-regulation in the face of challenge (Sroufe, 1996). In real-world terms, this could result in the child resorting to maladaptive behaviors within a task (e.g. throwing materials) or inappropriate behaviors prior to a task (e.g. task-avoidant behaviors, such as refusing to try a new activity).

To address these issues, we first offer ideas for facilitating the early development of exploratory behavior in this population, which may facilitate the acquisition of cognitive representations such as object affordances and causality. We then present more suggestions that specifically target goal-directedness.

Targeting motor exploration

Based on the argument presented in this chapter, we recommend that a primary goal of early intervention in DS includes the facilitation of early motor exploration of objects and the environment. Evidence for the malleability of early exploratory skills comes from a creative experiment conducted by Needham et al. (2002), who exposed three-month-old infants to a set of experiences that simulated reaching and grasping behavior, a skill that does not typically emerge until four or five months. These experiences involved at-home play sessions where the infant wore the sticky mittens that had Velcro covering their palms. During these sessions, the infants played with toys that had edges that were covered with the other side of the Velcro. When compared to their counterparts who had not had the simulated prehension experience, the three-month-old infants who had the sticky mitten experience swatted at objects more and looked more at objects in a follow-up session. Needham et al. (2002) concluded that "experience acting on objects is an important contributor to the increase in object attention and object exploration that is typically observed by 6 months of age" (p. 293). This suggests that exposure to the early motor experience of simulated reaching and grasping, even before such exploratory behaviors typically emerge, facilitates greater awareness and interest in objects, and leads to further object exploration in a sample of typically developing infants.

Similar facilitation can be achieved in real-world settings by providing specific supports to facilitate trunk stability, use of two hands together, hand/arm coordination, grasping, and other related motor skills. Physical and occupational therapists are important partners for identifying the adaptive physical supports a child may need in order to successfully facilitate exploratory behavior. Our view is that these supports need to be provided as early in development as possible so that the infant with DS has the opportunity to explore his/her environment in a manner that approximates that of an infant without motor impairments. Table 15.1 lists specific physical supports that could be useful for infants and young children with motor impairments, adapted from Finnie (1975) and Zeitlin and Williamson (1994).

Strategies to enhance goal-directedness

In addition to strategies that attempt to alter the atypical goal-directed behavior trajectory observed in this population, additional approaches may be effective for targeting issues such as persistence and goal-directedness once difficulties with avoidant patterns become pronounced. Early intervention can modify a child's orientation to challenge, particularly if it is delivered in a developmentally sensitive manner, with acute attention to the reasonable next steps (i.e. choosing intervention targets that are emerging skills for the child and not entirely new nor entirely familiar) and specification of the appropriate levels and types of support necessary for the child to experience mastery.

Early intervention aimed toward promoting improved goal-directedness may also need to focus on multiple domains of functioning, such that a sense of competence is achieved in social interactions, communication, motor skills, and emotional regulation. Thus, a comprehensive, integrative approach is necessary when trying to promote a temperamental tendency in an individual – goal-directedness may need to be experienced by a child in multiple domains in multiple learning opportunities in order to evolve into an overall orientation for an individual. Therefore, in the case of a child with DS, activities that promote a sense of mastery across several domains (e.g. communication, motor) are probably necessary to instill a sense of personal agency. With these ideas in mind, the following ideas for early intervention to promote goal-directedness in a child with DS are offered for consideration:

Table 15.1 Physical supports to promote early motor skills

Skill/Target	Physical support
Trunk stability	Place the child in adaptive and stable seating and blow bubbles above the child's head to encourage reaching with trunk extension
Using two hands together	Suspend toys of interest from strings of different lengths above the child's crib or adapted seat; make sure some are readily reachable
Hand/arm coordination	Finger-paint with pudding (or another substance that can be ingested safely) on surfaces that vary from flat to inclined positions to encourage more muscle action Provide remote-controlled switch toys so that when the child presses a large switch the toy is activated
Moving legs and arms intentionally	Place ribbons with bells attached to the child's ankles and wrists to reinforce movement attempts with pleasant sounds Use sloping wedge boards or bolsters to provide stability so that the child can lie on his stomach and use his hands to play with toys
Grasping	Use puzzles with large knobs on pieces Place preferred objects on a slightly inclined board with Velcro attachments so that the child can easily grasp and pull the object Use Velcro fasteners on clothes or as a way to store the child's favorite blanket or stuffed toy and encourage independent retrieval of the object
Standing	Provide a mounted bar on the wall or a stable chair and teach the child to grasp it to pull to stand

1 Embed challenging activities into highly engaging social games. For children with DS who are motivated by social interactions with caregivers, consider ways to develop play routines that provide a lot of very pleasant social interaction in coordination with some more challenging activities. Games such as peek-a-boo and hide-and-seek can be used to encourage reaching and crawling. Song play and simple turn-taking games that require basic hand movements can be enjoyable for the children and promote many important practice opportunities. Responding to the child's attempts to reach or crawl with high affect and enthusiasm can be very reinforcing for some children.

2 Develop a consistent work–break routine. The work of young children in early intervention is often defined as any activity that involves active engagement on the part of the child and is often chosen by an adult because it is important for facilitating the development of a skill. A break for a young child is defined as child-directed and may involve nonfunctional or passive exploration. At other times, break activities can be child-directed, functional practice of already mastered skills. For example, once a child has been taught how to activate a music-producing cause-and-effect toy, that toy can be moved from the work set to the break set. An interventionist or caregiver can develop a routine cycle of engaging in work for several seconds or a few minutes and then give the child a break for a similar amount of time. Keeping the child in the same physical location is usually best, to avoid difficulties transitioning to and from instructional areas. Keeping the work periods brief and practicing the shift from adult-directed to child-directed several times in a teaching interval can also help to build flexibility. The child's efforts and participation are reinforced with a preferred break activity, and the emphasis is not on performance but on engagement. Duration of work periods can be gradually increased, but maintaining consistency in the routine can help to promote

predictability and lessen task avoidance. Physical and visual supports are often integrated within the work and break activities.

3 Practice coping with frustration. During the preschool years, children are challenged to develop self-regulation strategies to tolerate frustration and distress. Building frustration tolerance can be especially difficult for children whose mouths, hands, and body are not working very efficiently. We hypothesize that actively teaching developmentally appropriate forms of coping to children with motor challenges could be very helpful in reducing task avoidance, increasing engagement in learning opportunities, and promoting goal-directed learning. Identify signs of distress and, when first observed, be ready to slow down tasks, provide more physical prompting, or use a back-chaining approach (i.e. providing full assistance in the beginning of a task sequence and only asking the child to complete the last step). Identify appropriate self-calming behaviors that the child can engage in when upset. If this involves objects (such as an oral stimulator or a soft blanket), try to keep these objects in a predictable location that is easily accessible by the child. Observe the child for changes in his/her activity level, facial expression, and quality of vocalizations for cues that indicate rising frustration. Try to intervene before the child is experiencing intense frustration by gently and unobtrusively prompting the child to reach for the calming object. Allow the child time to self-soothe and gradually transition to a new activity. It may also be helpful to identify patterns in the child's frustration and consider ways to minimize the distress by simplifying the task, adding more physical or visual structure, or providing help earlier in the task sequence. There may be some underlying skills (such as postural control) that if targeted may decrease frustration in many activities. If so, then consider enhancing intervention efforts on this domain. Coach caregivers and interventionists to model calm behavior, particularly when the infant or toddler is distressed.

It is critical to note that these treatment recommendations are suggested as a starting point for future research on this topic. Additional empirical treatment studies will be necessary in order to determine whether such approaches can alter the developmental trajectory associated with DS and strengthen goal-directed behavior in quantifiable ways. Nevertheless, there is mounting evidence that goal-directed behavior is a critical target for early intervention in the population of young children with DS. This outcome is likely the result of a dynamic, cascading process that begins with early compromised motor integrity, leading to altered exploratory and cognitive representations. Future work in this area should attempt to test and refine these theories in order to support the community of individuals with DS more effectively.

Summary

There is mounting evidence that individuals with Down syndrome (DS) show a disruption in the development of goal-directed behavior. In this chapter, we present a possible account of the atypical development of goal-directed behavior in young children with DS, including a discussion of hypothesized cascading effects of motor impairments onto early exploratory experiences and early cognitive representations. We specifically review relevant literature on the critical role of early exploratory motor behavior in the formulation of representations of: (1) object affordances; and (2) causality. We then identify how impairments in the formulation of those representations may directly impact on the goal-directed behavior outcomes observed in DS. We conclude the chapter with a discussion of intervention approaches that aim to alter this cascading pathway in order to increase task persistence and strengthen goal-directedness in this population.

References

Baer, D. M. & Pinkston, E. M. (1997). *Environment and Behavior*. Boulder: Westview Press.

Bandura, A. (1997*). Self-efficacy: The Exercise of Control*. New York: W.H. Freeman.

Barrett, K. C. & Morgan, G. A. (1995). Continuities and discontinuities in mastery motivation during infancy and toddlerhood: a conceptualization and review. In R. H. MacTurk & G. A. Morgan (eds.), *Mastery Motivation: Origins, Conceptualizations, and Applications*, pp. 57–93. Westport: Ablex Publishing.

Belsky, J. & Most, R. K. (1981). From exploration to play: a cross-sectional study of infant free play behavior. *Developmental Psychology*, **17**, 630–639.

Berk, L. (2001). *Awakening Children's Minds: How Parents and Teachers Can Make a Difference*. New York: Oxford University Press.

Block, M. E. (1991). Motor development in children with Down syndrome: a review of the literature. *Adapted Physical Activity Quarterly*, **8**, 179–209.

Bojczyk, K. E. & Corbetta, D. (2004). Object retrieval in the 1st year of life: learning effects of task exposure and box transparency. *Developmental Psychology*, **40**, 54–66.

Bourgeois, K. S., Khawar, A. W., Neal., S. A., Lockman, J. J. (2005). Infant manual exploration of objects, surfaces, and their interrelations. *Infancy*, **8**, 233–252.

Campos, J. J., Bertenthan, B. I., Kermoian, R. (1992). Early experience and emotional development: the emergence of wariness of heights. *Psychological Science*, **3**, 61–64.

Carlson, S. M. (2003). Executive function in context: development, measurement, theory and experience. *Monographs of the Society for Research in Child Development*, **68**, 138–151.

Chen, H. & Woolley, P. V. (1978). A developmental assessment chart for non-institutionalized Down syndrome children. *Growth*, **42**, 157–165.

Dunst, C. (1988). Stage transitioning in the sensorimotor development of Down's syndrome infants. *Journal of Mental Deficiency Research*, **32**, 405–410.

Fidler, D. J. (2006). The emergence of a syndrome-specific personality-motivation profile in young children with Down syndrome. In J. A. Rondal & J. Perera (eds.), *Down Syndrome Neurobehavioral Specificity*. West Sussex: Wiley Publishers.

Fidler, D. J., Hepburn, S., Mankin, G., Rogers, S. (2005). Praxis skills in young children with Down syndrome, other developmental disabilities, and typically developing children. *American Journal of Occupational Therapy*, **59**, 129–138.

Finnie, N. (1975). *Handling the Young Cerebral Palsy Child at Home*. New York: Dutton.

Fontenelle, S., Kahrs, B. A., Neal, S. A., Newton, A. T., Lockman, J. J. (2007). Infant manual exploration of composite substrates. *Journal of Experimental Child Psychology*, **98**, 153–167.

Gelman, R. & Cohen, M. (1988). Qualitative differences in the way Down syndrome and normal children solve a novel counting problem. In L. Nadel (ed.), *The Psychobiology of Down Syndrome: Issues in the Biology of Language and Cognition*, pp. 51–99. Massachusetts: MIT Press.

Gibson, E. J. (1988). Exploratory behavior in the development of perceiving, acting, and the acquiring of knowledge. *Annual Review of Psychology*, **39**, 1–41.

Harris, S. R. & Shea, A. M. (1991). Down syndrome. In S. K. Campbell (ed.), *Pediatric Neurologic Physical Therapy (2nd edn.)*, pp. 131–168. Melbourne: Churchill Livingstone.

Kasari, C. & Freeman, S. F. N. (2001). Task-related social behavior in children with Down syndrome. *American Journal on Mental Retardation*, **106**, 253–264.

Lockman, J. (2000). A perception-action perspective on tool use development. *Child Development*, **71**, 137–144.

MacTurk, R. H., Vietze, P. M., McCarthy, M. E., McQuiston, S., Yarrow, L. J. (1985). The organization of exploratory behavior in Down syndrome and nondelayed infants. *Child Development*, **56**, 573–581.

Needham, A. (2000). Improvements in object exploration skills may facilitate the development of object segregation in early infancy. *Journal of Cognition and Development*, **1**, 131–156.

Needham, A., Barrett, T., Peterman, K. (2002). A pick-me-up for infants' exploratory skills: early simulated experiences reaching for objects using 'sticky mittens' enhances young infants' object exploration skills. *Infant Behavior and Development*, **25**, 279–295.

Ohr, P. S. & Fagen, J. W. (1994). Contingency learning in 9-month-old infants with Down syndrome. *American Journal on Mental Retardation*, **99**, 74–84.

Piaget, J. (2001). *The Child's Conception of Physical Causality*. New Brunswick: Transaction Publishers.

Piaget, J. & Inhelder, B. (1987). The sensori-motor level. In J. Oates & S. Sheldon (eds.), *Cognitive Development in Infancy*, pp. 51–57. Hillsdale: Erlbaum.

Pitcairn, T. K. & Wishart, J. G. (1994). Reactions of young children with Down's syndrome to an impossible task. *British Journal of Developmental Psychology*, **12**, 485–489.

Rochat, P. (1987). Mouthing and grasping in neonates: evidence for the early detection of what hard or soft substances afford for action. *Infant Behavior and Development*, **10**, 435–449.

Rochat, P. (1989). Object manipulation and exploration in 2- to 5-month-old infants. *Developmental Psychology*, **25**, 871–884.

Ruskin, E. M., Kasari, C., Mundy, P., Sigman, M. (1994). Attention to people and toys during social and object mastery in children with Down syndrome. *American Journal on Mental Retardation*, **99**, 103–111.

Sommerville, J. A. (2007). Detecting causal structure: the role of interventions in infants' understanding of psychological and physical causal relations. In A. Gopnik & L. Schulz (eds.), *Causal Learning: Psychology, Philosophy, and Computation*, pp. 48–57. New York: Oxford University Press.

Sommerville, J. A., Hildebrand, E. A., Crane, C. C. (2008). Experience matters: the impact of doing versus watching on infants; subsequent perception of tool-use events. *Developmental Psychology*, **44**, 1249–1256.

Sroufe, L. A. (1996). *Emotional Development*. Cambridge: Cambridge University Press.

Wachs, T. (1999). The what, why, and how of temperament: a piece of the action. In L. Balter & C. S. Tamis-LeMonda (eds.), *Child Psychology: A Handbook of Contemporary Issues*, pp. 23–44. New York: Psychology Press.

Wishart, J. G. (1996). Avoidant learning styles and cognitive development in young children. In B. Stratford & P. Gunn (eds.), *New Approaches to Down Syndrome*, pp. 157–172. London: Cassell.

Woodward, A. L. (1998). Infants selectively encode the goal object of an actor's reach. *Cognition*, **69**, 1–34.

Zeitlin, S. & Williamson, G. G. (1994). *Coping in Young Children: Early Intervention Practices to Enhance Adaptive Behavior and Resilience*. Baltimore: Brookes.

Zelazo, P. & Cunningham, W. A. (2007). Executive function: mechanisms underlying emotion regulation. In J. J. Gross (ed.), *Handbook of Emotion Regulation*, pp. 135–158. New York: Guilford.

Chapter

16

The role of parents of children with Down syndrome and other disabilities in early intervention

Gerald Mahoney and Frida Perales

Contemporary early intervention has been closely tied to the proposition that interventions that directly involve parents are more effective at promoting children's learning and development than those that do not (White et al., 1992). This proposition was part of the rationale for the design of the federally mandated early intervention program in the United States, which required that every family in this program have an Individualized Family Service Plan (IFSP). While one of the purposes of the IFSP was to ensure that parents have the resources and supports they need to care for their children, an equally important purpose was to help parents become active participants in their children's intervention. The committee report for the 1986 amendments to the Education of the Handicapped Act (Public Law 99–457) stated,

The committee received overwhelming testimony affirming the family as the primary learning environment for children less than six years of age and pointing out the critical need for parents and professionals to function in a collaborative manner. (From House Report No. 99–860, as cited in Gilkerson et al., 1987, p. 20.)

The emphasis on involving parents in children's intervention services stems from ecological theories of child development (Bronfenbrenner, 1992, 1999; Dunst et al., 2000, 2006; Sameroff & Fiese, 2000). These theories postulate that early developmental learning is a continuous process that can be affected by each of the experiences children have in their daily environment. While developmental interventions that are provided by professionals in child care programs, schools, clinics, and home visits can provide important learning experiences, the ecological model stresses that children's opportunities for developmental learning are greater than this. Efforts to maximize children's developmental learning will be incomplete unless they include most, if not all, of children's natural learning opportunities. Because parents have far more opportunities to interact with their children than do early intervention professionals (Mahoney & MacDonald, 2007), a generally accepted assumption in early intervention is that parents must play an active role to maximize the developmental outcomes children attain in early intervention.

Despite the central role that parent involvement has in early intervention theory and policy as well as the widespread belief by professionals that parent involvement is critical, the actual practice of engaging parents in their children's intervention is controversial and challenging. Even when early intervention services are provided in children's homes, professionals have been reported to primarily work directly with the child, seldom focusing on helping parents learn how they can carry out intervention strategies and enhance

Neurocognitive Rehabilitation of Down Syndrome, eds. Jean-Adolphe Rondal, Juan Perera, and Donna Spiker. Published by Cambridge University Press. © Cambridge University Press 2011.

children's learning opportunities in the context of daily routines and activities (McBride & Peterson, 1997; Peterson et al., 2007).

In contemporary early intervention programs for children from three to six years of age, the overwhelming focus is on professionals providing direct services to children in preschools or child care centers (Mahoney et al., 2004). Little, if any, effort is made to coordinate the developmental services that professionals provide children with what parents are doing with their children at home or in other settings. Parent involvement is restricted primarily to participation in children's Individualized Educational Program (IEP) meetings. Seldom do programs for children in this age range devote substantial resources to parent involvement activities. When these activities do occur, they are often informal, supplementary activities initiated by individual teachers or interventionists, as opposed to ongoing and focal activities supported by the early intervention agency or school.

Parent involvement has been controversial because it is perceived by some as incompatible with family-centered service philosophy, one of the philosophical pillars of early intervention in the United States as well as in many other countries throughout the world (Turnbull et al., 1999). Family-centered service philosophy is clearly supportive of services that empower and enhance the competence of parents, such as occurs in parent involvement activities. Yet, this philosophy also asserts that parents should be given the right to choose their own level of participation, and that intervention should support parents and families and avoid burdening them with responsibilities that could increase their stress (Turnbull et al., 1999). As a result, when parents choose not to participate in their children's intervention, or when parents appear stressed and overwhelmed with their normal activities and routines, based on this philosophy interventionists often view their task as providing services to children in a way that causes the least amount of inconvenience or hardship to parents.

The challenges to parent involvement are numerous. They range from many intervention professionals having limited training and experience in working with parents, to parents having expectations that professionals should be directly responsible for addressing their children's developmental needs, to intervention service models that provide inadequate resources and opportunities to work with parents, to the difficulties of parents and professionals finding convenient times and places to work together (Mahoney et al., 1999).

However, given the philosophical commitment of early intervention to collaborating with parents, the controversies regarding parent involvement and the challenges of carrying this out should not impede this process, particularly if there were compelling evidence that parent involvement made a difference to the outcomes that children attain in early intervention. Until recently, however, there has been little scientific evidence to support the benefits of parent involvement.

A dramatic example of this comes from a study reported by White et al. (1992). These researchers conducted a meta-analysis of 88 high-quality early intervention studies to determine whether the effectiveness of interventions in promoting children's development improved as the level of parent involvement increased. As indicated in Table 16.1, these studies involved young disadvantaged children, children with disabilities, and children who had biological risks. Most of these programs were reported to have average effect sizes on children's development that were in the small to medium range. However, programs that had moderate to extensive levels of parent involvement did not have statistically greater effect sizes than programs that had little to no parent involvement. In fact, although the differences were not significant, the effect sizes of the developmental improvements reported for programs for children with disabilities that had little to no parent involvement were 50% greater

Table 16.1 Effect size of intervention programs as a function of level of parent involvement

Types of children	Degree of parent involvement	
	Extensive/moderate[1]	Little/none[1]
Disadvantaged children	0.52 89(14)	0.53 140(29)
Children with disabilities	0.43 41(8)	0.65 32(12)
At-risk	0.30	0.32
Children	10(4)	41(21)

[1] Number in first line is average effect size. Numbers below effect sizes indicate number of effect sizes and number of studies (in parentheses) on which calculation is based. (From White et al., 1992.)

than the effect sizes for interventions that had moderate to high levels of parent involvement (see Table 16.1).

At the time the White et al. (1992) study was published, it was criticized for assessing outmoded models of parent involvement, and for not giving an accurate account of more innovative approaches. More recently, several single subject and quasi-experimental research studies of parent-mediated interventions have been reported which indicate that parents can follow-through effectively with intervention procedures at home and that these procedures appear to result in significant changes in children's developmental and functional behaviors (Kaiser et al., 2000; Stahmer & Gist, 2001; Chandler et al., 2002). Nonetheless, a recent review of parent-implemented intervention studies with children with autism spectrum disorders (ASD) concluded that although parent-implemented intervention can improve the quality of interaction between parents and children and enhance children's use of social communicative behaviors, there is no reliable evidence that they enhance children's overall developmental functioning (McConachie & Diggle, 2007). In fact, a randomized control study reported by Smith et al. (2000) indicated that a group of children with ASD, whose parents implemented applied behavioral analysis (ABA) with them, made significantly lower developmental improvements than a control group of children who received intensive ABA services from tutors.

The parenting model of child development

For the most part, parent involvement has been conceptualized almost exclusively in terms of an educational or remedial model. That is, parents have been asked to participate in their children's interventions by implementing the types of educational or remedial strategies and activities that professionals implement with children. For example, White et al. (1992) reported that 85% of the parent involvement studies they examined asked parents to follow through with either behavioral instructional activities as prescribed in curricula, such as the Portage Guide (Shearer & Shearer, 1972), or to provide sensory stimulation activities to their children similar to what is prescribed in sensory integration therapy. McConachie and Diggle (2007) also commented that most of the studies they reviewed asked parents to carry out intensive behavioral intervention (IBI) strategies that were derived from ABA. Parent involvement appears to have been considered to be an additive process, in which parents' implementation of intervention activities was thought to augment the effects that they, as parents, naturally had on their children's development.

The parenting model of child development is a term coined by Goodman (1992). This model asserts that all parents normally play a substantial role in supporting and encouraging their children's development. Understanding the ways that parents either promote or inhibit their children's development can inform us about not only the psychosocial strategies that parents naturally use to enhance their children's development, but also the processes children use for developmental learning. This information can be used in one of two ways: (1) as a foundation for instructional or remedial procedures that can be implemented by professionals; or (2) as a basis for developing interventions that maximize the effects that parents have on their children's development.

The key to the parenting model is to identify the interactional processes used by parents that appear to influence children's developmental learning and social–emotional functioning and to understand how these processes work. This is an effort has that has been taking place in the context of parent–child interaction research studies that have been conducted over the past 30 years with typically developing children as well as children with a variety of developmental risks and disabilities including Down syndrome (DS).

Several years ago we reported a parent–child interaction study that included a sample of 60 parent–child dyads in which children were either 12, 24, or 36 months of age (Mahoney et al., 1985; Mahoney, 1988). Ninety percent of these children had DS. Parent–child interaction was assessed from observations of mothers and children playing together for a period of approximately 20 minutes. These observations were used to address two questions.

First, we were interested in determining how mothers' general style of interacting with their children was associated with their children's rate of cognitive functioning (Mahoney et al., 1985). In this study, mothers' overall pattern of interaction was rated with the Maternal Behavior Rating Scale (Mahoney et al., 1986). This scale consisted of 18 items that assessed three dimensions of mothers' style of interaction. One was called achievement/performance orientation. This dimension included the degree to which mothers attempted to encourage their children to learn and use advanced developmental skills. The second dimension was the amount of stimulation parents provided while playing with their children. This was reflected in the number of different activities parents did with their children, the amount they spoke to their children, as well as their general pace of interaction. The third dimension was responsiveness. This included the degree to which parents' behaviors were linked to previous child behaviors; whether parents responded to children in a way that supported and encouraged children's interests and intentions; and the amount of children's non-demand behavior that parents responded to.

We assessed the relationship of these three dimensions of mothers' interaction with their children's current rate of development as measured by the Bayley Scales of Mental Development (Bayley, 1969). Our findings indicated that mothers' style of interaction accounted for 23% of the variability in children's rate of development. Whether 12, 24, or 36 months old, children had higher Bayley Developmental Quotients when their mothers were rated high in responsiveness and low on achievement/performance orientation and amount of stimulation. Children with DS were more likely to have attained higher levels of developmental functioning the more their parents responded to and supported the behaviors that they were currently capable of doing and the less they stimulated their children and attempted to teach them advanced developmental skills. Surprisingly, the children with the lowest developmental scores had parents who focused most on stimulating their children, teaching advanced developmental skills.

Second, we were interested in determining how mothers' communications with their children were related to children's rate of communication and language development (Mahoney, 1988). We coded each of the 20,000 verbal and nonverbal communicative acts these mothers and children produced during these observations. Our results indicated that how much mothers communicated with their children and the semantic and syntactic quality of mothers' communication was not associated with children's rate of communication development. Instead, similar to cognitive development, children's communication development was associated primarily with the manner in which mothers responded to their children. The amount that children communicated with their mothers during these observations was highly associated with three qualities of mothers' communication. The first was the frequency that mothers responded to children's communication as if it were meaningful even if children were using lower forms of communication than typical for their chronological age. The second was the degree to which mothers communicated with short, simple phrases that were directly related to children's current actions, interests, or communications. The third was the degree to which mothers refrained from asking or otherwise pressuring their children to do or say specific actions and communications. The children with DS who communicated most frequently with their mothers had mothers' whose communication most reflected these three features. Furthermore, children's rate of language development, as measured by the Receptive and Expressive Emergent Language Scale, was also associated with these same features of their mothers' communication.

In general, there are at least two important observations to be made from these studies. First, the types of interactions that appeared to be associated with the effectiveness of parents at fostering the development of children with DS were quite different from the instructional and remedial activities that most intervention programs had been asking parents to do as part of their children's intervention. Intervention programs and professionals had been asking parents to engage in activities such as increasing the amount of stimulation they provided their children, teaching predetermined sets of developmental skills to their children, or modeling the words and phrases targeted as children's intervention objectives and prompting them to say them. Parents were being asked to use directive or didactic instructional strategies to encourage their children to use the advanced developmental skills and communications that they were being taught by professionals. Intervention programs either discouraged or de-emphasized the importance of parents engaging in the types of responsive and supportive interactions that characterized the more effective parents that were observed in our studies of parent–child interaction.

Second, the types of parental interactions that were associated with higher levels of cognitive and communication development among children with DS were very similar to the types of parental interactions associated with the development of all children. Research investigating how parents enhance their children's cognitive development shows that responsiveness is the only parenting quality that consistently predicts children's developmental age or intelligence quotient (IQ) scores (Beckwith & Cohen, 1989; Bradley, 1989; Beckwith et al., 1992; Fewell et al., 1996; Landry et al., 1997). Similarly, the patterns of communication that have been reported to facilitate the communication development of children with DS have also been identified as positive influences on typically developing children as well as children who have a wide range of developmental risks and disabilities (Nelson, 1973; Hoff-Ginsberg & Shatz, 1982; Bornstein et al., 1999). Children attain higher levels of communication the more often their parents respond to their communicative behaviors and interpret their attempts to communicate as though they were meaningful.

The parenting model and developmental intervention

Insofar as the parenting model assumes that parents play a substantial role in supporting and encouraging the development of their children, there are two important questions this model raises regarding the effectiveness of early intervention. The first is how does the effectiveness of parents at facilitating their children's development contribute to the effects of developmental intervention? Might the effectiveness of intervention be related to the effectiveness of parents, such that more responsive parents enhance the effectiveness of intervention while less responsive parents undermine or lessen the effectiveness of intervention? The second is could intervention be effective at promoting children's development by focusing primarily on increasing the effectiveness of parents at supporting their children's development?

Parenting and intervention effectiveness

There is little, if any, disagreement that parents play a significant role in promoting their children's development, and that parents vary greatly in their effectiveness at doing this. Nonetheless, for the most part, investigators have not examined how parents and intervention services each contribute to the effectiveness of intervention services. However, we have reported two studies that attempted to investigate this issue. In one study, we conducted a secondary analysis of 629 children and their parents who had participated in four different early intervention research studies (Mahoney et al., 1998). The sample included 298 parent–child dyads from the Infant Health and Development Program (IHDP) (Brooks-Gunn et al., 1994), 238 dyads from the Longitudinal Studies of Alternative Types of Early Intervention (White & Boyce, 1993), 42 subjects from the Play and Leaning Strategies Program (PALS) (Fewell & Wheeden, 1998), and 47 subjects from the Family-Centered Outcomes Study (Mahoney & Bella, 1998). The common elements of these four studies were that children began participating when they were under three years of age, and that observations of parent child interaction that could be used to determine how the effects of intervention were associated with mothers' style of interacting with their children were collected. In all four studies, mothers' style of interacting with their children was assessed with the same instrument, the Maternal Behavior Rating Scale (Mahoney, 1992).

These interventions differed from each other in terms of the developmental disabilities and risks of the children that were involved as well as the types and intensity of intervention services they received. The IHDP was an intensive and comprehensive intervention that involved low birthweight children and their parents. This intervention was initiated when children came home from neonatal intensive care units and continued until children were three years old. The first year of this intervention consisted primarily of weekly home visits in which parents received information about play activities they could do to support their children's development. During the second and third years, parents continued to receive monthly home visits, while children also received a high-quality preschool experience for 25 hours each week.

The Longitudinal Studies were conducted with children with disabilities who were enrolled in early childhood special education programs. This multi-site study compared different types of enhanced classroom-based early intervention services to standard classroom-based intervention services. Children received from two to five days per week of early intervention services. In some cases, parents also received parent education classes related to how to manage their children at home. As none of the early intervention enhancements varied in terms of their impact on children's development (White & Boyce, 1993) in this study, children who received enhanced classroom early interventions were compared to children who received standard early intervention services.

The PALS project evaluated the effects of a three-month parenting intervention (24 sessions, 30 minutes each) that was designed to teach teenaged mothers how to engage in more responsive interactions with their typically functioning children.

The Family Service Outcomes Study examined the impact of the family support services that were provided during weekly intervention sessions with children with disabilities who were enrolled in Part C early intervention programs over a 12-month period.

Data analyses attempted to focus on how improvements in children's developmental functioning that occurred during each of these interventions were associated with mothers' style of interaction. In two of the studies, IHDP and PALS, intervention had a statistically significant effect on children's rate of development. In addition, in both of these studies, mothers increased their level of responsiveness with their children while participating in the intervention. In the IHDP, mothers' level of responsiveness at 30 months was significantly associated with the gains that children made during intervention. In fact, mothers' responsiveness accounted for approximately 20% of the variability in children's rate of development when they were 24 and 36 months old, while the intervention services that children and parents received (e.g. home visiting and preschool) accounted for only 4% of the variance.

In the PALS program, after three months of intervention the children in the treatment group attained developmental quotients that were nine points higher than those of children in a no-treatment contrast group. In addition, consistent with the focus of this intervention, the responsiveness of mothers in the treatment group was significantly greater than for mothers in the contrast group. A regression analysis that examined the contributions of children's development at pretest and mothers' responsiveness at posttest to the developmental status of children at the end of intervention indicated that mothers' responsiveness was the only significant predictor of children's development, accounting for 10% of the variance.

In the other two intervention studies, Family-Centered Outcomes and the Longitudinal Studies, there were no significant changes in children's rate of development during intervention. In the Family-Centered Outcomes Study, children's developmental quotients changed from 62 at pretest to 63 at posttest; while in the Longitudinal Studies, developmental quotients for children in both the expanded and typical treatment groups were 67 at pretest and 68 at posttest. In addition, in both of these studies there were no significant pre-post changes in mothers' responsiveness with their children. It is interesting to note that in the Longitudinal Studies, even though mothers' responsiveness did not change during intervention, this was the only factor that was significantly associated with children's rate of development both at the beginning and end of intervention. Neither the type nor intensity of intervention services children received in this project had any influence on the rate of development children attained during intervention.

In another study (Mahoney et al., 2004), we examined the impact of preschool special education over the course of one school year on a sample of 70 children with disabilities. These children were between three and five years of age (mean chronological age = 41 months) at the beginning of the school year and had moderate levels of developmental delay [mean developmental quotient = 59 (Bayley Scales of Mental Development)]. The children came from 41 classrooms, which operated four half-days each week for a total of

36 weeks. We classified these classrooms according to the type of instructional model teachers were implementing. Approximately 27 children were receiving services in developmentally oriented classrooms in which teachers focused on providing developmentally appropriate activities in child-selected play and instructional activities; 15 children were receiving services in which teachers focused on didactic instruction related to children's individualized educational objectives in teacher-directed individual and group activities; and 28 children received naturalistic intervention services in which teachers blended child-selected developmental activities with teacher-directed instructional activities. We then examined the impact of these instructional models on children's rate of developmental growth and parents' style of interaction. Results indicated that there were no significant improvements in children's level of developmental functioning over the course of this intervention. Children's developmental quotients averaged 59 at the beginning of intervention and 60 at the end of intervention. While the three types of instructional models clearly affected the classroom experiences children received, there were no differences between these models in terms of their impact on children's development. Pre-post comparisons also indicated that parents' style of interacting with their children did not change during the course of the school year. This result was not surprising, because these preschools had little if any direct involvement with parents and they made no effort to influence parents' interactions with their children. They are also consistent with several research reports which indicate that, in the absence of interventions designed to change parents' style of interacting with their children, parents' style of interacting with their children appears to be stable over time (Masur & Turner, 2001). Despite this, parents' level of responsiveness with their children was the only variable investigated in this study that was associated with children's development at the end of intervention. That is, while the preschool classroom experience had no effect on children's development regardless of the type of instructional model that was used, parents' level of responsiveness accounted for 10% of the variability of their children's developmental quotients.

Overall these findings, which are based on studies that included nearly 700 children and parents, provide evidence that is highly consistent with the parenting model of child development. They suggest that: (1) parents continue to be the major influence on their children's development even when their children participate in intervention, and (2) the effectiveness of intervention is highly associated with the effectiveness of parents at manifesting those interactive processes that have been reported to influence the development of children who are not involved in intervention.

That is, findings from these studies indicated that children's rate of development while they participated in intervention was highly associated with how effective their parents were at engaging in responsive interactions with them. The level of responsiveness of mothers or other primary caregivers had a much stronger relationship with children's rate of development during intervention than did the services that children received, regardless of the type or intensity of these services. Intervention appeared to accelerate children's development when it was also successful at enhancing mothers' responsiveness with their children. When interventions did not affect mothers' responsiveness, children's rate of development during intervention was similar to their rate of development prior to intervention, which was also associated with mothers' level of responsiveness. The effects of mothers' responsiveness on children's development during intervention appeared to occur among all children, and did not vary according to the nature or etiology of children's developmental disabilities.

These results suggest that developmental interventions that are provided directly to children can augment the effects that parents have on their children's development, but that even when interventions are high quality and intensive, their influence is still not as great as the influence that parents have on their children. For example, the center-piece of the IHDP was the 25-hour per week, high-quality, preschool experience that children received when they were between 12 and 36 months of age. Yet results from our analyses indicated that improvements in parents' responsiveness, which were an unintended consequence of the home-visiting component of the IHDP, accounted for nearly five times more variability in children's developmental outcomes than the high-intensity preschool experience. In addition, however, our results also indicated that high-quality child-directed intervention services do not impact children's rate of development if they do not also enhance the effectiveness of parents. In the Longitudinal Studies as well as in the investigation of preschool special education classes reported by Mahoney et al., 2004, intervention did not enhance the effectiveness of parents at interacting with their children. In both studies, regardless of the quality and intensity of the child-directed services, children failed to show improvements in their rate of development during intervention.

Parenting as intervention

If parenting can have a significant impact on children's development, then one likely possibility is that children's rate of developmental growth can be enhanced by primarily focusing intervention efforts on increasing the effectiveness of parents at engaging in responsive interactions with their children. This approach to developmental intervention has been referred to as relationship-focused intervention because it is derived from research on parent–child interaction. For the past 30 years, from when the apparent effects of parental responsiveness began to be reported, several studies have investigated the potential effects of this type of intervention (McCollum & Hemmeter, 1997; Trivette, 2003). In general, this research has produced some very promising results. First, this research has clearly established that relationship-focused intervention strategies can be effective at encouraging parents to modify their style of interacting with their children through the use of responsive interaction strategies which are described below (McCollum, 1984; Girolametto, 1988; Hemmeter & Kaiser, 1994). Second, enhancements in parents' interactions with their children, particularly as reflected in increases in their level of responsiveness, are often associated with improvements in the quality of children's involvement or participation in interactions with their parents (McCollum, 1984; Hemmeter & Kaiser, 1994). Third, when relationship-focused intervention is carried out for approximately six months or longer, it can result in improvements in children's cognitive and language development as well as social–emotional functioning (Mahoney, 1988; Seifer et al., 1991; Landry et al., 2003, 2006). In the following, we will describe results from a relationship-focused intervention study with a sample of young children with disabilities and their parents that we reported.

Responsive Teaching (Mahoney & MacDonald, 2007) is a developmental intervention that is designed to enhance the development and social–emotional functioning of children by encouraging parents to engage in highly responsive interactions with them. Parents are taught to use several Responsive Teaching strategies as a means of increasing their level of responsiveness with their children during routine interactions. These strategies help parents increase five dimensions of responsiveness. These include reciprocity (e.g. take one turn and wait), contingency (e.g. respond immediately to little behaviors), shared control (e.g. follow my child's lead; playful obstruction), affect (e.g. interact for fun), and interactive match (e.g. do what my child can do). These strategies are usually taught to parents in weekly individual parent–child sessions, in which the professional describes and demonstrates the strategy with the child and then coaches parents in their use of the strategy. While interventionists may recommend that parents spend brief periods of time practicing to learn how to implement these strategies with their children, the focus of this intervention is to encourage parents to use these strategies during each of the routine interactions that they normally have while caring for and socializing or playing with their children.

Mahoney and Perales (2005) reported an evaluation of Responsive Teaching with a sample of 50 children and their parents. The average age of the children at the start of intervention was 30 months. Twenty of the children were diagnosed with ASD while the other 30 had a variety of neurodevelopmental delays (ND) including DS. The intervention took place over a one-year period during which the sample received an average of 32 Responsive Teaching sessions that lasted approximately one hour each.

Pre-post comparisons indicated that the intervention promoted: (1) significant increases in parents' responsiveness; and (2) significant and dramatic improvements in children's cognitive, communication, and social–emotional functioning. On average, children's rate of cognitive development increased by 64% during the course of intervention, while their rate of language development increased by approximately 150%. In addition, this intervention had a significant impact on children's social–emotional functioning, although this effect was stronger for children with ASD who were showing many more problems in this domain than children with other types of disabilities. Similar to reports described previously in this chapter, improvements in parental responsiveness accounted for between 10% and 20% of the variability in the developmental improvements that children made during intervention.

Some of the children who participated in this intervention were receiving other child-directed early intervention services in addition to Responsive Teaching. Yet for the majority of children, responsive teaching was the only intervention they received. The effects of intervention on children's development were not associated with the number of other interventions they were receiving. Instead, the key to the effectiveness of this intervention was the degree to which primary caregivers learned and integrated Responsive Teaching strategies into their routine interactions with their children. When parents were successful at doing this, children made significant developmental gains, and the magnitude of their developmental improvements was associated with the changes in responsiveness that parents made with their children. If parents did not change their responsiveness during intervention, children made no or minimal developmental improvements.

Long-term effects of responsive parenting

A reasonable question to ask regarding the effects of relationship-focused intervention is what effect these interventions have on children's development over the long term. At this point, no studies have been reported that have conducted long-term follow-ups that could be used to address this question. However, Fewell and Deutscher (2004) reported the effects of parental responsiveness on 543 children who participated in the IHDP when they were five and eight years of age. In this study, regression analyses were used to determine if mothers' level of responsiveness, which was assessed when children were 30 months old, was associated with children's verbal IQ scores when children were five and eight years as well as their reading achievement scores when they were eight years old. In conducting these analyses, these authors controlled for the effects of children's IQ when they were three years old, which was a variable that was highly associated with ratings of maternal responsiveness as reported in a previous section of this chapter. Yet despite this very conservative statistical procedure, mothers' responsiveness still accounted for 7% of the variance of children's verbal IQ when they were five years old and 4% of variance in their verbal IQ and reading achievement scores when they were eight years old. While the effect sizes of responsiveness were small, they were nonetheless statistically significant. More importantly, the classroom-based intervention services that children received when they were between 12 and 36 months of age was reported to be unrelated to any of these developmental outcomes. Once again these data provide evidence to indicate that parental responsiveness, which was enhanced through the IHDP, had far greater effect on the long-term developmental outcomes of the children who participated in this intervention than did the high-quality intensive preschool intervention that they received.

Making sense of the role of parents in intervention

In this chapter, we have presented information which indicates that parents are perhaps the most important psychosocial influence on the development of all children, including children with disabilities such as DS, at least during the early childhood period. In particular, the effectiveness of parents at promoting their children's development is related to how responsive they are when they engage in routine play and social interactions with their children. We presented evidence that suggests that the influence parents have on their children's development does not diminish when children are receiving early intervention services. In fact, just the opposite appears to be true. How well children do in various types of interventions appears to be highly associated with parents' level of responsiveness with their children. When children participate in early intervention, the developmental outcomes attained by children with disabilities whose parents are highly responsive are generally greater than those attained by children with similar disabilities whose parents are less responsive.

In intervention studies that have evaluated the effects of both parents and formal intervention services on children's development, interventions appear to have a significant influence on children's development only if they are also successful at enhancing parents' level of responsiveness with their children. We described some evidence which indicates that child-directed intervention activities can add to the effects that parents have on their children's development, but that the amount that these interventions enhance children's development appears to be far less than the effects of parents. However, if interventions do not enhance parents' responsiveness with their children, the studies we reviewed indicated that child-directed services may have little if any impact on children's rate of development.

These findings raise two important questions: (1) why do parents appear to have a greater effect on children's development than do child-directed intervention activities; and (2) how does responsive interaction foster children's developmental growth?

Why parents are so important to children's development

There are at least three major reasons why parents play a critical role in their children's development. First, all parents, whether they are biological or adoptive parents, have a special social–emotional bond or attachment to their children that no other people can, or should even try to replace (Bowlby, 1969). This bond places parents in the unique role of being the most powerful influence in the lives of their young children, even if their time with their children may be limited because of work or other responsibilities. Not only is this bond the reason why young children prefer to be with their parents, it is also what makes the things that parents say or do more influential on young children than whatever any other adults say or do.

Second, children's learning and development is a continuous process that can occur in any situation in which children are actively engaged. When or where children learn new developmental information or skills is determined by what children pay attention to and what interests or excites them. It has little, if anything, to do with whether adults are actively trying to teach or provide children with special experiences to help them learn. Young children are as likely to learn new information or skills when they are waking up in the morning, eating breakfast, taking a bath, playing with their parents, or riding in a car as they are in a preschool or child care classroom, or when they receive special instruction from therapists or other child development specialists. The unique capability that parents have to influence their children's developmental learning comes from the fact that they are the ones most likely to be there when their children are ready to learn.

Third, the opportunities parents have to interact with and influence their children's development are far greater than the opportunities that any other professionals or adults could ever have. This effect is accentuated by the fact that most parents are a constant influence in their children's lives throughout the early childhood years.

To illustrate this last point, we conducted a hypothetical analysis of the opportunities parents have to influence their children's development compared to teachers, therapists, or intervention specialists when children are in preschool special education or early intervention (Mahoney & MacDonald, 2007). Based on the types of early intervention services that are commonly provided in the United States, we assumed that when children are enrolled in preschool special education, the classes they attend last about two-and-a-half hours per day, four days a week for approximately 30 weeks each year. If children also receive therapy, such as speech or physical therapy, these therapy sessions last approximately 30 minutes each and are usually provided one day a week for approximately 35 weeks a year. In addition, we assumed that most parents spend at least one hour per day in one-to-one contact with their children.

When we analyzed classrooms in terms of the total amount of time teachers interact with children (assuming two teachers in a classroom divided among 12 children and distributed among group instruction, management activities, and one-to-one interactions), we estimated that children receive approximately 33 minutes of one-to-one interaction with their teachers each week. This can be contrasted with approximately 25 minutes of one-on-one time with therapists and 420 minutes with parents each week.

However, as parents are with children 52 weeks each year, while teachers and therapists average between 30 and 35 weeks, the greater amount of one-to-one time parents spend with their children each week is magnified by the number of weeks they are with their children over the course of a year. Assuming that most adults engage in 10 interactions per minute, parents engage in at least 220,000 discrete interactions with their children each year; while early intervention teachers engage in approximately 9900 and therapists 8750 interactions in the same period.

As illustrated in Figure 16.1, if a child were enrolled in a special education classroom or early intervention playgroup and also received therapy once each week, in one year parents would have at least 200,000 more interactions with their children, or 10 times more opportunities to influence their children's development than teachers and therapists combined.

This is an extremely conservative estimate of the opportunities parents have to influence their children's development. If parents spend two, three, or more hours each day interacting

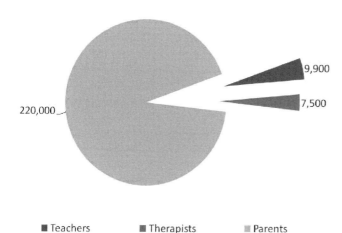

Figure 16.1 Opportunities of teachers, therapists, and parents to interact with children in one year's time. (From Mahoney and MacDonald, 2007.)

9,900

7,500

220,000

■ Teachers   ■ Therapists   ▨ Parents

with their children, as many parents do, the discrepancy between the opportunities parents have to interact with their children compared with the opportunities of teachers and therapists would be magnified by two or three times. Thus, our example illustrates how the opportunities parents have to influence their children's development are substantially greater than professionals could ever have, even when parents have limited time to be with their children because of work or other responsibilities.

Given the relatively limited opportunities that professionals have to interact with and provide stimulation to children, why would professionals be expected to have a greater capacity to alter the developmental life course of any child than parents do, particularly if a child has significant disabilities? Given the fact that parents have at least ten times more opportunities to interact with their children than professionals do, it should not be surprising that, as the studies reviewed in this chapter indicate, the developmental outcomes children attain are primarily related to the effectiveness of parents, not professionals, at influencing children's development. Parents' influence on their children's development comes from the enormous number of opportunities they have to interact with their children. They do not relinquish their developmental role because either their children have disabilities or are receiving early intervention services (Figure 16.1).

Why responsiveness is so important to children's development

Although numerous studies have reported that parental responsiveness plays an important role in promoting children's rate of development, far less research has attempted to determine the reasons why responsiveness has these effects. One of the most common explanations for this phenomenon is that parental responsiveness contributes to the quality of the relationship between children and their parents, such that children are likely to become more securely attached to high responsive versus low responsive parents (Bowlby, 1969). Children who are more securely attached to their parents (or other adult caregivers) are thought to have two factors that contribute to their developmental learning. First, they are less fearful and more prone to interact with and explore the objects and people in their world (van Ijzendoorn et al., 1999; Velderman et al., 2006). Second, they are likely to be more receptive or reactive to the stimulation and supports provided by their parents and other adult caregivers (Landry et al., 2006).

While there is considerable merit to these explanations, we recently reported a study (Mahoney et al., 2007) which suggested that responsiveness may also impact on development by enhancing the rate that children use pivotal developmental behaviors, which are the behaviors that are the foundations for developmental learning. This study included 45 mother–child dyads in which each of the children had developmental delays and were less than three years of age. Videotaped observations of these dyads were used to assess mothers' responsiveness and children's use of behaviors such as attention, initiation, persistence, interest cooperation, joint attention, and affect. Two interesting findings were reported from this study. The first was that mothers' level of responsiveness was related to the frequency that their children used these behaviors. Children whose mothers were rated as being high on responsiveness had significantly higher ratings on each of the seven behaviors that we assessed than children whose mothers had lower responsiveness ratings. The second finding was that the frequency that children used these behaviors (e.g. attention, initiation, persistence, interest cooperation, joint attention, and affect) was related to children's rate of social, communication, and cognitive development, as assessed by two developmental measures, the Vineland Adaptive Behavior Scale (Sparrow et al., 1984) and the Transdisciplinary Play Based Assessment (Linder, 1993).

These research findings suggest that the behaviors parents encourage when they interact responsively with their children are the learning processes that are the foundations for developmental learning. Following the work of Koegel and his colleagues (Koegel et al., 1999), we refer to these as pivotal behaviors, which are "behaviors that are central to wide areas of functioning such that a change in the pivotal behavior will produce improvement across a number of behaviors" (p. 579) (Koegel et al., 1999).

Based upon these research findings, we proposed the pivotal behavior model of developmental learning to explain how responsiveness promotes children's early developmental learning (Mahoney et al., 2007). This model postulates that the behaviors that are most critical to this process are pivotal behaviors or learning processes that are the foundation for developmental learning. By interacting responsively, adults influence children's developmental learning less by teaching the skills and behaviors that are the benchmarks of higher levels of development or social–emotional functioning, and more by encouraging children to use the pivotal behaviors, or learning processes, that are needed to learn from each of the children's routine social and nonsocial activities. The more responsively adults interact with children, the more likely are children to use their pivotal behaviors.

The critical role that parents play in promoting children's development is largely attributable to the number of opportunities they have to engage in one-to-one interaction with them. Insofar as parents' style of interacting transcends each of the 220,000 interactions they have with their children each year, parents who are highly responsive repeatedly encourage their children to use higher frequencies of pivotal behavior. Over time, this repetitive pattern of parent–child interaction helps children learn to become habitual users of pivotal developmental behaviors (i.e. more effective learners) such that the high levels of pivotal behavior use that children experience with their parents carries over into their daily routine activities. As a result, children of responsive parents learn more not only when they interact with their parents but also when they play by themselves and interact with others. Over time, this results in their attaining higher levels of cognitive and communication functioning.

In this chapter we have argued that parents play a critical role in supporting and nurturing their children's development, and that this role continues even when children are receiving early intervention services. We presented data from several studies that indicated that the developmental outcomes children attain while participating in early intervention are strongly associated with their parents' level of responsiveness. We described studies which indicated that when intervention did not enhance parents' responsiveness with their children, intervention did not appear to be successful at enhancing children's rate of development, regardless of the type or intensity of services children received. We also described studies which indicated that when parents' responsiveness increases during intervention, regardless of whether this is an intended or untended outcome, intervention appeared to be effective at accelerating children's developmental growth. In addition, we reported that relationship-focused interventions that attempt to directly enhance parents' level of responsiveness with their children have been reported to be successful at promoting children's rate of development, and that the developmental improvements children make in these interventions are related to the degree to which parents improved their responsiveness with their children.

We argued that the type of parent involvement that we have described in this chapter is very different from the way that many intervention programs have asked parents to follow through with instructional activities with their children. Nonetheless, the notion of encouraging parents to interact more responsively with their children is very reasonable when interpreted within the context of the parenting model of child development. This model asserts that parents are the primary influence on the early development of young children. Parents' influence derives from both the unique bond that they have with their children, as well as from the numerous opportunities they have to engage in one-to-one interactions with their children. We also argued that parental responsiveness plays a critical role in promoting development, not so much by teaching children the developmental skills and behaviors that they are lacking, but more by encouraging children to become more efficient learners by increasing their use of pivotal developmental behaviors such as attention, persistence, initiation, and cooperation.

There are some who maintain that the unique effects that DS has on children's learning, and social and communication abilities may require that these children have different types of psychosocial supports or educational experiences than children with other types of disabilities. Although the research reviewed in this chapter was not conducted exclusively with children with DS, children with DS were highly represented in most of the studies reviewed. The studies reported by Mahoney et al. (1985) and Mahoney (1988) consisted primarily of children with DS. These studies provided strong support for two of the basic premises of the argument presented in this paper: (1) parents play a substantial role in promoting the early development of their children; and (2) parental responsiveness is one of the main parenting qualities that enhances children's learning and development. The studies which indicated that intervention was not effective unless it promoted parents' responsiveness with their children (e.g. Mahoney et al., 1998, 2004) and that children's development can be enhanced by encouraging parents to interact more responsively with their children (Mahoney & Perales, 2005), all included children with DS. None of these studies reported any evidence to indicate that their findings did not apply to children with DS. Thus, while it is possible that children with DS may require specialized educational or intervention experiences to address some of their unique learning and social needs, we feel confident that our conclusion that parent involvement is critical to the success of early intervention has as much empirical support for children with DS as it does for children with other types of disabilities.

As a concluding note, we observed earlier in this chapter that although parent involvement is highly valued by most of the professionals in early intervention and is a core component of early intervention policy, the actual practice of interventionists working collaboratively with parents occurs only sporadically. The emerging research evidence regarding the critical role that parents play in intervention means not only that parents need to demand greater involvement in their children's intervention, but also that intervention agencies and programs must begin to address those factors that have prevented this practice from occurring. A strong commitment to parent involvement will require that the field of early intervention engage in several activities including: reexamining models for providing services; ensuring that professionals are well trained to carry out this mission; and utilizing intervention curriculi and instructional strategies that have been demonstrated to be effective in working with parents.

Summary

This chapter argues that parent involvement is essential to the success of developmental interventions with young children with Down syndrome (DS) and other disabilities. A major turning point in contemporary views of parent involvement has been related to recent efforts to conceptualize this from the framework of the parenting model of child development. The parenting model emphasizes intervention activities that maximize parents' use of those interactive qualities that research has shown to be associated with children's development. Research indicates that parental responsiveness is a critical influence on the development and social–emotional well being of children with DS and other disabilities. We describe how interventions that enhance parents' responsiveness have resulted in substantial improvements in children's development.

References

Bayley, N. (1969). *Bayley Scales of Infant Development*. New York: Psychological Corporation.

Beckwith, L. & Cohen, S. E. (1989). Maternal responsiveness with preterm infants and later competency. In M. H. Bornstein (ed.), *Maternal responsiveness: characteristics and consequences. New Directions for Child Development*, **43**, 75–87.

Beckwith, L., Rodning, C., Cohen, S. (1992). Preterm children at early adolescence and continuity and discontinuity in maternal responsiveness from infancy. *Child Development*, **63**(5), 1198–1208.

Bornstein, M. H., Tamis-LeMonda, C. S., Haynes, O. M. (1999). First words in the second year: continuity, stability, and models of concurrent and predictive correspondence in vocabulary and verbal responsiveness across age and context. *Infant Behavior and Development*, **22**(1), 65–85.

Bowlby, J. (1969). *Attachment and Loss*. New York: Basic Books.

Bradley, R. (1989). HOME measurement of maternal responsiveness. In M. H. Bornstein (ed.), Maternal responsiveness: characteristics and consequences. *New Directions for Child Development*, **43**, 63–74.

Bronfenbrenner, U. (1992). Ecological systems theory. In Vasta, R. (ed.), *Six Theories of Child Development*, pp. 3–28. Philadelphia: Jessica Kingsley.

Bronfenbrenner, U. (1999). Environments in developmental perspective: theoretical and operational models. In S. L. Freidman & T. D. Wachs (eds.), *Measuring Environment Across the Lifespan: Emerging Methods and Concepts*. Washington, DC: American Psychological Association.

Brooks-Gunn, J., McCarton, C. M., Casey, P. H., et al. (1994). Early intervention in low birthweight, premature infants. *Journal of the American Medical Association*, **272**, 1257–1262.

Chandler, S., Christie, P., Newson, E., Prevezer, W. (2002). Developing a diagnostic and intervention package for 2- to 3- year olds with autism. *Autism*, **6**(1), 47–69.

Dunst, C. J., Hamby, D. W., Trivette, C. M., Raab, M., Bruder, M. B. (2000). Everyday family and community life and children's naturally occurring learning opportunities. *Journal of Early Intervention*, **23**, 151–164.

Dunst, C. J., Trivette, C. M., Hamby, D. W., Bruder, M. B. (2006). Influences of contrasting natural learning environment experiences on child, parent and family well-being. *Journal of Developmental and Physical Disabilities*, **18**(3), 235–250.

Fewell, R. R., Casal, S. G., Glick, M. P., Wheeden, C. A., Spiker, D. (1996). Maternal education and maternal responsiveness as predictors of play competence in low birth weight, premature infants: a preliminary report. *Developmental and Behavioral Pediatrics*, **17**(2), 100–104.

Fewell, R. R. & Deutscher, B. (2004). Contributions of early language and maternal facilitation variables to later language and reading abilities. *Journal of Early Intervention*, **26**(2), 132–145.

Fewell, R. & Wheeden, C. A. (1998). A pilot study of intervention with adolescent mothers and their children: a preliminary examination of child outcomes. *Topics in Early Childhood Special Education*, **17**(4), 18–25.

Gilkerson, L., Hilliard, G. A., Schrag, E., Schonkoff, J. P. (1987). *Report accompanying the Education of the Handicapped Act Amendments of 1986* (House Report No. 99–860). Washington, DC: National Center for Clinical Infant Programs.

Girolametto, L. (1988). Improving the social conversational skills of developmentally delayed children: an intervention study. *Journal of Hearing and Speech Disorders*, **53**, 146–157.

Goodman, J. F. (1992). *When Slow is Fast Enough: Educating the Delayed Preschool Child*. New York: Guilford.

Hemmeter M. L. & Kaiser A. P. (1994). Enhanced milieu teaching – effects of parent-implemented language intervention. *Journal of Early Intervention*, **18**(3), 269–289.

Hoff-Ginsberg, E. & Shatz, M. (1982). Linguistic input and the child's acquisition of language. *Psychological Bulletin*, **92**, 3–26.

Kaiser, A. P., Hancock, T. B., Neitfeld, J. P. (2000). The effects of parent-implemented enhanced milieu teaching on the social communication of children who have autism.

Early Education and Development, **11**(4), 423–446.

Koegel, R. L., Koegel, L. K., Carter, C. M. (1999). Pivotal teaching interactions for children with autism. *School Psychology Review*, **28**(4), 576–594.

Landry, S. H., Smith, K. E., Miller Loncar, C. L., Swank, P. R. (1997). Predicting cognitive-language and social growth curves from early maternal behaviors in children at varying degrees of biological risk. *Developmental Psychology*, **33**(6), 1040–1053.

Landry, S. H., Smith, K. E., Swank, P. R. (2003). The importance of parenting during early childhood for school-age development. *Developmental Neuropsychology*, **24**(2–3), 559–591.

Landry, S. H., Smith, K. E., Swank, P. R. (2006). Responsive parenting: establishing early foundations for social, communication, and independent problem-solving skills. *Developmental Psychology*, **42**(4), 627–642.

Linder, T. W. (1993). *Transdisciplinary Play-based Assessment: A Functional Approach to Working with Young Children*. Baltimore: Brookes.

Mahoney, G. J. (1988). Maternal communication style with mentally retarded children. *American Journal on Mental Retardation*, **92**, 352–359.

Mahoney, G. (1992). *The Maternal Behavior Rating Scale-Revised*. Available from the author, Family Child Learning Center, 143 Northwest Ave. (Bldg A), Tallmadge, Ohio 44278, USA.

Mahoney, G. & Bella, J. (1998). The effects of family-centered early intervention on child and family outcomes. *Topics in Early Childhood Special Education*, **18**(2), 83–94.

Mahoney, G., Boyce, G., Fewell, R., Spiker, D. Wheeden, C. A. (1998). The relationship of parent-child interaction to the effectiveness of early intervention services for at-risk children and children with disabilities. *Topics in Early Childhood Special Education*, **18**(1), 5–17.

Mahoney, G. J., Finger, I., Powell, A. (1985). The relationship between maternal behavioral style to the developmental status of mentally retarded infants. *American Journal of Mental Deficiency*, **90**, 296–302.

Mahoney, G., Kaiser, A., Girolametto, L., et al. (1999). Parent education in early intervention: a call for a renewed focus. *Topics in Early Childhood Special Education*, **19**(3), 131–140.

Mahoney, G. J., Kim, J. M., Lin, C. S. (2007). The pivotal behavior model of developmental learning. *Infants and Young Children*, **20**(4), 311–325.

Mahoney, G. & MacDonald, J. (2007). *Autism and Developmental Delays in Young Children: The Responsive Teaching Curriculum for Parents and Professionals*. Austin: PRO-ED.

Mahoney, G. & Perales, F. (2005). A comparison of the impact of relationship-focused intervention on young children with pervasive developmental disorders and other disabilities. *Journal of Developmental and Behavioral Pediatrics*, **26**(2), 77–85.

Mahoney, G., Powell, A., Finger, I. (1986). The maternal behavior rating scale. *Topics in Early Childhood Special Education*, **6**, 44–56.

Mahoney, G., Wheeden, C. A., Perales, F. (2004). Relationship of preschool special education outcomes to instructional practices and parent-child interaction. *Research in Developmental Disabilities*, **25**(6), 493–595.

Masur, E. F. & Turner, M. (2001). Stability and consistency in mothers' and infants' interactive style. *Merrill-Palmer Quarterly*, **47**(1), 100–120.

McBride, S. L. & Peterson, C. (1997). Home-based intervention with families of children with disabilities: who is doing what? *Topics in Early Childhood Special Education*, **17**(2), 209–233.

McConachie, H. & Diggle, T. (2007). Parent-implemented early intervention for young children with autism spectrum disorder: a systematic review. *Journal of Evaluation of Clinical Practice*, **13**, 120–129.

McCollum, J. A. (1984). Social interaction between parents and babies: variation of intervention procedure. *Child Care, Health, and Development*, **10**, 301–315.

McCollum, J. A. & Hemmeter, M. L. (1997). Parent-child interaction intervention when children have disabilities. In M. J. Guralnick (ed.), *The Effectiveness of Early Intervention*, pp. 549–576. Baltimore: Brookes.

Nelson, K. (1973). Structure and strategy in learning to talk. *Monograph of the Society for Research in Child Development*, **38**(1–2 serial), 149.

Peterson, C. A., Luze, G. J.. Eshbaugh, E. M., Jeon, H., Kantz, K. R. (2007). Enhancing parent-child interactions through home visiting: promising practice or unfulfilled promise? *Journal of Early Intervention*, **29**(2), 119–140.

Sameroff, A. J. & Fiese, B. H. (2000). Models of development and developmental risk. In C. H. Zeanah (ed.), *Handbook of Infant Mental Health*, pp. 3–13. New York: Guilford.

Seifer, R., Clark, G. N., Sameroff, A. J. (1991). Positive effects of interaction coaching and infants with developmental disabilities and their mothers. *American Journal on Mental Retardation*, **96**, 1–11.

Shearer, M. S. & Shearer, D. E. (1972). The Portage project: a model of early childhood intervention. In T. J. Tjossen (ed.), *Intervention Strategies for High Risk Infants and Young Children*. Baltimore: University Park Press.

Smith, T., Groen, A. D., Wynne, J. W. (2000). Randomized trial of intensive early intervention for children with pervasive developmental disorder. *American Journal on Mental Retardation*, **105**(4), 269–285.

Sparrow, S., Balla, D., Cicchetti, D. (1984). *Vineland Adaptive Behavior Scales*. Circle Pines: American Guidance Service.

Stahmer, A. & Gist, K. (2001). The effects of an accelerated parent education program on technique mastery and child outcome. *Journal of Positive Behavioral Interventions*, **3**, 75–82.

Trivette, C. (2003). Influence of caregiver responsiveness on the development of children with or at-risk for developmental disabilities. *Bridges*, **1**(6), 1–13.

Turnbull, A. P., Blue-Banning, M., Turbiville, V. (1999). From parent education to partnership education: a call for a transformed focus – response. *Topics in Early Childhood Special Education*, **19**(3), 164–172.

van Ijzendoorn, M. H., Schuengel, C., Bakermans-Kranenburg, M. J. (1999). Disorganized attachment in early childhood: meta-analysis of precursors, concomitants, and sequelae. *Development and Psychopathology*, **11**(2), 225–249.

Velderman, M. K., Bakermans-Kranenburg, M. J., Juffer, F., van Ijzendoorn, M. H. (2006). Effects of attachment-based interventions on maternal sensitivity and infant attachment: differential susceptibility of highly reactive infants. *Journal of Family Psychology*, **20**(2), 266–274.

White, K. R. & Boyce, G. C. (eds.) (1993). Comparative evaluations of early intervention alternatives [Special issue]. *Early Education and Development*, **4**(4).

White, K. R., Taylor, M. J., Moss, V. D. (1992). Does research support claims about the benefits of involving parents in early intervention programs? *Review of Educational Research*, **62**(1), 91–125.

17

Perspectives of hybrid therapeutic strategies in intellectual disabilities and Down syndrome

Jean-Adolphe Rondal and Juan Perera

Major progress in molecular genetics over the last decades has made it possible to chart a number of mammalian genotypes including the human one composed of approximately 23,000 genes distributed over 23 pairs of chromosomes. Although the particular locations of these genes are known, their exact roles in cell functioning have not been specified yet except for a few hundred. However, the available knowledge is sufficient to support the definition of animal analogs to some conditions leading to intellectual disabilities in humans, such as fragile-X (etiologically linked to a mutation of the gene FMR-1 or FMR-2 on chromosome X) and Down syndrome (DS) (trisomy 21). For example, trisomy 21 in humans is mimicked (genotypically and phenotypically) in mice by experimentally induced trisomy 16. Recent work suggests that it is possible to ameliorate, at least partially, FMR-1 knockout (KO) mice, an animal model of fragile-X syndrome (FXS), at both cellular and behavioral levels in inhibiting the catalytic activity of p21-activated kinase (PAK), a kinase known to play a critical role in actin polymerization and dendritic spine morphogenesis (Hayashi et al., 2007). Greater spine density and elongated spines in the cortex, morphological synaptic abnormalities commonly observed in FXS, are partly restored by postnatal expression of a dominant negative PAK transgene in the forebrain. Likewise, the deficit in cortical long-term potentiation observed in FMR-1 KO mice is fully restored by the PAK transgene. Several behavioral abnormalities associated with FMR-1 KO mice, including those in locomotor activity, stereotypy, and anxiety are also partly ameliorated or eliminated by the PAK transgene. Particularly interesting is the fact that in vivo data in mice suggest that PAK inhibition is still possible after the appearance of the FXS symptoms. FMR-1 KO mice exhibit abnormalities as early as the first postnatal week. In human patients with FXS, developmental delay appears as early as 9–12 months of age and diagnosis usually follows shortly. Current data suggest that PAK inhibition could still be an effective therapy for infants with FXS, even during the first year of life.

Other gene-based strategies exist, targeting either gene products or downward pathways (Delabar, 2007; and Chapter 4 of this book). Extending the action of the gene material (deoxyribonucleic acid – DNA), outside the cell nucleus is messenger RNA (ribonucleic acid). Any excess in DNA products (for example, in trisomy 21) is thought to determine an increase of the corresponding messenger RNA. The use of a restricted class of small RNAs, the interfering RNAs or siRNAs, is one of the strategies allowing the decrease in, first, the amount of the targeted RNA and, second, the amount of encoded proteins. siRNA molecules

Neurocognitive Rehabilitation of Down Syndrome, eds. Jean-Adolphe Rondal, Juan Perera, and Donna Spiker. Published by Cambridge University Press. © Cambridge University Press 2011.

can selectively silence any gene in the genome. Applied to a mouse model of amyotrophic lateral sclerosis, a mutated form of the gene superoxide dismutase 1 (SOD1) has been experimentally targeted, reducing its expression, improving survival of vulnerable motor neurons, and mediating an improved motor performance in mice (Delabar, 2007).

A second strategy is to target the protein product of the candidate gene. For example, antibodies can be used to decrease the amount of amyloid-beta peptides derived from the amyloid precursor protein. In mice, by direct hippocampal perfusion, researchers were able to restore hippocampal acetylcholine release and reduced impaired habituation learning (Pritchard & Kola, 2007). This work offers hope for the therapeutic potential of targeting amyloid-beta peptide overproduction in Alzheimer patients or in patients with DS in the early stages of developing Alzheimer's disease.

A third possibility is to use chemical compounds that serve to modify the activity of the target protein or the targeted physiological pathway. For example, minibrain kinase/dual-specificity tyrosine phosphorylation-regulated kinase (Mnb/DYRK1A) is a kinase encoded by a gene located within the DS critical region of chromosome 21 (region DSCR1; Korenberg et al., 1997). Its expression is elevated in individuals with DS and it is thought to be involved in the control of neurogenesis. In vitro research shows that this type of kinase is inhibited by a natural molecule that is the main component of the polyphenols in green tea. Delabar (2007; and Chapter 4 of this book) has reported successful in vivo attempts to partly correct the alterations in the brain morphogenesis of transgenic mice, using a diet rich in polyphenols given to pregnant females and continued in the offspring postnatally until magnetic resonance imaging (MRI) was performed between two and four months of age. These results suggest that it is possible to improve a brain phenotype by the use of some particular molecules without affecting the rest of the organism.

Two general hypotheses have been proposed to explain the DS phenotype at the genetic level: (1) the amplified developmental instability hypothesis suggesting that DS is the result of a disturbance of chromosome balance owing to additional chromosome material; and (2) the gene dosage hypothesis proposing that the DS phenotype stems from the effects of the overexpression of a number of particular genes on a portion of chromosome 21 (HSA21), and/or indirectly through the interaction of these genes with the whole genome, transcriptome (transcription events from DNA to RNA), or proteome (protein synthesis following the instructions listed in the genes). Evidence from murine models points to specific genes affecting phenotypes rather than non-specific effects of the amount of extragenetic material (Pritchard & Kola, 2007). It appears, however, that the comprehensive DS phenotype cannot be accounted for on the basis of gene dosage effects alone. In fetuses or adults with DS, a number of genes across the genome are expressed at either higher or lower transcriptional levels than normal (Jenkins & Velinov, 2001). In this respect, it is interesting to note that some murine approaches have introduced large foreign DNA pieces with homologies with HSA21 in the animals' genome. Such approaches overcome some of the limitations of single-gene transgenics as the models involve the utilization of overlapping or contiguous parts that cover a significant part of the chromosome.

Targeting specific genes or fragments of the genome in animal models is now possible. However, the corrective interventions may create negative side effects that have to be controlled or suppressed. Rescuing strategies with a larger scope are also being considered. For example, Pritchard and Kola (2007) have investigated the effects of a transcription factor known as Ets2. This factor regulates the expression of numerous genes involved in cell cycles, cell survival, and tissue remodeling. In mice, overexpression of Ets2 produces some of the skeletal abnormalities characteristic of DS, as well as a smaller thymus similar to that seen in persons with DS, and increases neuronal apoptosis. It would appear that Ets2 up-regulates pro-apoptotic genes and down-regulates the anti-apoptotic genes analog to the corresponding HSA21 genes in mice. This trend in research supplies an initial picture of the cellular function of transcription factors regulating the cellular effects of genes. They open the door to new drug therapies that will act specifically on the pathways disrupted by chromosome imbalances.

The genetic conditions etiologically linked to a single gene mutation (such as fragile-X or Rett syndromes) will likely be the first to witness rescuing altered brain phenotypes within the span of a few years. Syndromes characterized by missing genetic material (such as Williams syndrome, Cri du Chat syndrome, or Turner syndrome 45XO) will be harder to come by. Progress has been made in recent years in inserting new or modified genes into a person's cells to treat or prevent disease (e.g. Hemophilia B and X-linked immunodeficiency; Seppa, 2000). Already in advanced clinical trials in the USA, there are treatments of hereditary disorders such as cystic fibrosis by delivering functional copies of missing genes to cells that need them. Heart treatment of this kind is also under consideration. Immune cells are helping to hunt down cancer cells and make the system resistant to infection. Scientists currently use modified viruses (e.g. retroviruses – viruses without DNA only RNA, adenoviruses – viruses with DNA) as vectors to deliver gene therapy. Viruses are good at delivering genetic payloads to cells. After all, that is what they do naturally. The strategy is to strip viruses of their own genetic material and replace it with therapeutic genes that they will deliver to the target cells. However, ensuring that the gene reaches its target is no small feat. Retroviruses can also induce mutations in the cells, which lead to cancer (Wenner, 2008). Researchers tend to prefer the less dangerous adenoviruses. There is another problem, however; our immune system evolved to reject viruses. Thus, even if a virus reaches its target, one must ensure that the receptive body does not attack the re-engineered cells as they might be identified by the immune system as infected cells. There are a number of particular strategies that can be used to annihilate or at least reduce this sort of complication (e.g. lowering therapy doses, pretreating patients with immunosuppressive drugs, making viral vectors so immune that the immune system will not detect them). Some approaches are developing naked (vectorless) DNA and genes packaged in other and less intrusive ways. Clearly, a lot of basic research is still needed in terms of the safety of these procedures.

In utero gene transfer can be achieved. Various successful ex vivo and in vivo techniques have been reported (Ye et al., 2001). Ex vivo techniques require the removal of the target cells from the fetus. The cells are infected with the virus carrying the foreign gene and re-infused into the fetus. In the in vivo technique, the vector is administered directly to the fetus and infection/transduction occurs within the fetus in utero. Gene transfer introduces certain risks to both mother and fetus, but more to the fetus (e.g. damage impacted on fetal development in addition to adverse immune reactions and possible tumor formation, as indicated previously), which need to be carefully checked. Again additional research is needed in order to ensure that these therapeutic strategies can be carried out in a secure way. What makes gene therapy so promising also makes it extremely challenging. It can target only those biological structures that need it, which is in major contrast to traditional pharmacotherapy where usually only a small portion of the injected product ends up at the site that needs it most.

In addition, aneuploidies such as trisomy 21 will be harder to come by for another reason: the large number of genes, the protein products of which have to be corrected. The DNA sequencing of HSA21 has been completed (Hattori et al., 2000). Chromosome 21 is the second smallest human autosome extending for a total of 33.8 Megabases (Mb). It is predicted to contain from 261 to 364 protein-coding genes involved in 87 different biological processes. The exact function of many of these genes remains unknown, as does their individual contribution, if any, to the DS phenotype. However, it is known that numerous proteins encoded by genes located on HSA21 can affect the structure and/or the function of the brain. A short list containing 25 entities is already available (Wisniewsky et al., 2006). Based on the analysis of human individuals with partial segmental trisomy 21, it has been possible to identify a DS critical region (DSCR) located in the q part of chromosome 21 and encompassing a 1.2 Mb region around D21S55 (Peterson et al., 1994). This is the part of HSA21 where genetic loci presumably display genes with major effects regarding the DS phenotype (e.g. somatic features, developmental delays, cognitive disability). There is no a priori way to determine the exact number of genes involved in the genesis of a complex phenotype. Assuming linear distribution of the genes along HSA21, one could speculate that the DSCR contains something like a dozen genes. One should not forget, however, that interactions between DSCR genes and other genes located on chromosome 21 as well as perhaps on other chromosomes may and probably do contribute to the phenotype. Additionally, not all genes on HSA21 may be dosage sensitive, that is, potentially harmful when triplicated (which increases expression by 50% at the RNA and protein levels). Nevertheless, the number of candidate genes for genetic intervention provides for unique complexities in the case of DS. Partial human trisomies 21 will be relatively easier to compare with the mice models consisting of corresponding trisomies. The mouse orthologs of the human genes located on HSA21 are on chromosomes 10, 16, and 17. Mice trisomic for fragments of chromosome 16, corresponding to 132 genes on HSA21 in one case and to 85 genes in another case, are available (Davisson et al., 1990; Sago et al., 1998). The transgenic mice present a series of features of DS: cranial abnormalities, developmental delay, learning difficulties, neuronal reduction in some parts of the brain, reduction in cerebellar volume (Baxter et al., 2000).

Rescuing the complete phenotype in DS appears a formidable task today. However, given that strategies targeting specific genes are already yielding promising results, a pragmatic approach consisting of inhibiting particular gene products and cautiously avoiding possible negative effects is something that could soon be on the clinical agenda. The immediate objective would not be to cure DS as such, but to gradually improve the phenotype. "It is probably not essential that we know all the genes on chromosome 21 before rational therapies can be considered" (Epstein, 1999, p. 221). Early diagnosis will then possibly become an event with positive consequences for the fetus and the infant, and no longer be a death sentence. Phenotypic plasticity is greatest in the early years (which does not mean that it is restricted to these periods; the brain remains a plastic and highly malleable organ throughout life; Bailey et al., 2001). The sooner phenotypic development can be rescued, the better for the rest of the ontogenesis, given its highly cumulative character.

As genomic science moves forward, we will increasingly be in a better position to determine the precise effects of neurobehavioral interventions on gene expression (Reiss & Niederhiser, 2000). Genetic factors alone account for only a fraction of variance in human behavior. To account for the remaining variance, one must move toward analyses of functional interactions between biology, environment, and behavior (Rutter, 2002). Probably the greatest potential of the neurosciences today and tomorrow resides in its integration with the expanding knowledge of genomics. We should be heading toward hybrid intervention approaches (Warren, 2002), that is, approaches in which neuroscientists will focus more on how genes express themselves in terms of brain functions and behaviors. This will require an unprecedented degree of interdisciplinary understanding and collaboration. The knowledge currently generated and future developments in the life sciences will tremendously enhance the possibilities of better outcomes for individuals with intellectual and developmental disabilities.

Future changes in the prognosis of DS, for example, could have an impact on the way lay people conceptualize the condition. If it can be improved markedly through the application of the strategies envisaged here and/or some new breakthroughs in future years, the social pressures will no longer play in favor of terminating a pregnancy because the fetus was diagnosed with a severe form of developmental disability, but in the opposite sense, that of keeping alive a baby whose developmental prognosis is much better assuming efficient hybrid intervention right from the start, because it would be a terrible shame on all grounds to deprive a human being so close to normality of the right to live.[1] In future, our already enhanced ability to scan an individual's DNA at birth will be applied before birth with the objective of launching therapeutic action as early as possible.

The frequency of aneuploidies following human conception is high. Trisomy 21 is not the most frequent form of aneuploidy recognized during gestation. There are other forms that are much more frequent. It is estimated that roughly 20% of known conceptions are spontaneously aborted and that half of these are genetically abnormal. If one looks, earlier in gestation, at conceptions that last no more than a couple of weeks, the frequency of aneuploidies is even higher. No predisposing factor except maternal age has been identified. Epstein (1999) speculates that there seems to be something inherent in human reproduction that causes or allows the rate of meiotic non-disjunction to remain at a high level. Evolution should have worked the other way around in reducing this rate as it decreases the ability of the species to reproduce successfully. It could be that the relative fragility of human meiosis is related to some vital cell process of which we know nothing, as it is unlikely that evolution would have kept a failing reproductive mechanism for no biological reason.

Because people will continue to be conceived with trisomy 21 (or other aneuploidies) no matter what we do, we would like to be able to prevent the central nervous system deficits from occurring in the first instance. The techniques for efficient neurobehavioral intervention are with us today and they have begun to be widely used in developed countries. There is little doubt that they can be improved and specified further, as suggested in the preceding chapters of this book. Early neurobehavioral intervention is not and will not be in competition with genetic therapeutic approaches. That is why, while waiting longer for the human genetic therapeutic approach to materialize safely, scientists must continue improving the early intervention approach on the grounds that the efforts and energies spent are well directed not only for the present but also for the future.

Summary

An analysis is proposed of what we see as a near-future convergence between genetic therapies in human beings with intellectual disabilities and neurobehavioral interventions. This will lead to a radical modification in the life prospect of these people, changing their biological status into a condition that can be substantially improved with refined knowledge and more powerful technical tools. Such a change, in the longer term, could impact favorably on

---

[1] We are not implying that it is not terrible to terminate the life of a fetus, regardless of her/his medical status.

the general public's conceptions and attitudes regarding the persons with severe intellectual disabilities.

References

Bailey, D., Bruer, J., Symons, F., Lichtman, J. (2001). *Critical Thinking about Critical Periods*. Baltimore: Brookes.

Baxter, L., Moran, T., Richtmeier, J., Troncoso, J., Reeves, R. (2000). Discovery and genetic localization of Down syndrome cerebellar phenotype using the Ts65Dn mouse. *Human Molecular Genetics*, **9**, 195–202.

Davisson, M., Schmidt, C., Akeson, E. (1990). Segmental trisomy of murine chromosome16: a new model system for studying Down syndrome. *Progress in Clinical Biological Research*, **360**, 263–280.

Delabar, J. (2007). Perspective on gene-based therapies. In J. A. Rondal & A. Rasore Quartino (eds.), *Therapies and Rehabilitation in Down Syndrome*, pp. 1–17. Chichester: Wiley.

Epstein, C. (1999). The future of biological research on Down syndrome. In J. A. Rondal, J. Perera, L. Nadel (eds.), *Down Syndrome. A Review of Current Knowledge*, pp. 210–222. London: Whurr.

Hattori, M., Fujiyama, A., Taylor, D., et al. (2000). The DNA sequence of human chromosome 21. *Nature*, **405**, 311–319.

Hayashi, M., Rao, S., Seo, J., et al. (2007). Inhibition of p21-activated kinase rescues symptoms of fragile X syndrome in mice. *Proceedings of the National Academy of Sciences of the United States of America*, **104**(27), 11489–11494.

Jenkins, E. & Velinov, M. (2001). Down syndrome and the human genome. *Down Syndrome Quarterly*, **6**, 1–12.

Korenberg, J., Aaltonen, J., Brahe, C., et al. (1997). Report and abstracts of the 6th International Workshop on Human Chromosome 21 Mapping 1996. Cold Spring Harbor, New York, USA. May 6–8, 1996. *Cytogenetic Cell Genetics*, **79**(1–2), 21–52.

Peterson, A., Patil, N., Robins, C., et al. (1994). A transcript map of the Down syndrome critical region of chromosome 21. *Human Molecular Genetics*, **3**, 1735–1742.

Pritchard, M. & Kola, I. (2007). The biological bases of pharmacological therapies in Down syndrome. In J. A. Rondal & A. Rasore Quartino (eds.), *Therapies and Rehabilitation in Down Syndrome*, pp. 18–27. Chichester: Wiley.

Reiss, D. & Niederhiser, J. (2000). The interplay of genetic influences and social processes in developmental theory: specific mechanisms are coming into view. *Development and Psychopathology*, **12**, 357–374.

Rutter, M. (2002). Nature, nurture, and development: from evangelism through science toward policy and practice. *Child Development*, **73**, 1–21.

Sago, H., Carlson, E., Smith, D., et al. (1998). Ts1Cje, a partial trisomy 16 mouse model for Down syndrome, exhibits learning and behavioral abnormalities. *Proceedings of the National Academy of Sciences of the United States of America*, **95** (14), 6256–6261.

Seppa, N. (2000). Bubble babies thrive on gene therapy. *Science News Online* (retrieved from www.science online.org).

Warren, S. (2002). Presidential address 2002 – Genes, brains, and behavior: the road ahead. *Mental Retardation*, **40**(6), 471–476.

Wenner, M. (2008). Regaining lost luster. New developments and clinical trials breathe life back into gene therapy. *Scientific American*, January, 9–10.

Wisniewski, K., Kida, E., Golabeck, A., et al. (2006). Down syndrome: from pathology to pathogenesis. In J. A. Rondal & J. Perera (eds.), *Down Syndrome. Neurobehavioural Specificity*, pp. 17–33. Chichester: Wiley.

Ye, X., Mitchell, M., Newman, K., Batshaw, M. (2001). Prospects for prenatal gene therapy in disorders causing mental retardation. *Mental Retardation and Developmental Disabilities Research Review*, 7, 65–72.

Conclusions

More states and governments are promulgating laws and regulations ensuring that early education and care for the child with a congenital handicap and her/his family is readily available on an equal basis for everybody. Conceptually and technically, major progress has been made in the last decades particularly in the industrialized countries. What is still missing, however, is a fully fledged translational science of neurocognitive rehabilitation. We have been concerned with the various facets of early rehabilitation directed particularly toward the infants and children with Down syndrome (DS). The basic methodological principles and recommendations are likely to be valid for other congenital genetic syndromes of intellectual disabilities, however, pending further research on development in these syndromes. One of the objectives of this book has been to reunite, in a single opus, technical contributions from a variety of fields bearing on the general problem; that is, given the present biological limitations, how to improve the abilities of the child with DS to a maximal extent in a variety of aspects relevant to her/his place as an active member of society. As stressed in the various chapters, it has become clear that the best chances to achieve such a goal are through early (even very early), intensive, and systematic intervention, conducted by competent operators in close collaboration with the parents and the schools. Quite clearly, efficient rehabilitation does not terminate at six or seven years of age. In addition, stressing the need to develop better and more systematic early intervention programs does not mean that the following periods of time until adolescence and adulthood are not equally important. However, further progress at later stages is likely to be easier when based on strong foundations. The need for adequate operators and teachers, and to correctly inform and involve parents has been acknowledged. One of the difficulties in this respect is to make sure that the knowledge gathered in research works on a large number of issues, as reflected in this book and the current literature, and is put into practice by the practitioners.

As explained in several chapters, genetic therapy is no longer regarded as science fiction, although practically still some time away, particularly for chromosomal conditions such as DS. We must prepare mentally, ethically, and socially for this perspective that will allow gradual improvement (probably gene-by-gene or gene product-by-gene product, in the first place) of some of the most negative aspects of the DS phenotype. It is important to keep in mind, however, that we need to maintain and even increase the synergy between genetic and organic therapies and neurocognitive interventions. The latter will always be necessary in order to obtain the best possible outcome in improving the biological and psychological status of people with DS and other congenital genetic conditions leading to intellectual disability. Once more we find ourselves facing the issue of DS at the cross-road between genotypic and phenotypic disciplines and the necessity to develop genuine interdisciplinary relationships and collaboration, as centrally advocated in this book.

Neurocognitive Rehabilitation of Down Syndrome, eds. Jean-Adolphe Rondal, Juan Perera, and Donna Spiker. Published by Cambridge University Press. © Cambridge University Press 2011.

Index